AF184088

Ernest E. Moore Shock Trauma Center at Denver Health Illustrated Tips and Tricks in Trauma Surgery

Ernest E. Moore Shock Trauma Center at Denver Health Illustrated Tips and Tricks in Trauma Surgery

Editors

Ernest E. Moore, MD
Distinguished Professor of Surgery
Ernest E. Moore Shock Trauma Center at Denver Health
University of Colorado School of Medicine
Denver, Colorado

Charles J. Fox, MD
Associate Professor of Surgery
Division of Vascular Surgery
University of Maryland School of Medicine
Director, Vascular Surgery, University of Maryland Capital Region
Attending Surgeon, University of Maryland Medical Center
Attending Surgeon, R Adams Cowley Shock Trauma Center
Baltimore, Maryland

Fredric M. Pieracci, MD, MPH
Professor of Surgery
University of Colorado School of Medicine
Director of Surgery
Ernest E. Moore Shock Trauma Center at Denver Health
Denver, Colorado

Wolters Kluwer

Philadelphia • Baltimore • New York • London
Buenos Aires • Hong Kong • Sydney • Tokyo

Senior Acquisitions Editor: Keith Donnellan
Senior Development Editor: Ashley Fischer
Editorial Coordinator: Vinodhini Varadharajalu
Marketing Manager: Kirsten Watrud
Production Project Manager: Matt West
Manager, Graphic Arts & Design: Stephen Druding
Manufacturing Coordinator: Lisa Bowling
Prepress Vendor: Aptara, Inc.

Copyright © 2024 Wolters Kluwer.

All rights reserved. This book is protected by copyright. No part of this book may be reproduced or transmitted in any form or by any means, including photocopies or scanned-in or other electronic copies, or utilized by any information storage and retrieval system without written permission from the copyright owner, except for brief quotations embodied in critical articles and reviews. Materials appearing in this book prepared by individuals as part of their official duties as U.S. government employees are not covered by the above-mentioned copyright. To request permission, please contact Lippincott Williams & Wilkins at Two Commerce Square, 2001 Market Street, Philadelphia, PA 19103, via e-mail at permissions@lww.com, or via Website at shop.lww.com (products and services).

9 8 7 6 5 4 3 2 1

Printed in Singapore

Library of Congress Cataloging-in-Publication Data
Names: Moore, Ernest Eugene, editor. | Fox, Charles J. (Vascular surgeon) editor. | Pieracci, Fredric M., editor.
Title: Ernest E. Moore Shock Trauma Center at Denver Health illustrated tips and tricks in trauma surgery / editors, Ernest E. Moore, Charles J. Fox, Fredric M. Pieracci.
Other titles: Illustrated tips and tricks in trauma surgery
Description: Philadelphia, PA : Wolters Kluwer, [2024] | Includes bibliographical references and index.
Identifiers: LCCN 2022052636 (print) | LCCN 2022052637 (ebook) | ISBN 9781975109516 (paperback) | ISBN 9781975109530 (ebook)
Subjects: MESH: Ernest E. Moore Shock Trauma Center at Denver Health. | Wounds and Injuries–surgery | Surgical Procedures, Operative | Critical Care–methods | BISAC: MEDICAL / Surgery / General
Classification: LCC RD93 (print) | LCC RD93 (ebook) | NLM WO 700 | DDC 617.1–dc23/eng/20230119
LC record available at https://lccn.loc.gov/2022052636
LC ebook record available at https://lccn.loc.gov/2022052637

This work is provided "as is," and the publisher disclaims any and all warranties, express or implied, including any warranties as to accuracy, comprehensiveness, or currency of the content of this work.

This work is no substitute for individual patient assessment based upon healthcare professionals' examination of each patient and consideration of, among other things, age, weight, gender, current or prior medical conditions, medication history, laboratory data and other factors unique to the patient. The publisher does not provide medical advice or guidance and this work is merely a reference tool. Healthcare professionals, and not the publisher, are solely responsible for the use of this work including all medical judgments and for any resulting diagnosis and treatments.

Given continuous, rapid advances in medical science and health information, independent professional verification of medical diagnoses, indications, appropriate pharmaceutical selections and dosages, and treatment options should be made and healthcare professionals should consult a variety of sources. When prescribing medication, healthcare professionals are advised to consult the product information sheet (the manufacturer's package insert) accompanying each drug to verify, among other things, conditions of use, warnings and side effects and identify any changes in dosage schedule or contraindications, particularly if the medication to be administered is new, infrequently used or has a narrow therapeutic range. To the maximum extent permitted under applicable law, no responsibility is assumed by the publisher for any injury and/or damage to persons or property, as a matter of products liability, negligence law or otherwise, or from any reference to or use by any person of this work.

shop.lww.com

MKO823

Contributors

Eric Campion, MD
Associate Director of Surgery
Ernest E. Moore Shock Trauma Center at Denver Health
Associate Professor of Surgery
University of Colorado School of Medicine
Denver, Colorado

Charles J. Fox, MD
Associate Professor of Surgery
Division of Vascular Surgery
University of Maryland School of Medicine
Director, Vascular Surgery, University of Maryland Capital Region
Attending Surgeon, University of Maryland Medical Center
Attending Surgeon, R Adams Cowley Shock Trauma Center
Baltimore, Maryland

Thomas J. France, MD
Resident
Department of Orthopedics
University of Colorado
Aurora, Colorado

Michael Hines, MD
Senior Staff Physician
Adult and Pediatric Congenital Cardiac Surgery
ECMO Director
Ochsner Clinic Foundation
New Orleans, Louisiana

Ryan A. Lawless, MD
Trauma Medical Director
Director, Extracorporeal Life Support Service
Ernest E. Moore Shock Trauma Center at Denver Health
Assistant Professor of Surgery
Department of Surgery
University of Colorado School of Medicine
Denver, Colorado

Ernest E. Moore, MD
Distinguished Professor of Surgery
Ernest E. Moore Shock Trauma Center at Denver Health
University of Colorado School of Medicine
Denver, Colorado

Hunter B. Moore, MD, PhD
Transplant Surgery
University of Colorado Anschutz
Assistant Professor of Surgery
University of Colorado School of Medicine
Aurora, Colorado

Fredric M. Pieracci, MD, MPH
Professor of Surgery
University of Colorado School of Medicine
Director of Surgery
Ernest E. Moore Shock Trauma Center at Denver Health
Denver, Colorado

Elizabeth A. Pomfret, MD, PhD
Director of Transplant Surgery
University of Colorado Anschutz
Professor of Surgery
University of Colorado School of Medicine
Aurora, Colorado

Meryl Singer, MD
Private Practice
Denver, Colorado

Krystle R. Tuaño, MD
Hand & Upper Extremity Fellow
Department of Orthopaedic Surgery
Massachusetts General Hospital
Boston, Massachusetts

Daniel VanDerPloeg, MD
Assistant Professor of Surgery
University of Colorado School of Medicine
Chief of Thoracic Surgery
Ernest E. Moore Shock Trauma Center at Denver Health
Denver, Colorado

Nicole L. Werner, MD
Acute Care Surgeon
Assistant Professor of Surgery
University of Wisconsin School of Medicine and Public Health
Madison, Wisconsin

Daniel Dante Yeh, MD, MHPE
Professor of Surgery
Chief of Emergency General Surgery
Department of Surgery
Ernest E. Moore Shock Trauma Center at Denver Health
Denver, Colorado

Preface

Established in 1860, fittingly one of the first patients treated at the Denver General Hospital (DGH) was Dr Stone who was shot in a duel by the acting Governor Bliss. In 1967, over a century later, Ben Eiseman, MD became the first academic Chief of Surgery at DGH and recruited Ernest E. Moore, MD as the first Chief of Trauma a decade later. Together they emphasized the necessity to develop operative skills to be successful in academic trauma surgery. DGH became nationally renowned as the original "Knife and Gun Club" (Eugene Richards) during the drug/gang wars that were occurring in many large cities during the 1980s. This text describes the technical skills learned over the past 50 years to manage the critically injured, with an emphasis on thoracic and vascular injures. While most of the operative techniques are routine procedures employed by many trauma centers throughout the United States, several were studied extensively at DGH. These include emergency department thoracotomy, left heart bypass for torn thoracic aorta, damage control surgery, preperitoneal pelvic packing, resuscitative endovascular aortic occlusion, and surgical stabilization of rib fractures. As standardized for this series of texts, the focus is on operative technical details. Each chapter provides a list of essential equipment, patient positioning, and step-by-step operative steps, written by experienced trauma surgeons. The DGH became Denver Health (DH) in the 1990s, and more recently the trauma center has been named the Ernest E. Moore Shock Trauma Center at DH.

We hope you find these "tips and tricks" useful in your care of the seriously injured.

Ernest E. Moore, MD
Charles J. Fox, MD
Fredric M. Pieracci, MD

Contents

SECTION IV: ABDOMINAL INJURIES

SECTION V: PELVIC INJURIES

SECTION VI: SPINAL INJURIES

SECTION VII: EXTREMITY VASCULAR INJURIES

SECTION I Resuscitation

Chapter 1

Emergency Department Thoracotomy

ERNEST E. MOORE AND FREDRIC M. PIERACCI

PERIOPERATIVE CONSIDERATIONS

Procedure Rationale

Resuscitative thoracotomy performed in the emergency department (ED) was proposed by cardiac surgeons at the Ben Taub Hospital in Houston a half century ago, who documented improved survival for patients presenting in extremis with cardiac wounds. The objectives of the procedure were expanded subsequently to include (1) release of pericardial tamponade, (2) access for cardiorrhaphy, (3) mechanical control of intrathoracic bleeding, (4) pulmonary hilar clamping to prevent bronchoalveolar air embolism, (5) internal cardiac massage, and (6) aortic cross-clamping to increase perfusion to the heart and brain, and reduce subdiaphragmatic bleeding. The specific indications continue to be debated, but critical factors include (1) injury mechanism, (2) primary site of injury, (3) duration of prehospital cardiopulmonary resuscitation (CPR), and (4) presenting cardiac rhythm.

Essential Equipment

Emergency Department Thoracotomy Tray

- Scalpel with 10 blade
- Curved Mayo scissors
- Lebsche knife with mallet
- Finochietto chest retractor (ensure the device is assembled correctly)
- Large-toothed forceps
- Large Satinski clamps (aortic cross-clamping)
- Crawford vascular clamps × 2 (control lung bleeding and air leak)
- Standard needle holder
- Sutures: 3-0 Prolene with needle
  - 3-0 silk with needle
  - 3-0 silk ties
  - Teflon pledgets precut 2 × 2 cm
- Internal cardiac defibrillator

TIP

The emergency department thoracotomy (EDT) tray (Fig. 1.1) should be opened on a separate sterile covered stand before patient arrival, positioned on the patient's left side of the ED gurney. The instruments should be limited to those essential and arranged front to back according to their anticipated use.

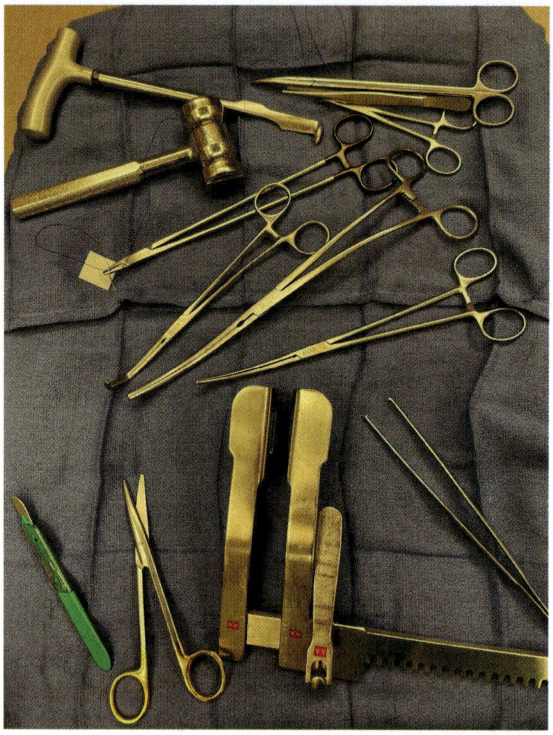

FIGURE 1.1 ▎The emergency department thoracotomy (EDT) tray should contain the minimal number of instruments to facilitate rapid access to the chest.

Patient Positioning and Prepping

- Upon transfer to the ED gurney, the patient's left arm should be raised above the head to optimize exposure of the left chest wall. Betadine solution should be applied generously to the entire anterior and left lateral thorax.
- The operator should wear personal protective equipment (PPE) and be careful with sharp instruments.

SURGICAL TECHNIQUE

Left Anterolateral Thoracotomy

- The skin incision is made in the inframammary crease, elevating the breast in women (Fig. 1.2).
- The skin incision begins on the right border of the sternum and continues into the posterior axilla, following the curvature of the ribs. Failure to curve the incision into the axilla will hinder exposure and may result in entering the chest too inferiorly.

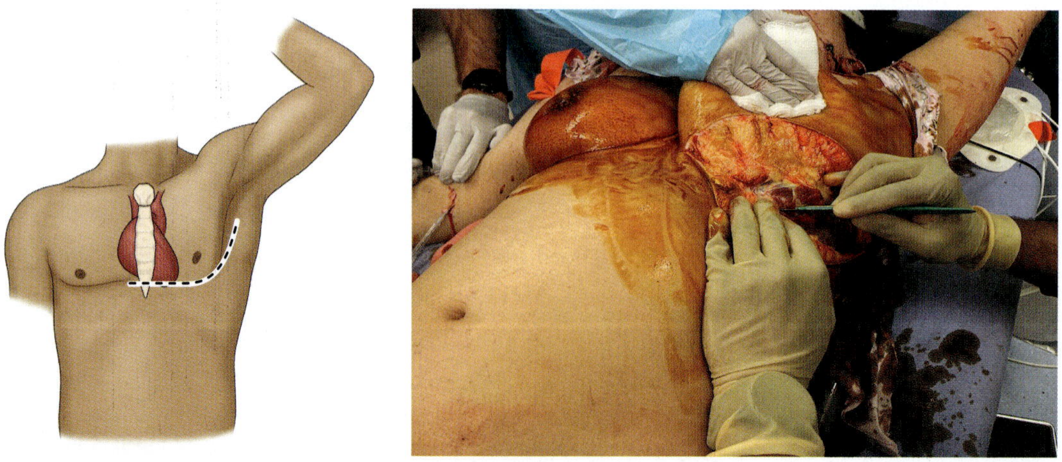

FIGURE 1.2 ▎The patient is positioned with the left arm elevated above the head. The incision is initiated on the right border of the sternum and extended along the curvature of the ribs into the axilla.

- The scalpel should be used to traverse the chest wall to the level of the ribs.
- The thorax is entered in the fifth intercostal space with the curved Mayo scissors along the superior margin of the rib to avoid the neurovascular bundle beneath the inferior edge (Fig. 1.3).
- The rib space should be opened extensively from the axilla to the left border of the sternum, and widened sufficiently to permit placing the operator's hands into the left chest.
- A Finochietto chest retractor is placed between the ribs with the handle positioned posteriorly (Fig. 1.4).

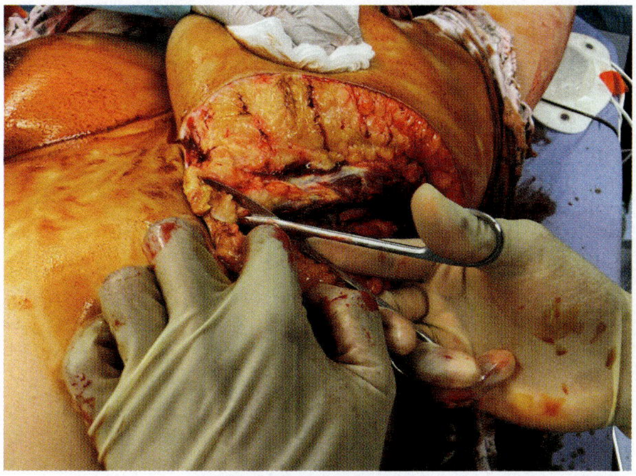

FIGURE 1.3 ▌ The incision is made with a scalpel to the ribs, and Mayo scissors are used to enter the intercostal space.

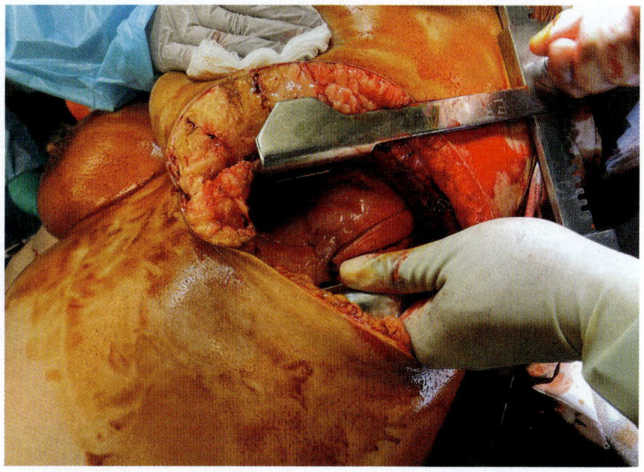

FIGURE 1.4 ▌ The Finochietto chest retractor is positioned between the ribs with the handle directed posteriorly.

- If the rib space opening is insufficient, a Lebsche knife is used to divide one or two costal margins along the sternum.
- Clot should be evacuated and the source of bleeding identified.
- The pericardium is opened vertically anterior to the phrenic nerve (Fig. 1.5) for patients with pulseless electrical activity (PEA) to assess cardiac contractility. Furthermore, the pericardium should be opened promptly if there is possible intrapericardial blood.

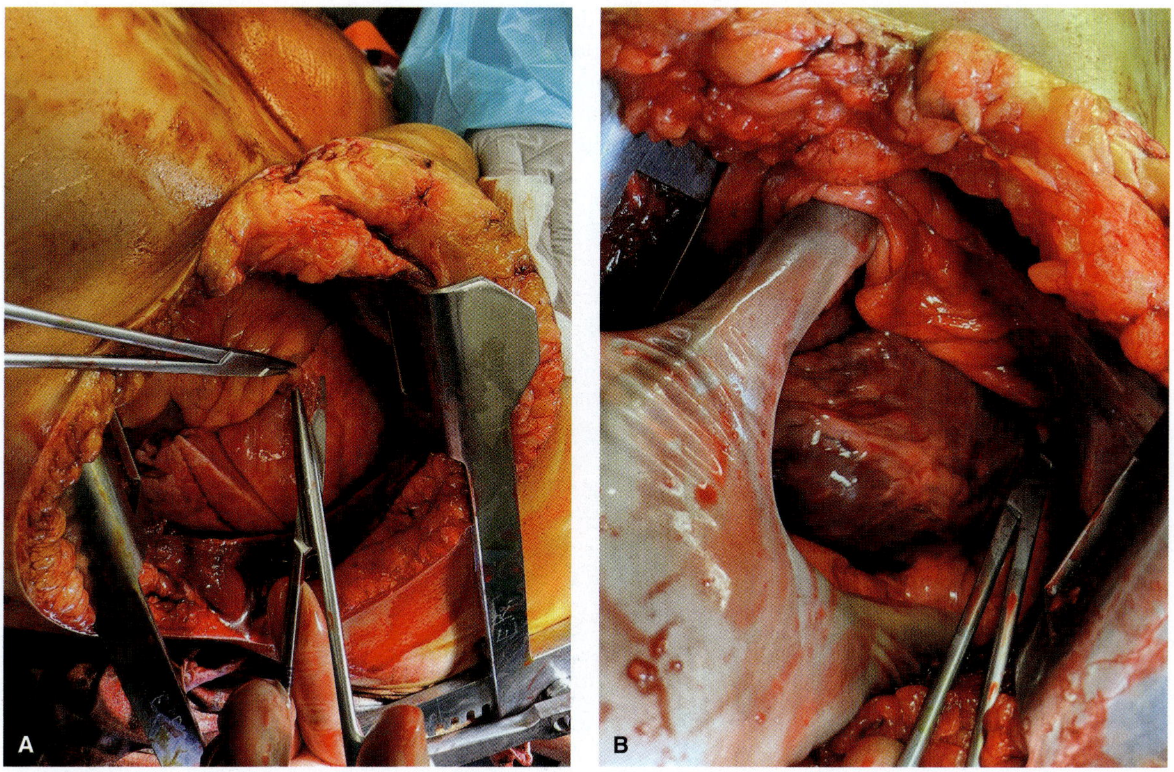

FIGURE 1.5 ▌ The pericardium is opened anterior to the phrenic nerve, and extended the full distance of the pericardial sac.

TIP

The pericardium can be tense with blood and, in this scenario, it is best opened with a scalpel.

- The pericardium is elevated with toothed forceps and opened widely with Mayo scissors, allowing the heart to be delivered into the left chest (Fig. 1.6).

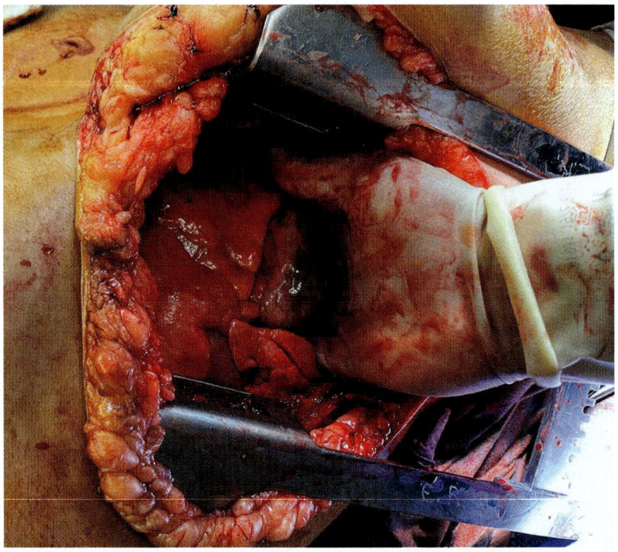

FIGURE 1.6 ▮ With the pericardium opened widely, the heart can be delivered into the left thorax for inspection and internal massage.

- Clot should be removed from the pericardial and the bleeding site(s) identified.
- Active bleeding from the ventricles is controlled digitally, and a medium Satinsky clamp is applied for atrial bleeding (see Chapter 9)
- Air leak and bleeding from the lung is controlled with large Crawford clamps to minimize blood loss and, more importantly, prevent bronchovenous air embolism (Fig. 1.7). Increased airway pressure due to positive ventilation combined with low venous pressure due to hypovolemia facilitates air embolism into the left heart and then systemically. Coronary air migrates preferentially into the right system and is difficult to extract.

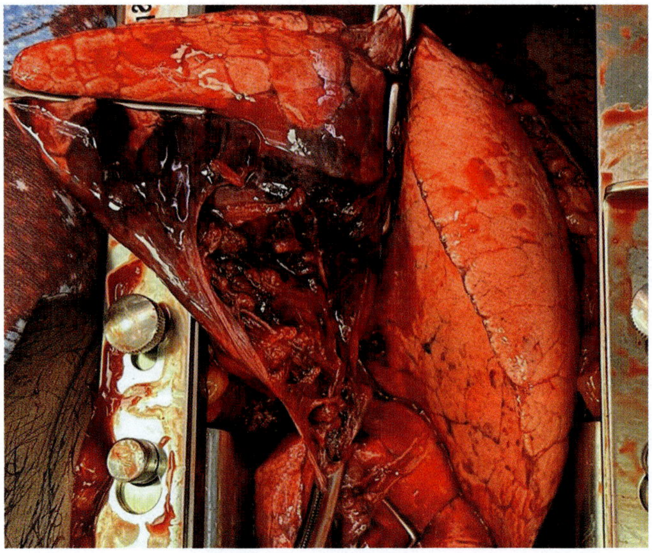

FIGURE 1.7 ▮ Active bleeding or air leak from the lung is controlled with large Crawford clamps to avoid air embolism.

Bilateral Anterolateral Thoracotomy ("Clamshell")

- If a right thoracic penetrating wound exists, the operator's right hand should be advanced under the sternum into the right chest, creating a "buffalo" mediastinum. Alternatively, a concurrent right tube thoracostomy can be used to assess for right thoracic bleeding.
- If bleeding is confirmed in the right thorax or a complex cardiac wound is encountered, the thoracotomy is extended across the sternum into a "clamshell" thoracotomy (Fig. 1.8).

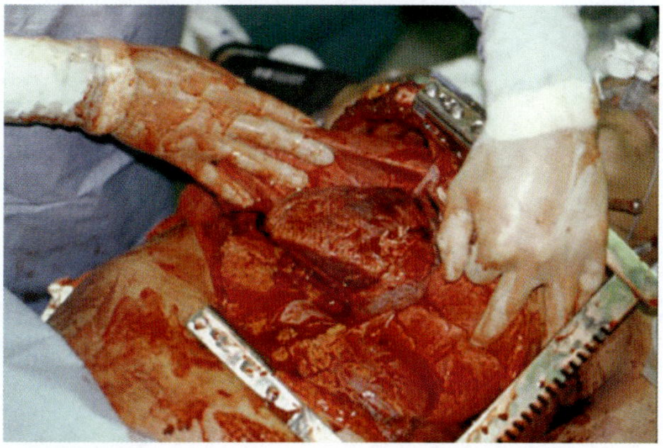

FIGURE 1.8 ▌ If bleeding is from the right thorax or a complex cardiac wound is encountered, the thoracotomy is extended across the sternum into a "clamshell" thoracotomy.

Descending Thoracic Aortic Occlusion

The rationale for clamping the descending thoracic aorta is to (1) redistribute limited circulating blood volume to enhance coronary and cerebral perfusion, and (2) reduce ongoing bleeding below the diaphragm.

- The thoracic aorta is occluded as close to the diaphragm as possible to minimize ischemia to the spinal cord due to interrupting the artery of Adamkiewicz, which can exit the aorta from the level of thoracic vertebral body 3 (T3) to lumbar vertebra body 4 (L4). The typical location, however, is from the left side of the aorta between T8-L1.
- The thoracic aorta is immediately anterior to the spine and lateral to the esophagus (Fig. 1.9). To access the aorta for cross-clamping, a window should be made by bluntly dissecting the

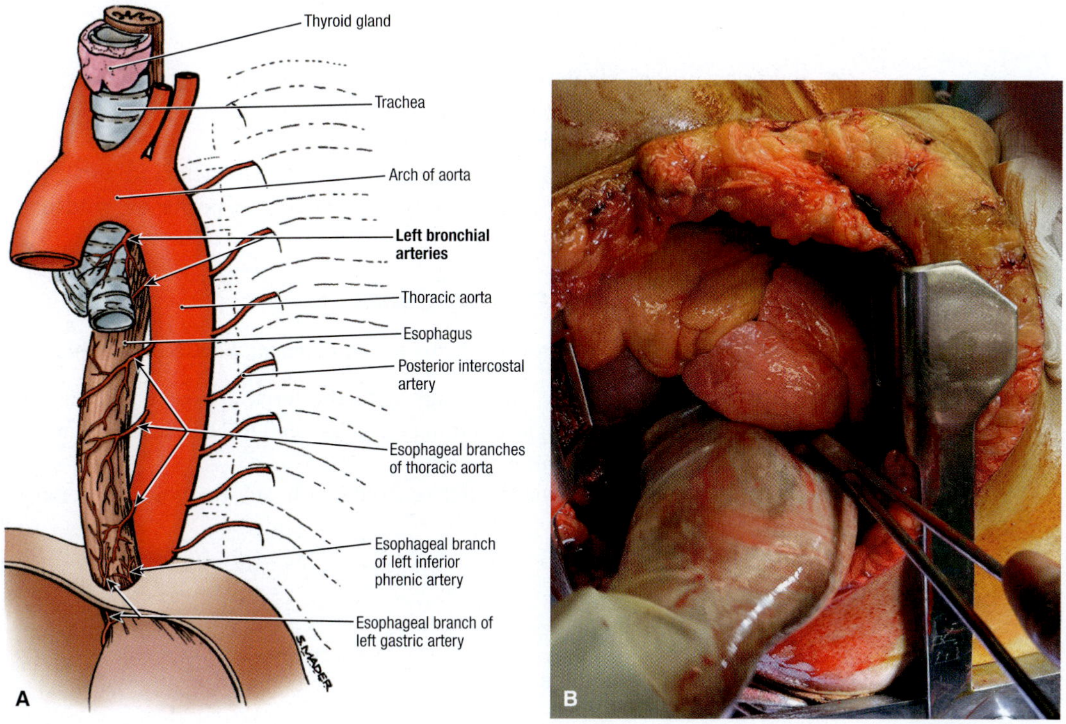

FIGURE 1.9 ▌ The descending thoracic aorta is immediately anterior to the spine (**A**), and should be clamped just above the diaphragm (**B**).

mediastinal pleura posterior to the aorta using the thumb and index finger to mobilize the aorta from the spine.

- The aorta is occluded with a large Satinsky clamp advanced via the mediastinal opening. If there is no improvement in upper extremity blood pressure, the clamp should be visualized to confirm appropriate position.
- The aortic occlusion time should be minimized to avoid visceral ischemia and reperfusion injury, as well as increased left ventricular afterload. Occlusion times exceeding 30 minutes produce organ dysfunction and thus intermittent occlusion should be employed if this time limit is exceeded.

Pulmonary Hilar Occlusion

The rationale for pulmonary hilum occlusion is predominantly to avoid bronchovenous air embolism. With a persistent major air leak or central lobar bleeding, the pulmonary hilum should be occluded with a large Satinski clamp (Fig. 1.10).

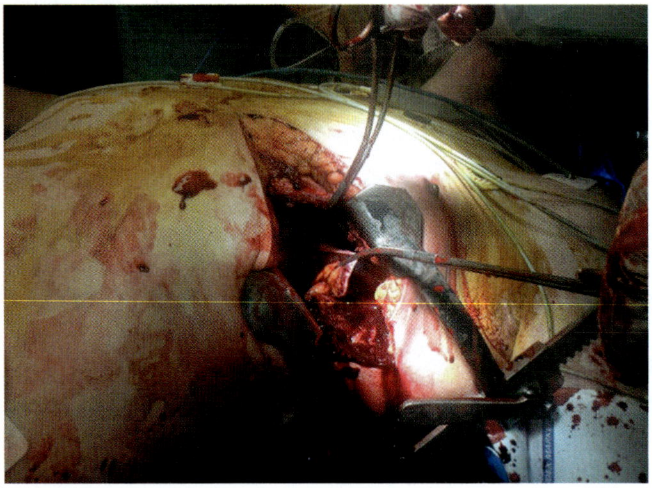

FIGURE 1.10 ▌ The pulmonary hilum is occluded with a major air leak to prevent bronchovenous air embolism.

- Pulmonary hilar clamping may not be tolerated due to right heart strain, and the hilar clamp may need intermittent release until selective lobar stapling can be accomplished in the operating room (OR). (See Chapter 11.)
- If air embolism is suspected, the apex of the left ventricle and aortic arch should be aspirated to remove air. A 27-gauge needle should be used to aspirate air if visualized within the coronary artery.

Internal Cardiac Compression

Internal cardiac massage is more effective than external, particularly when there is hypovolemia.

- Cardiac massage is done bimanually with the wrist apposed, forcing blood from the wrist to the fingertips (Fig. 1.11). Single-hand massage can lead to ventricular puncture with the thumb, the risk is increased by a stiff ventricular wall.
- Epinephrine is injected via the left ventricle with care to avoid a coronary artery.

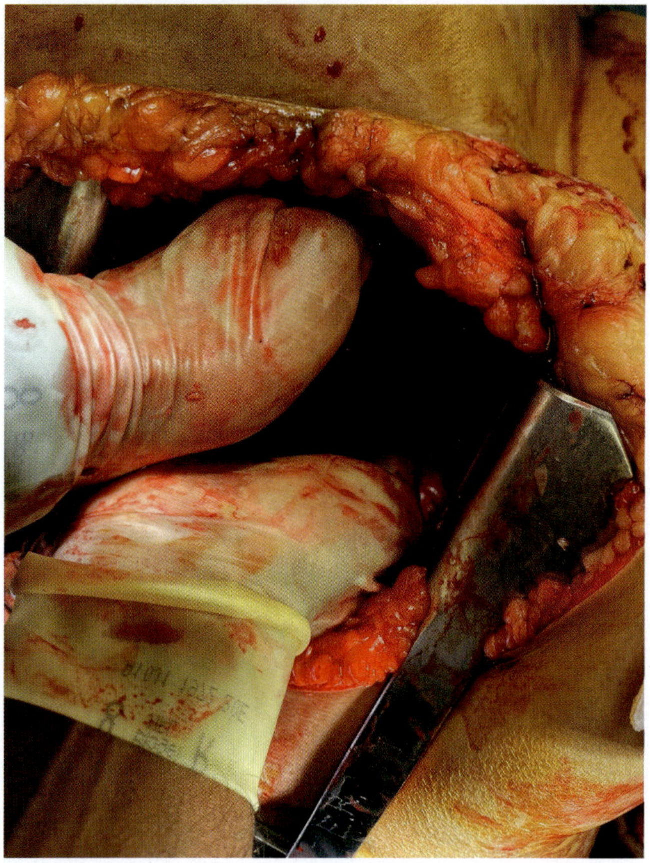

FIGURE 1.11 ▌ Internal cardiac massage is done bimanually with the wrist apposed.

Thoracotomy Closure

The anterolateral thoracotomy is closed using standard technique.

- A 28-Fr thoracostomy tube is placed via the eighth intercostal space, midclavicular line, and positioned in the posterior sulcus under direct vision. A second tube, positioned anteriorly, may be warranted with extensive intrathoracic tissue injury or persistent coagulopathy.
- We use # 1 PDS for the pericostal sutures, and muscle closure in layers with 2-0 PDS. The skin is stapled.
- We use # 5 wire suture to reapproximate the sternum.

TIP

When closing a trans-sternal extension or clam-shell thoracotomy, suture ligate proximal and distal ends of the internal mammary arteries

POSTOPERATIVE CARE

- The postoperative management following ED thoracotomy is based primarily on the underlying life-threatening injury. Patients are monitored in the surgical intensive care unit (SICU) and may require continued resuscitation.
  - The priorities are to reverse metabolic acidosis and restore normal coagulation as soon as possible.
  - Bleeding is the most common complication from resuscitative thoracotomy, and is usually indicated by thoracostomy or mediastinal tube output. But there are a number of additional serious complications that include herniation of the heart and torsion of the lung that demand immediate reoperation.

Suggested Readings

Beall AC Jr, Diethrich EB, Cooley DA, DeBakey ME. Surgical management of penetrating cardiovascular trauma. *South Med J.* 1967;60(7):698–704.

Moore EE, Knudson MM, Burlew CC, et al; WTA Study Group. Defining the limits of resuscitative emergency department thoracotomy: a contemporary Western Trauma Association perspective. *J Trauma.* 2011;70(2):334–339.

Moore HB, Moore EE, Burlew CC, et al. Establishing benchmarks for resuscitation of traumatic circulatory arrest: success-to-rescue and survival among 1,708 patients. *J Am Coll Surg.* 2016;223(1):42–50.

Seamon MJ, Haut ER, Van Arendonk K, et al. An evidence-based approach to patient selection for emergency department thoracotomy: a practice management guideline from the Eastern Association for the Surgery of Trauma. *J Trauma Acute Care Surg.* 2015;79(1):159–173.

Chapter 2

Resuscitative Endovascular Balloon Occlusion of the Aorta

CHARLES J. FOX AND ERNEST E. MOORE

PERIOPERATIVE CONSIDERATIONS

Procedure Rationale

Resuscitative endovascular balloon occlusion of the aorta (REBOA) is an endovascular adjunct designed to improve cerebral and coronary perfusion during shock from noncompressible torso hemorrhage. Early arterial access and deployment of the aortic occlusion balloon are crucial for resuscitative success. In cases of full cardiac arrest, emergency department thoracotomy may be preferable. Novel methods such as intermittent and partial REBOA are being explored to extend occlusion time and prevent ischemic complications. The treatment algorithm carefully selects the right patient in the right place at the right time to respond favorably to an aortic balloon occlusion during hemorrhagic shock from noncompressible torso hemorrhage.

Treatment Algorithm

- An endovascular method for temporary control of torso and lower junctional hemorrhage and is an alternative to resuscitative thoracotomy (RT) for descending aortic cross-clamping.
- RT is the procedure of choice, for patients with thoracic or cardiac injuries, and many believe is preferred when the patient is undergoing cardiopulmonary resuscitation (CPR).
- Optimal position of the REBOA is based on three zones of the aorta and determined by the anticipated injury pattern (Fig. 2.1).

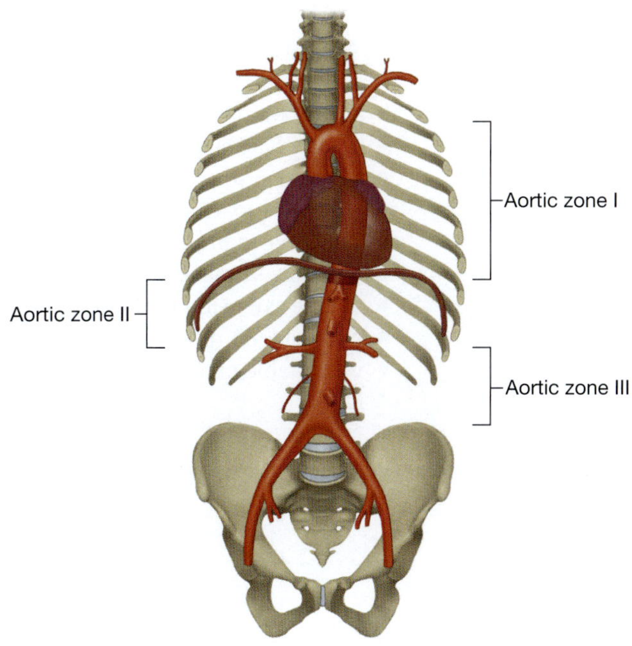

FIGURE 2.1 | Aortic zones related to REBOA. Zone I is from the origin of the left subclavian artery to the celiac artery. Zone II extends from the celiac artery to the lowest renal artery. Zone III is from the lowest renal artery to the aortic bifurcation and is favored for zone of occlusion for unstable pelvic ring fractures. (Redrawn from Stannard A, Eliason JL, Rasmussen TE. Resuscitative endovascular balloon occlusion of the aorta (REBOA) as an adjunct for hemorrhagic shock. *J Trauma*. 2011;71(6):1869–1872.)

  - Zone I is from the left subclavian artery to the celiac artery.
  - Zone II (never occluded) is from the celiac artery to the lowest renal artery.
  - Zone III is from the lowest renal artery to the aortic bifurcation.
- Occlusion time should be limited to 30 (zone I) and 120 minutes (zone III), but the newly approved partial REBOA should allow more extended occlusion times.

Essential Equipment

TIP

The trauma surgeon in charge should inventory all the essential items with the emergency department staff periodically. A portable cart is a useful way to ensure all supplies are available in any trauma room during an urgent situation.

- 18-gauge arterial access needle.
- 11-cm 7-French sheath
  - Cook, Arrow, and St. Jude Medical are not compatible introducer sheaths.
- 0.035-inch stainless steel guidewire, 45 cm.
- There are a number of commercially available occlusion balloons; we prefer the ER-REBOA catheter, Prytime Medical, Inc., Arvada, CO (Fig. 2.2).

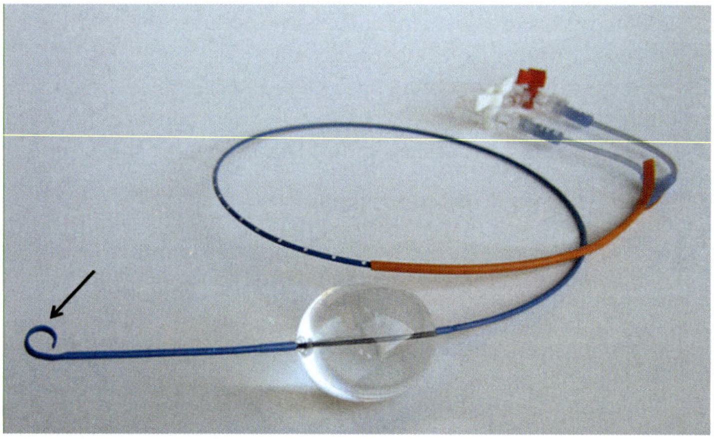

FIGURE 2.2 ▮ ER-REBOA Catheter with P-Tip (*arrow*). (Courtesy of Prytime Medical, Inc., Arvada, CO.)

- Contrast agent 50 mL (Omnipaque-240, GE Healthcare, Inc., Chicago, IL).
- 50-mL injectable saline, and optimally heparinized saline (50 U/mL) for line flushing.
- 5-, 10-, and 30-cc syringes × 2 each.
- Sutures 2-0 silk or nylon to secure catheter.
- Tegaderm to secure catheter.
- Linear 5- to 15-MHz Doppler probe.
- Ultrasound probe cover.
- Portable ultrasound machine.
- A-line extension tubing to monitor arterial pressure proximal to balloon.
- Scalpel (#11 or #15).
- A portable cart for immediate access and ease of restocking (Fig. 2.3).

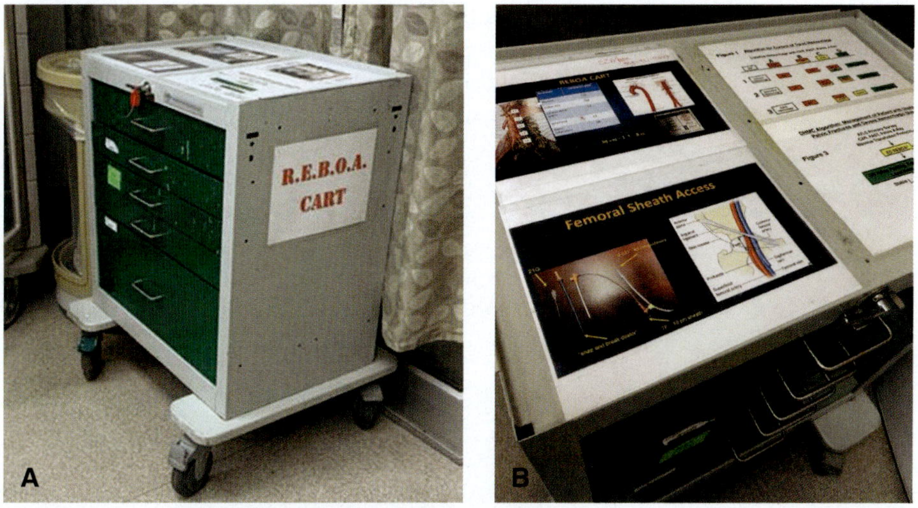

FIGURE 2.3 ▌ A portable REBOA cart (**A**) is kept in the emergency department trauma room. The top (**B**) is labeled with the algorithm, instructions for use, and tips for successful arterial access.

Anatomy

TIP

The inguinal skin crease can vary with body habitus and is not a reliable marker for the common femoral artery.

- Using surface landmarks, the inguinal ligament is identified between the anterior superior iliac spine (ASIS) and the pubic symphysis. The common femoral artery (CFA) is approximately midpoint between these bony landmarks and is accessed 2 cm below the inguinal ligament (Fig. 2.4A).

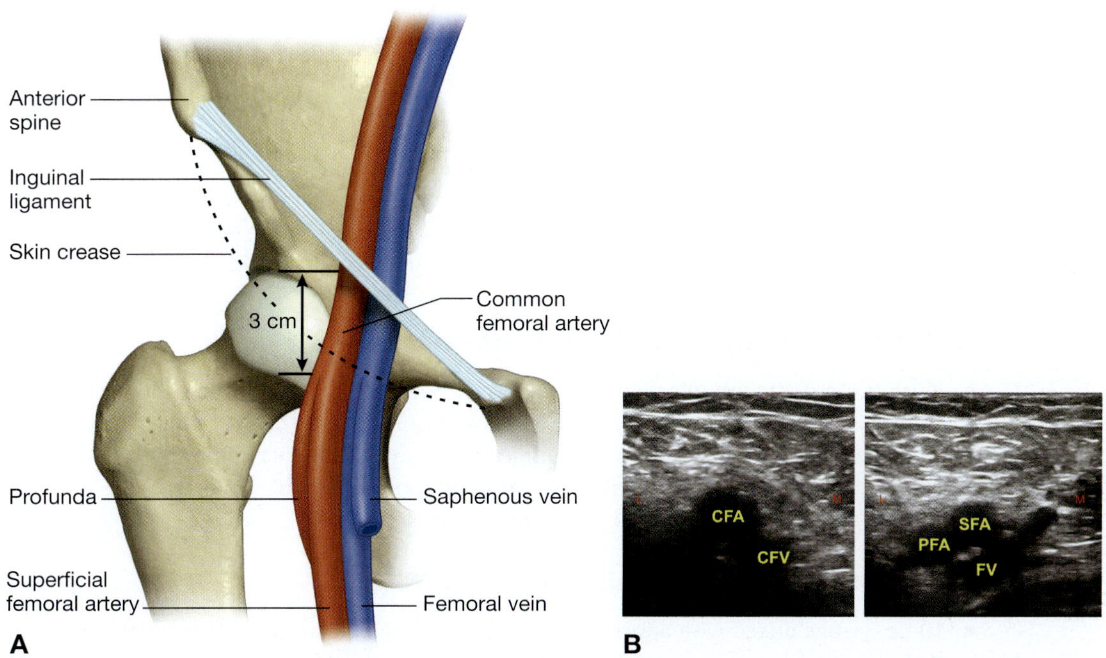

FIGURE 2.4 ▌ Anatomic landmarks used to identify the common femoral artery for percutaneous access at approximately 2 to 3 cm below the inguinal ligament where it overlies the middle third of the femoral head (**A**) and the ultrasound landmarks used to identify the common femoral artery for percutaneous access by viewing the femoral bifurcation and accessing above this level but below the inguinal ligament (**B**). (CFA, common femoral artery; CFV, common femoral vein; SFA, superficial femoral artery; PFA, profunda femoris artery; FV, femoral vein; M, medial; L, lateral.) (Reproduced from Yi J, Fox CJ, Moore EE. Resuscitative endovascular balloon occlusion of the aorta (REBOA). In: Rasmussen T, Tai N, eds. *Vascular Trauma*. 4th ed. Elsevier; 2021.)

- It is important to access the CFA, cephalad entry into the external iliac artery may preclude external compression following sheath removal, whereas caudal entry into the superficial femoral artery may lead to arterial thrombosis. A useful sonographic landmark for the borders of the CFA is the inferior epigastric artery proximally and profunda/superficial femoral bifurcation distally (Fig. 2.4B).

TECHNIQUE

Arterial Access

- The inner dilator is inserted snug into the 7-French sheath (Fig. 2.5).

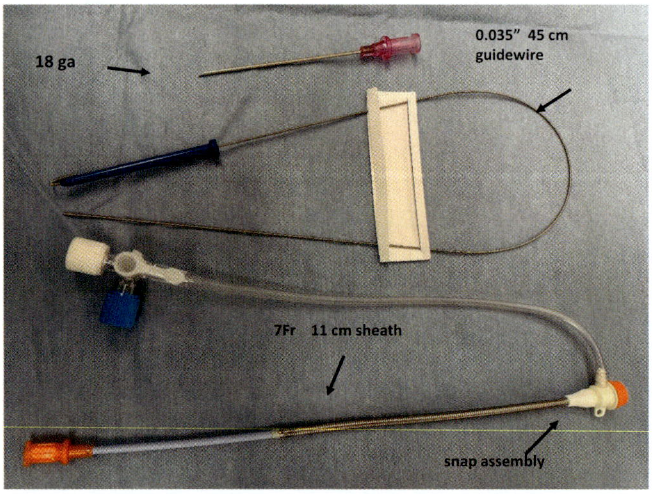

FIGURE 2.5 ▌ Optional arterial access supplies include an arterial entry needle, soft stainless-steel guidewire, and a 7-French sheath that comes with an inner dilator that must be reinserted and fit snug into the sheath to ensure smooth delivery into the vessel.

- A linear ultrasound probe is used to visualize the CFA.
- Access can be obtained on either CFA, but the least injured side is preferred.
- With bevel up, insert the needle at 45 degrees—arterial blood should return but may not be pulsatile if the patient is hypotensive.
- Advance the wire and if any resistance, stop, pull back, and spin forward.
- Ideally, intra-arterial location of the wire within the CFA should be confirmed by ultrasound.
- Remove the 18-gauge needle and insert the 7-French sheath over the 0.035 wire.
- Similarly, the sheath should be advanced cautiously and reinserted if there is any resistance.

Balloon Preparation and Insertion

- Flush the system with injectable saline and withdraw any air from the balloon.
- Slide the orange peel away over the P-tip to straighten the catheter for insertion.
- Measure the bottom of balloon to xiphoid (zone I) or umbilicus (zone III).
  - Typical insertion for zone I is 46 cm and for zone III 28 cm.
  - May also use P-tip at sternal notch for zone I.

Inflation and Confirmation of Position

- 10-cc syringe mixed with approximately 75/25 saline and contrast with the following guidelines:
  - 5-cc inflation volume = 15-mm balloon diameter
  - 8-cc inflation volume = 20-mm balloon diameter
  - 13-cc inflation volume = 25-mm balloon diameter
  - 20-cc inflation volume = 30-mm balloon diameter
  - 24-cc inflation volume is the maximum = 32-mm balloon diameter

- Tactile feedback during inflation may not occur, inflation volumes and the systolic blood pressure response should be your guide for optimal inflation. **Do not overinflate the balloon.**
- Secure the catheter and obtain a digital radiograph to verify position. (T4-L1-zone I or L2/L4-zone III, Fig. 2.6).

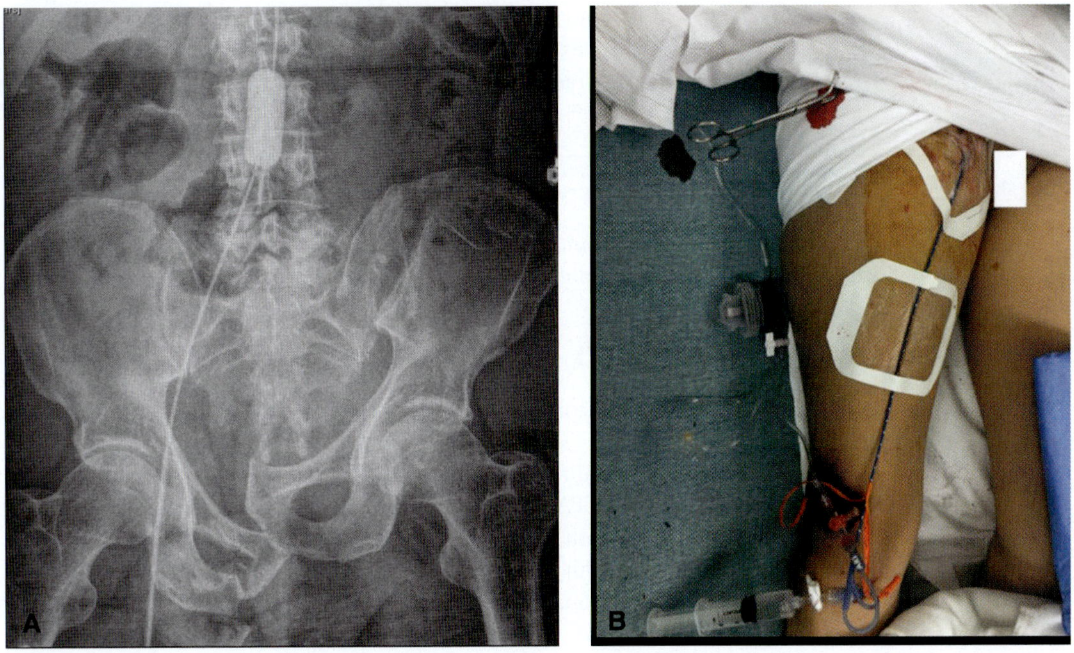

FIGURE 2.6 ▌ Plain x-ray in emergency department demonstrating REBOA balloon inflated in REBOA zone III (**A**). Patient with pelvic sheeting and REBOA catheter in right common femoral artery (**B**). (Reproduced from Campion EF, Fox CJ. Prehospital hemorrhage control and REBOA. *Curr Trauma Rep*. 2019;5:129–136.)

- The balloon must be deflated before repositioning.
- It is important to document the time of inflation, zone location, volume in balloon, as well as changes over time. The most secure method for documentation of the hemodynamic response is to use a marker and transcribe directly onto the patient (Fig. 2.7).

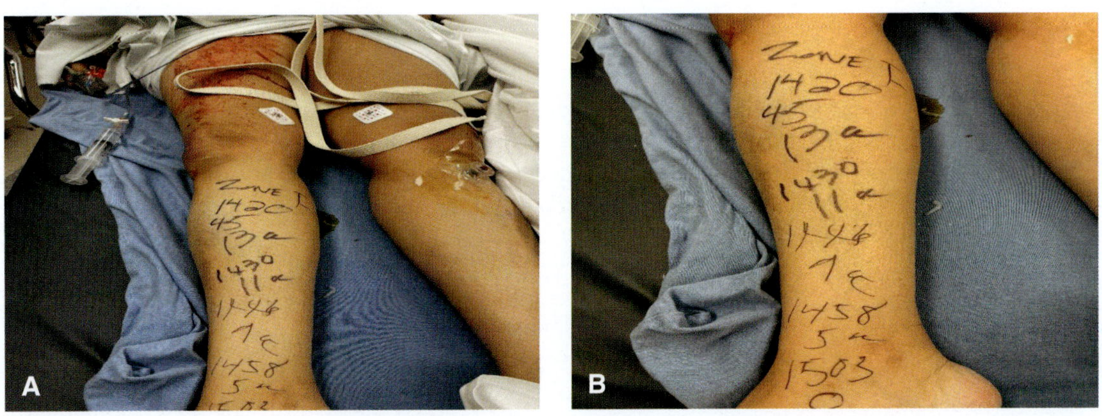

FIGURE 2.7 ▌ ER-REBOA catheter (Prytime Medical, Inc., Arvada, CO) inserted into a 7-French sheath and secured with a nylon suture. The time of aortic occlusion is annotated on the skin with a surgical marking pen.

BALLOON DEFLATION

- Overzealous filling of balloon can impede deflation.
- Deflation can have the same physiologic response as removing an aortic clamp.
- Anesthesia should be prepared to treat acidosis, hyperkalemia, and sudden cardiac deterioration.
- Do not withdraw the catheter before complete deflation of the balloon to prevent vessel injury.

POSTOPERATIVE CARE

- Reverse coagulopathy and remove as soon as normal coagulation is reestablished, but at the latest within 24 hours.
- If the sheath is left in place for >4 hours, the sheath should be infused with heparinized saline.
- 30 minutes of manual pressure is sufficient.
- For sheaths >8 Fr, consider an open repair or a percutaneous closure device.
- Document the pulse examination and ankle brachial index (ABI) comparing to the opposite leg.
- Perform a duplex ultrasound in the hospital and clinic for occult pseudoaneurysm at the puncture site.

TIP

Always have an assistant hold the catheter in place to prevent migration during inflation. Never reinflate without ensuring proper zone of aortic occlusion.

PEARLS AND PITFALLS

- Anticipate the need for REBOA, success is much lower when access is performed in a last-ditch effort.
- Ensure optimal visualization of the femoral artery, and adjust gain and depth accordingly.
- Insertion is via the CFA, use the inguinal ligament not skin creases as a surface landmark.
- If devices (wire, sheath, catheter) will not advance, abort, and go to the other side and consider the presence of vessel injury or occlusive plaques.
- To avoid bleeding from the side port of the sheath after the dilator is removed, place the stopcock in the "off" position.
- If the catheter cannot be withdrawn, deflate the balloon again, flush the sheath, and reattempt using fluoroscopy.

COMPLICATIONS

TIP

Access site complications are the most prevalent and can be avoided by using ultrasound guidance and taking note of key anatomical landmarks.

- Access related.
  - Incidence is 1% to 9% of all percutaneous interventions and is reduced with ultrasound.
  - Hematoma and pseudoaneurysm are the most common complications.
  - Arteriovenous fistulae may resolve spontaneously.
  - Arterial dissection is a complication that can be avoided with careful technique.
  - Arterial thrombosis requires early recognition and treatment (Fig. 2.8).

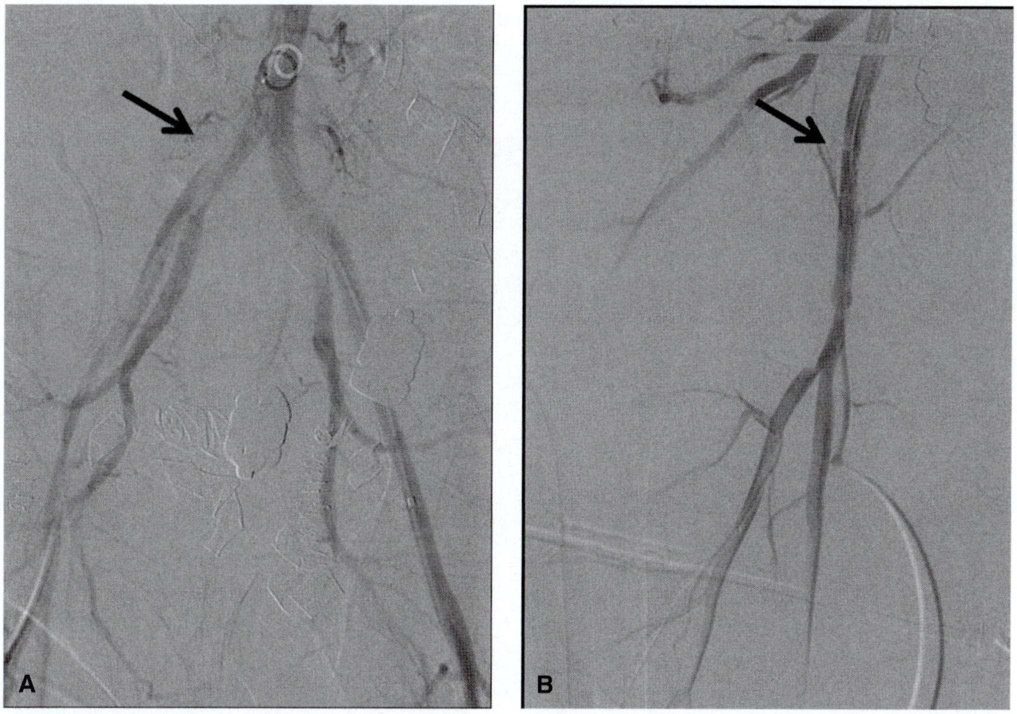

FIGURE 2.8 ❙ A digital subtraction angiogram demonstrated a filling defect (*arrow*) compatible with thrombus in the right common and external iliac arteries (**A**) and extensive clot with right femoral artery dissection (**B**, *arrow*) that resulted in transfemoral amputation. (Reproduced from Yi J, Fox CJ. Complications of endovascular and hybrid surgery. In: Horer T, DuBose JJ, Rasmussen TE, et al., eds. *Endovascular Resuscitation and Trauma Management*. Springer International; 2019.)

- Ischemic reperfusion injury
  - Total occlusion time in zone I should be <30 minutes; tolerance in zone III is unknown but likely >2 hours.
  - Renal embolization and infarction secondary to zone II malpositioning.
  - Coagulopathy, hyperkalemia, and acidosis from prolonged occlusion times.
  - Cardiovascular collapse and recurrent hypotension.
- Balloon inflation/deflation
  - Malposition into unintended anatomic zones (Fig. 2.9).

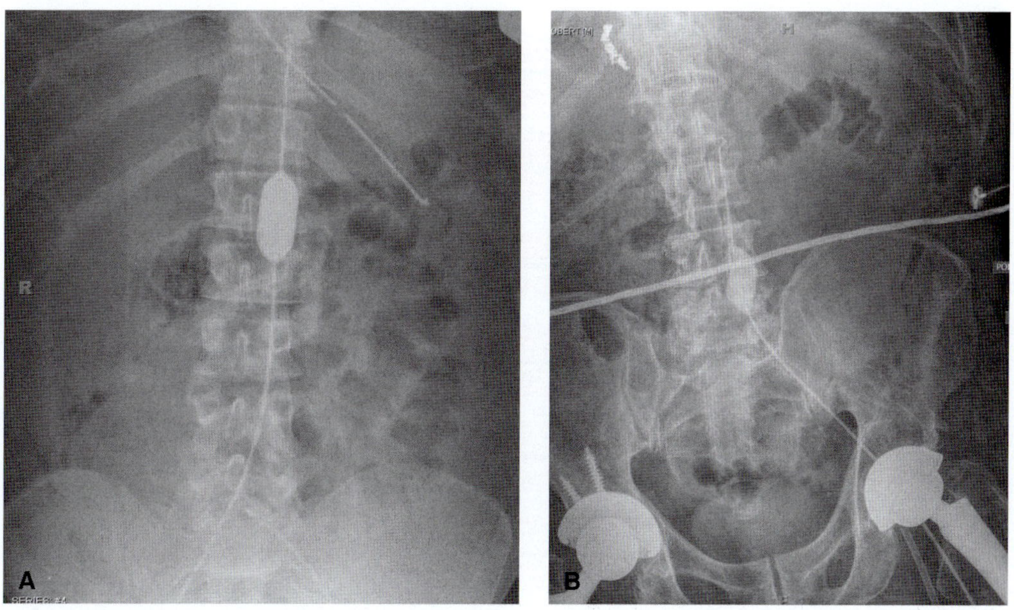

FIGURE 2.9 ❙ Inflation of an aortic occlusion balloon in the wrong location such as zone II (**A**) or the aortic bifurcation (**B**) can have catastrophic consequences.

- Balloon migration from inadequately securing the catheter.
- Arterial rupture from overinflation.
- Thromboemboli.

REBOA MODIFICATIONS

TIP

Aortic occlusion time should be carefully monitored to prevent ischemic complications. Variations of aortic occlusion may reduce the ischemic risk of end-organ malperfusion.

- Partial REBOA (pREBOA-Pro)
  - A wireless fluoroscopy free 7-Fr catheter designed for continuous inflation without full occlusion permitting distal flow (Fig. 2.10).

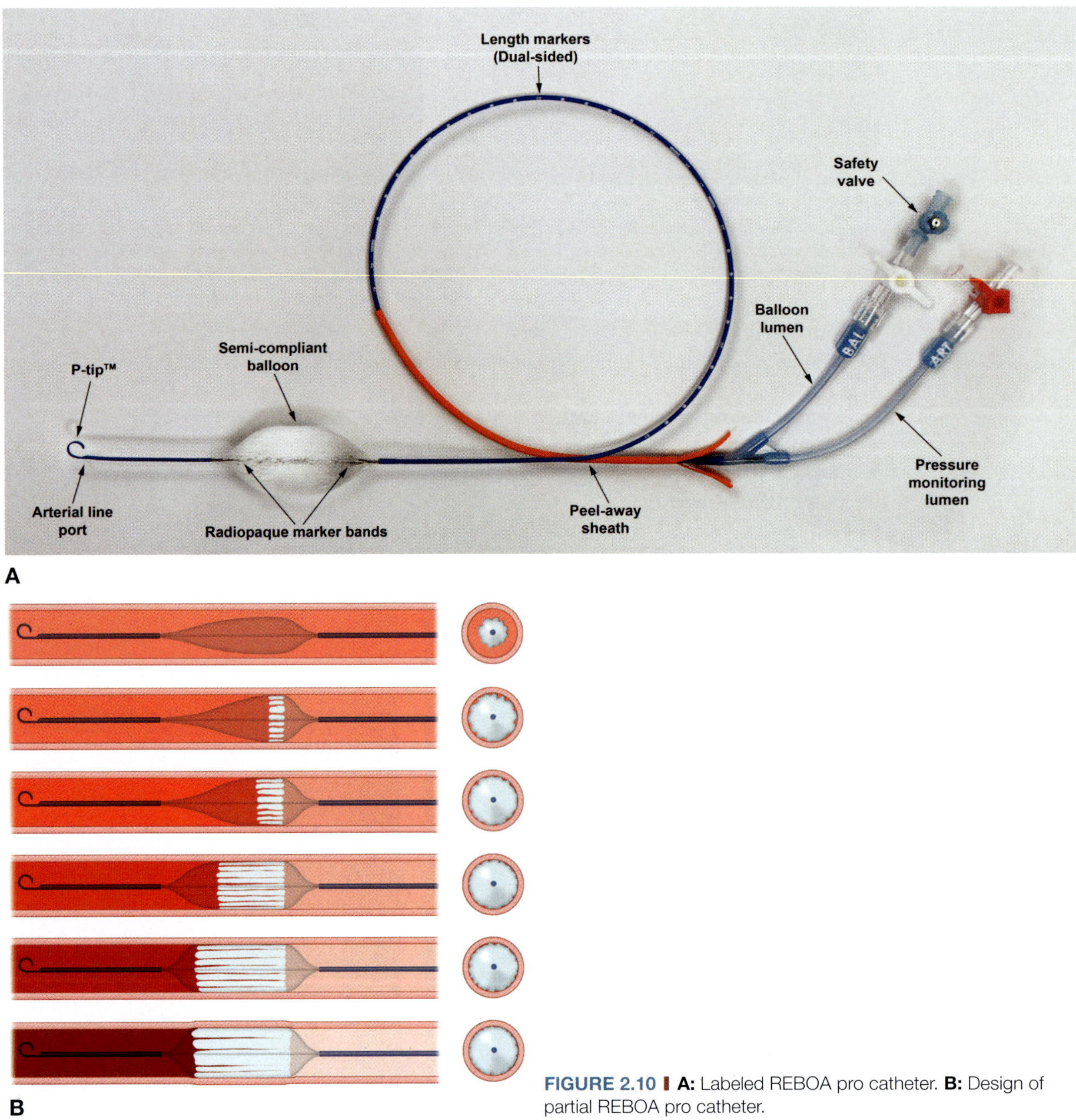

FIGURE 2.10 ▍**A:** Labeled REBOA pro catheter. **B:** Design of partial REBOA pro catheter.

- Semicompliant balloon with flow channels—functions like a "dimmer switch."
- Arterial monitoring above and below the balloon.
- 0.025-inch wire compatible for follow on procedures.
- Has pressure relief safety valve.
- Use 30-cc syringe for the whole procedure to ensure full deflation.
- "Testing" the balloon before insertion is not recommended.

- Intermittent REBOA
  - Full deflation followed by an interval of full inflation to achieve response.
  - Typically, withdrawal 1 mL per minute.

Suggested Readings

Adnan SM, Wasicek PJ, Crawford A, et al. Endovascular control of pelvic hemorrhage: concomitant use of resuscitative endovascular balloon occlusion of the aorta and endovascular intervention. *J Trauma Acute Care Surg*. 2019;86(1):155–159.

Biffl WL, Fox CJ, Moore EE. The role of REBOA in the control of exsanguinating torso hemorrhage. *J Trauma Acute Care Surg*. 2015;78(5):1054–1058.

Ordoñez CA, Rodríguez F, Parra M, et al. Resuscitative endovascular balloon of the aorta is in penetrating chest trauma with major hemorrhage: proposal of a new institutional deployment algorithm. *J Trauma Acute Care Surg*. 2020;89(2):311–319.

Stannard A, Eliason JL, Rasmussen TE. Resuscitative endovascular balloon occlusion of the aorta (REBOA) as an adjunct for hemorrhagic shock. *J Trauma*. 2011;71(6):1869–1872.

Chapter 3
Tube Thoracostomy

RYAN A. LAWLESS AND ERNEST E. MOORE

PERIOPERATIVE CONSIDERATIONS

Procedure Rationale

Evacuation of air or blood from the chest is the most common procedure performed in the acutely injured patient. There are a number of technical options for tube thoracostomy, we describe what we believe is the standard to ensure effective decompressive. Knowing the technique to properly place a tube thoracostomy is essential for anyone providing care for an injured patient. High rates of infection and malpositioning of a tube thoracostomy have been documented with tube thoracostomy performed in the emergency department. Thus, proper sterile preparation and careful tube placement are important.

Essential Equipment

TIP

Become self-sufficient. Learn to set up the equipment, including the local anesthetic, in such a manner that assistance is not required to minimize time. Be familiar with the institutional chest drainage system and know how to troubleshoot it.

- See Figure 3.1

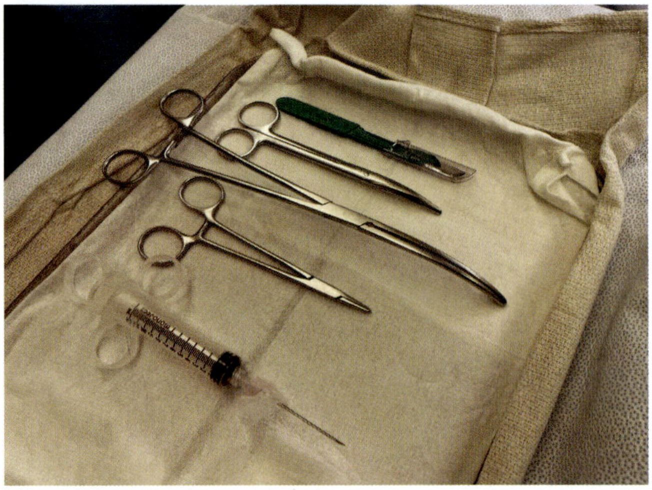

FIGURE 3.1 | Equipment should be limited to essential instruments.

- Surgical skin prepping solution of choice
- Sterile towels × 4
- Sterile drape, full length with central hole
- Personal protective equipment

- Sterile gown
- Sterile surgical gloves
- 10-cc syringe
- 1% local anesthesia
- Scalpel with a #10 Blade
- 18-gauge needle
- 21-gauge needle
- Mayo scissors
- Large Kelly clamp
- Tube thoracostomy: 24 Fr to 32 Fr, straight
- Polyester on a cutting needle
- Chest drain system
- Vaseline gauze/xeroform
- 4 × 4 gauze
- Tape

Positioning (Fig. 3.2)

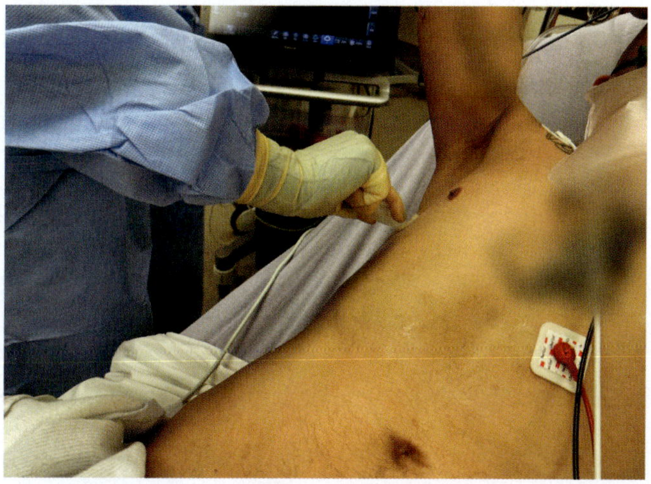

FIGURE 3.2 ▌ Positioning with ipsilateral arm abducted and over the head. Ultrasound is helpful for optimal chest tube placement.

- Extremis: Supine with ipsilateral arm over the head
- Hemodynamically stable: Supine with a slight bump under the ipsilateral shoulder/back and ipsilateral arm above the head

TIP

Use a wrist restraint or gauze wrap to secure the ipsilateral arm above the patient's head.

TECHNIQUE

Landmarks

- Anterior axillary line
- Nipple
- Inframammary fold

Surgical Approach (Fig. 3.3)

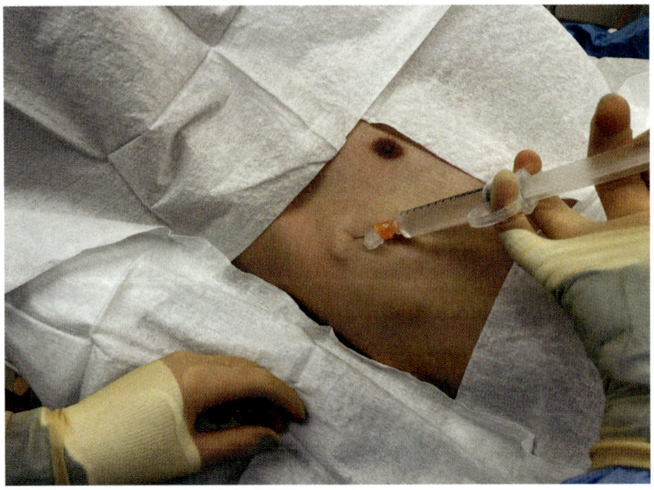

FIGURE 3.3 ▌The correct interspace is identified and a 21-gauge needle for delivery of local anesthetic.

- Position the patient as described previously
- Prepare the skin from the sternum to the bed and from the clavicle to the bottom of the rib cage
- Place the sterile towels to square off the operative field
  - Be sure to include the appropriate landmarks
- Place the sterile drape
- Identify the fifth intercostal space along the anterior axillary line
- Anesthetize the skin and planned track of the chest tube over the intended rib
  - Injecting generous local anesthesia, within the maximum recommended dose, is critical (Fig. 3.4)
  - Make a 1.5- to 2.0-cm incision perpendicular to the anterior axillary line (Fig. 3.5)

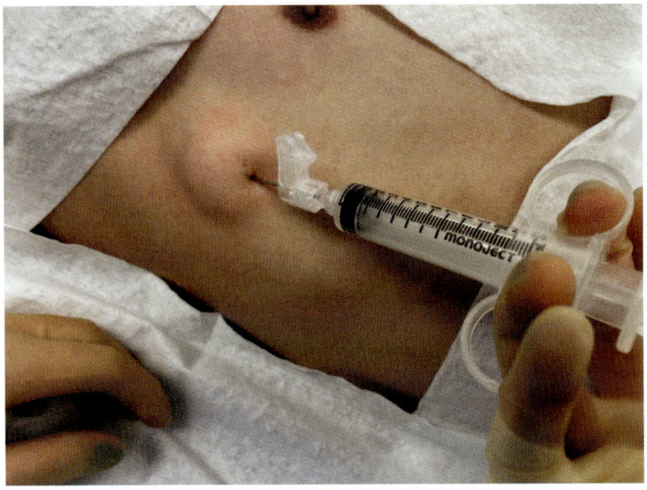

FIGURE 3.4 ▌Generous local anesthesia is injected into the planned surgical site.

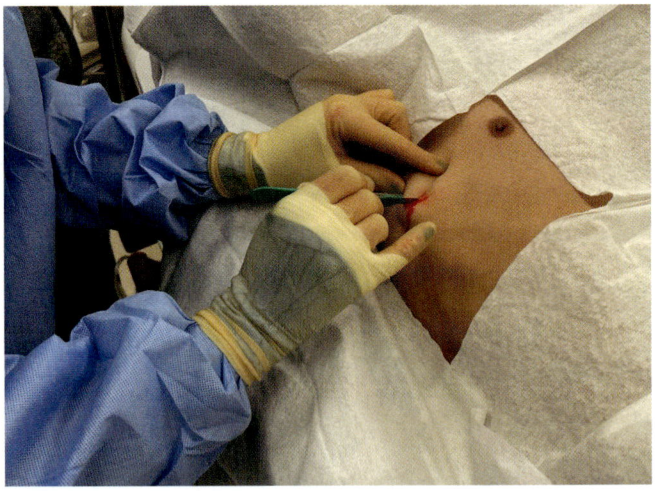

FIGURE 3.5 ▌A transverse incision is made over the fifth intercostal space.

- Enter the intrathoracic space with the Mayo scissors (Fig. 3.6)

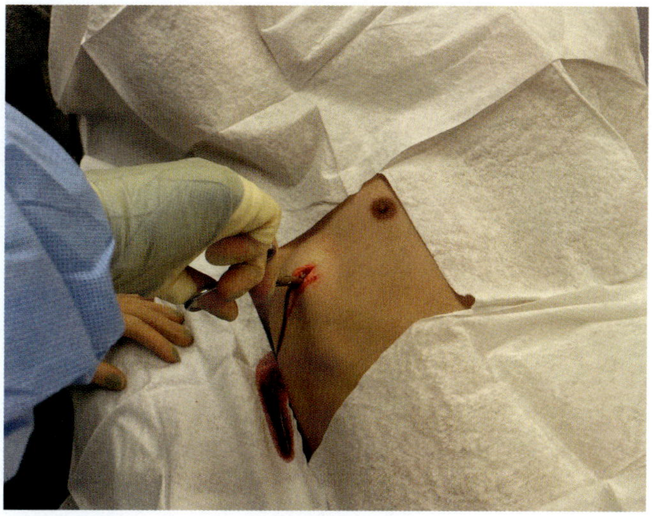

FIGURE 3.6 | The subcutaneous tissue is traversed over the top of the rib to enter the rib space over the rib.

TIP

Holding the clamp at the pivot point allows for better control of the clamp to avoid plunging the clamp into the chest.

- Leave the Mayo scissors in the chest and open along the direction of the rib to spread the intercostal muscles
- Remove the instrument and confirm entry into the chest with a finger (Fig. 3.7)

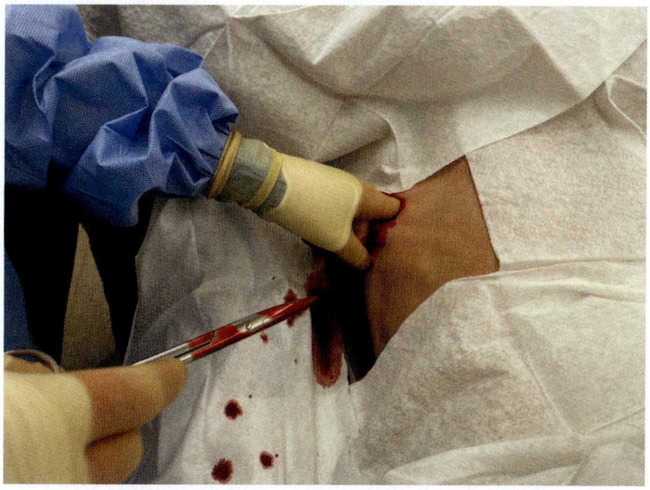

FIGURE 3.7 | Digital confirmation of entry into the thoracic cavity is essential.

TIP

Some providers will perform a sweeping motion, but rib fractures can lead to glove punctures and lacerations. Confirmation of chest entry is all that is necessary to appropriately place a tube thoracostomy unless there is evidence of previous thoracic disease.

- Clamp the end of the tube with the back of the curve of the large Kelly clamp with both tips facing the same direction (Fig. 3.8)

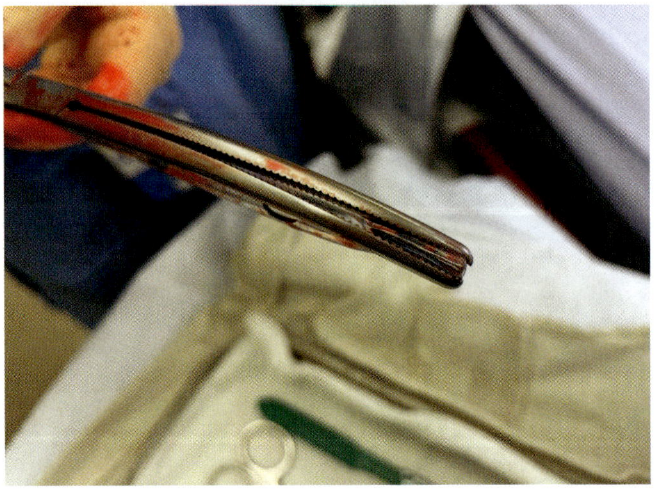

FIGURE 3.8 ▌ Clamp the tip of the thoracostomy tube in order to guide the tube into the thoracic cavity.

- Clamp and occlude the back of the tube with a separate clamp
- Insert the tube and Kelly clamp through the incision and hole in the intercostal muscles into the chest and direct the tube superior and posterior (Fig. 3.9)

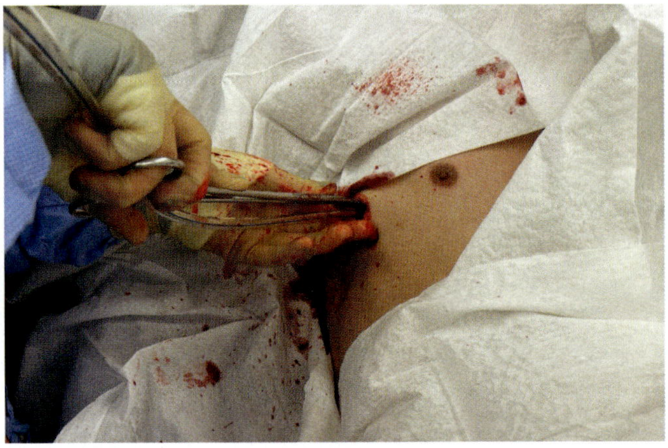

FIGURE 3.9 ▌ Insert the thoracostomy tube with a large Kelly clamp.

- Hold the tube with the left hand and remove the Kelly clamp with the right hand
- Insert the tube, directing it superior and posterior, 12–16 cm in depth
  - Spin the tube during insertion

TIP

A spinning tube will not bend. A bent tube will not spin.

- Approximate the incision if it is too large, meaning a finger can easily fit in the incision with the tube in place
- Secure the tube with the suture (Fig. 3.10)

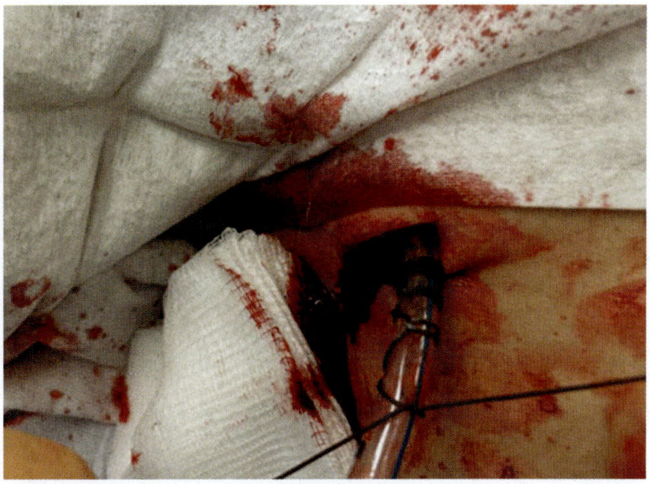

FIGURE 3.10 | Suture the tube thoracostomy to the skin by wrapping the tails around the tube in a Roman-sandal style manner.

TIP

The U-stitch technique is useful, particularly in thin patients to help prevent postpull pneumothoraxes.

- Dress the insertion site by placing the Vaseline gauze/xeroform at the insertion site around the tube (Fig. 3.11), followed by a folded 4 × 4 and tape (Fig. 3.12)

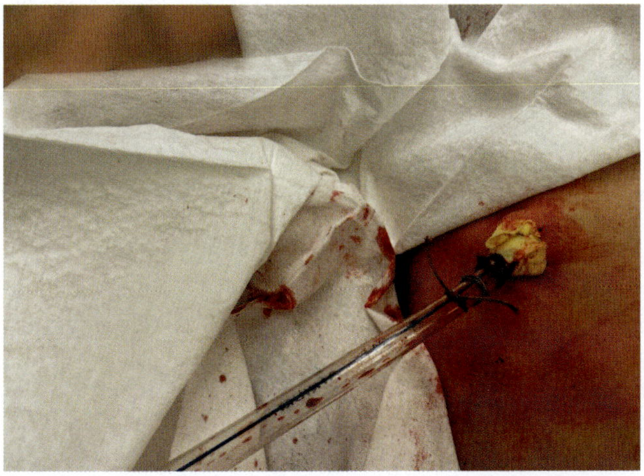

FIGURE 3.11 | Wrap Vaseline gauze, or xeroform, around the tube at the skin opening to improve the seal at the incision site.

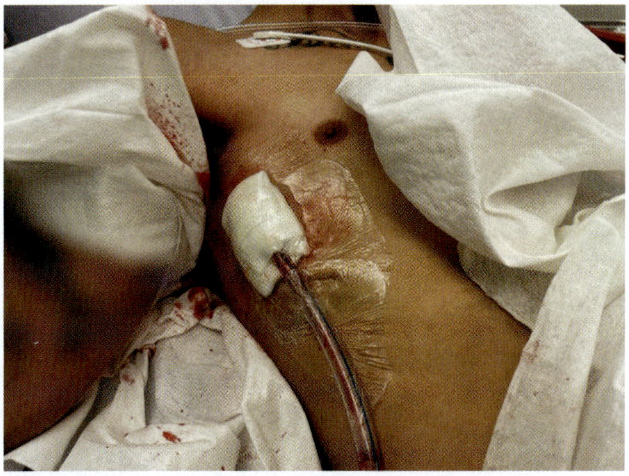

FIGURE 3.12 | Dress the site with a folded 4 × 4 beneath and on top of the tube. Place an occlusive dressing over the area.

- Attach the tube thoracostomy to the chest drainage system and secure the connection with tape (Fig. 3.13)

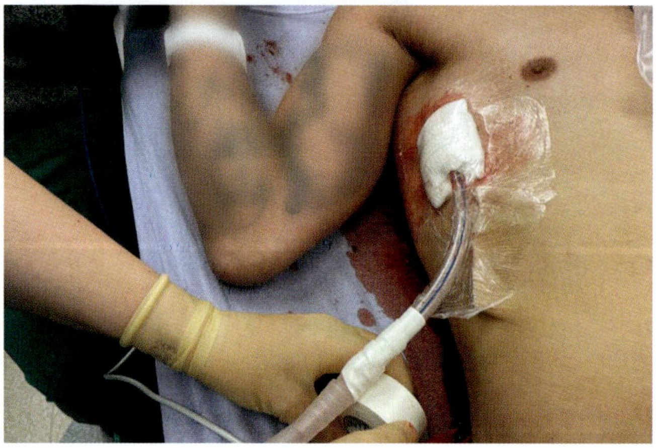

FIGURE 3.13 ▮ Tape the connection between the thoracostomy tube and the drainage system.

- Obtain a chest radiograph to confirm tube position and resolution of the indication for the tube thoracostomy

POSTOPERATIVE CARE

Postinsertion Troubleshooting

- Indication for the tube thoracostomy does not resolve
  - Is the tube in the chest?
    - Check imaging
    - Could the tube be laying between the chest wall and the scapula?
- Look for a bend in the tube at the level of the rib
- When in doubt, replace the tube
  - Is the chest drainage system assembled correctly?
    - Wet systems versus dry systems are assembled differently. Know the type and review the steps of setting up the system
- Persistent air leak is present
  - Is it the system?
    - Sequentially clamp the tubing from the chest drainage system to the chest wall and evaluate the air leak at every level
    - This will determine if the leak is from the chest or from somewhere in the system
- Sentinel eye is outside the thorax but within the subcutaneous tissue
  - Pneumothorax/hemothorax resolved
    - Management per usual pathway
  - Pneumothorax/hemothorax NOT resolved or air leak is present
    - Replace the tube thoracostomy versus placing a second tube thoracostomy

Suggested Readings

Bozzay JD, Walker PF, Ronaldi AE, Elster EA, Rodriguez CJ, Bradley MJ. Tube thoracostomy management in the combat wounded. *Am Surg*. 2018;84(4):1355–1362.

Hernandez MC, El Khatib M, Prokop L, Zielinski MD, Aho JM. Complications in tube thoracostomy: systematic review and meta-analysis. *J Trauma Acute Care Surg*. 2018;85(2):410–416.

Patel NJ, Dultz L, Ladhani HA, et al. Management of simple and retained hemothorax: a practice management guideline from the eastern association for the surgery of trauma. *Am J Surg*. 2021;221(5):873–884.

Platnick C, Witt CE, Pieracci FP, et al. Beyond the tube: can we reduce chest tube complications in trauma patients? *Am J Surg*. 2021;222(5):1023–1028.

SECTION II Cervical Injuries

Chapter 4
Carotid Arterial Injury

CHARLES J. FOX AND ERNEST E. MOORE

PERIOPERATIVE CONSIDERATIONS

Procedure Rationale

Vascular trauma to the neck may result in either life-threatening hemorrhage or severe neurologic deficit if not recognized promptly and treated appropriately. Advancements in imaging technology have improved the ability to detect injury and plan an operation that in the past would obligate exploration. Endovascular technology now offers additional therapeutic options for treating inaccessible regions of the neck. The wide variety of presentations and the spectrum of injuries that range from mild blunt injury to destructive penetrating wounds with exsanguination and airway compromise continue to stimulate refinements in the management of carotid arterial injury. In general, penetrating trauma undergoes prompt exploration for patients with hard signs (bleeding, expanding hematoma, thrill), whereas blunt injuries are usually surgically inaccessible and undergo multidetector CT angiography in preparation for medical therapy or endovascular repair.

Anatomic Zones of the Neck (Figs. 4.1 and 4.2)

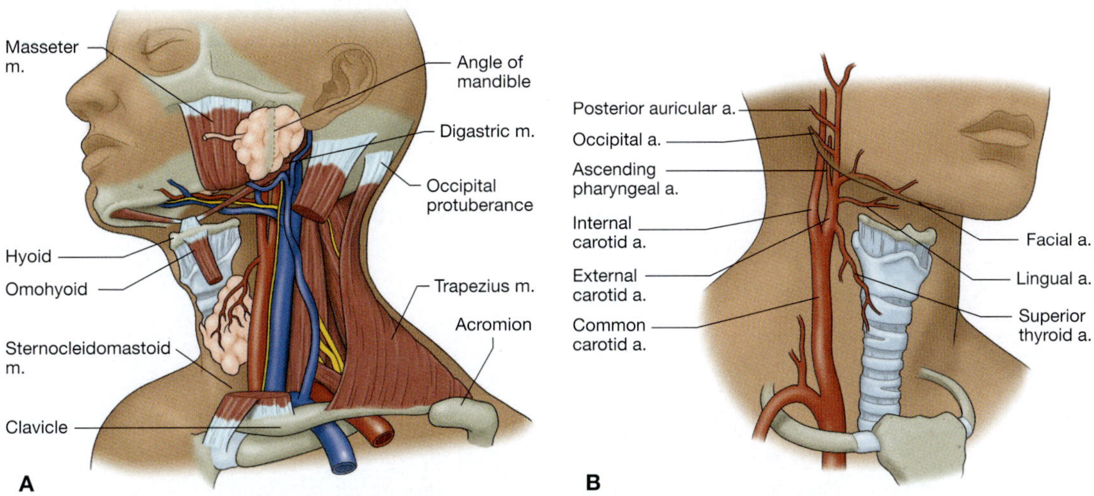

FIGURE 4.1 ❚ Anatomy of the cervical region (**A**) with named branches of the external carotid artery (**B**).

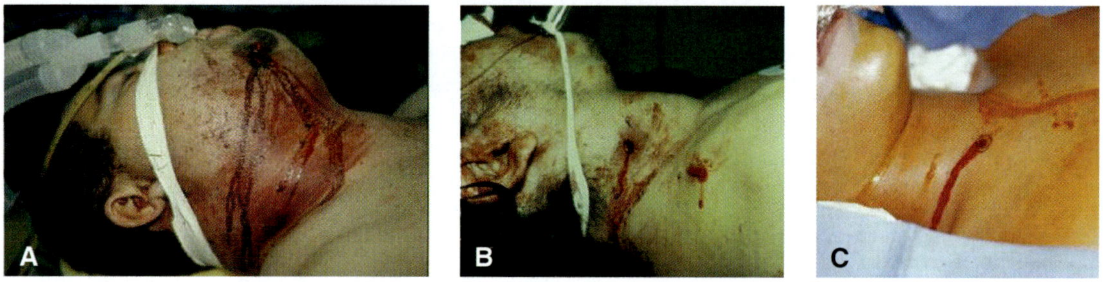

FIGURE 4.2 ▮ The three zones of the neck with penetrating injuries in descending order: **zone III, zone II, and zone I** (**A–C**). Patients with hard signs of vascular injury should proceed directly to the operating room for exploration and repair following airway control, a chest radiograph to diagnose occult hemopneumothorax and a thorough neurologic assessment.

- Zone I is below the cricoid cartilage.
- Zone II is from the cricoid cartilage to the angle of the mandible.
- Zone III is above the angle of the mandible.
- Zones I and III are hindered by difficult surgical access; obtaining preoperative “road-map” images in stable patients may delineate the trajectory and avoid a complicated operation (Fig. 4.3).

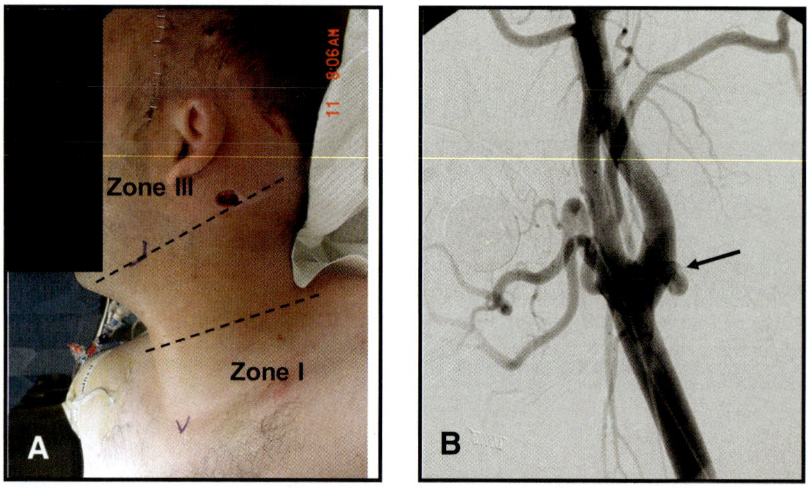

FIGURE 4.3 ▮ A young male with a penetrating left neck wound (**A**) underwent digital subtraction angiography (**B**) demonstrating a pseudoaneurysm (*arrow*) at the carotid bifurcation and repaired using a saphenous vein patch. Preoperative imaging is helpful when a zone II injury is not obvious.

- Penetration of zone II with violation of the platysma is the most common indication for routine exploration.

Essential Equipment

TIP

During the OR preparation, essential equipment must be immediately available because bleeding may be massive, and ischemia is tolerated poorly. Ensure that the Doppler box is charged and that the Doppler probe is functional. Flush and de-air the shunts.

- Headlight
- Loupe magnification 2.5
- Self-retaining retractor

- Castroviejo needle driver
- Microvascular forceps
- Vessel loops
- Rummel tourniquet (red rubber catheter and umbilical tape)
- Profunda vascular clamps (angled and straight)
- One pack of 6-in Argyle (8,10,12,14 French) shunts
- 31-cm Pruitt-Inahara shunt (with T port) 8- to 10-mm balloon diameter
- Sutures
  - 6-0 Prolene on a C1 or BV1 needle
  - 3-0 silk plain and stick ties
  - 3-0 Vicryl sutures
- Heparinized saline 50 to 100 units in 1,000 mL saline
- 10-cc syringes of heparinized saline on 18-gauge IV catheter
- Fogarty embolectomy catheters no. 2, no. 3, no. 4
- Bulldog soft vascular clamps
- Three-way stopcock and A-line extension tubing
- 10-cc syringes of heparin saline on 18-gauge IV catheter
- 21-gauge butterfly needle or angiocatheter
- Contrast agent 50 mL (Omnipaque-240, GE Healthcare, Inc., Chicago, IL)
- Linear 8- to 10-MHz Doppler probe
- Linear or footprint 5- to 20-MHz ultrasound probe
- Ring reinforced 6- or 8-mm polytetrafluoroethylene (PTFE)
- Polyester or bovine pericardial patch
- Vein graft solution containing heparin saline, papaverine, etc.

Positioning

TIP

When cervical spine injury has been ruled out a shoulder roll to extend the neck may facilitate better exposure.

- Prep an assistant into field with temporary digital or Foley catheter occlusion (Fig. 4.4).

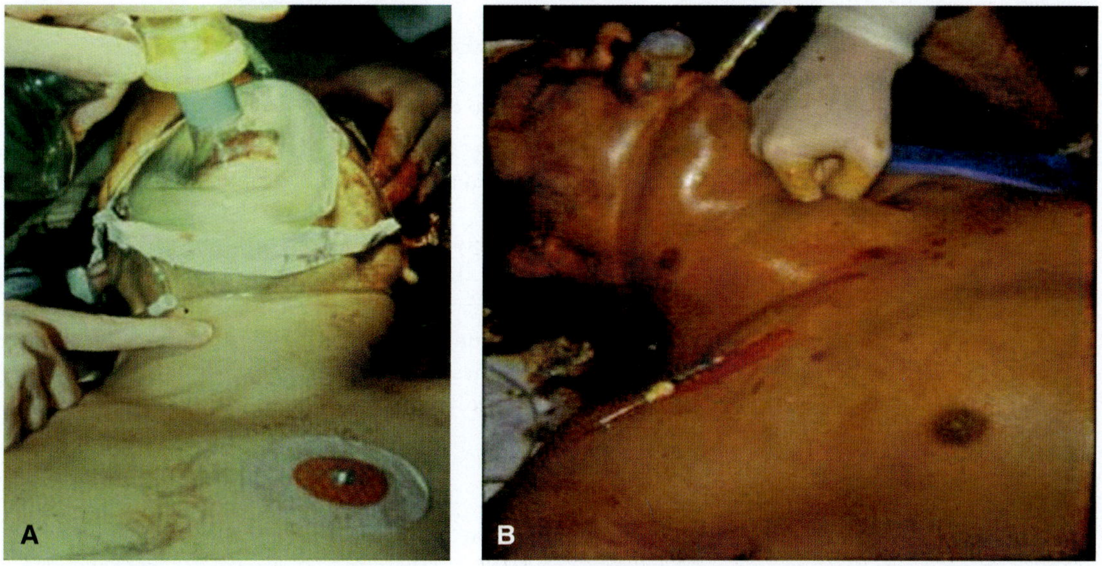

FIGURE 4.4 ▌ Prep an assistant into field with temporary **digital control (A) zone IIII and (B) zone II**.

- Supine with cervical spine maintained in neutral alignment.
- Drape from skull base to knees with anticipation of saphenous vein harvest.
- Radial arterial line is recommended for continuous hemodynamic monitoring.
- A careful neurologic assessment is documented prior to induction of general anesthetic.

TECHNIQUE

Surgical Approach

TIP

Take extra time to fully dissect, mobilize all structures, and completely explore the injury. Divide the posterior belly of the digastric muscle and mobilize the hypoglossal nerve and use a rongeur to resect the styloid process when high carotid exposures are necessary.

- An 8-cm oblique cervical incision along the sternocleidomastoid muscle (SCM), extending to the sternal notch or behind the ear as needed (Fig. 4.5).

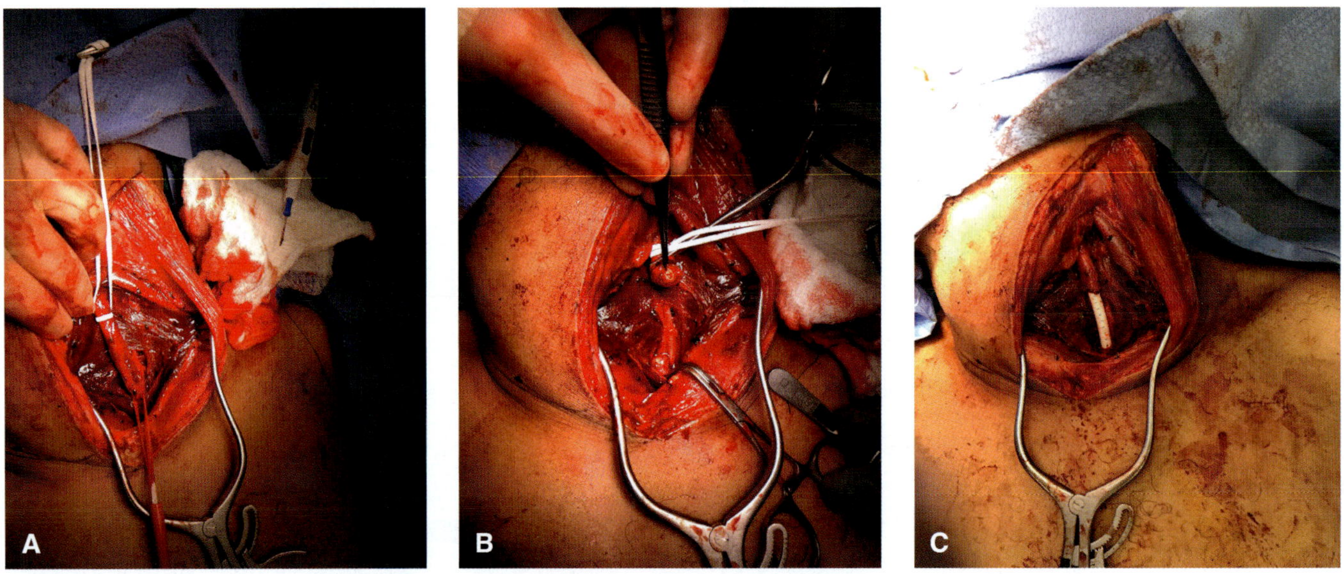

FIGURE 4.5 ▌ Left neck zone II stab wound showing the exposure using an oblique cervical incision (**A**). The transected CCA (**B**) is repaired with a prosthetic interposition graft due to the extent of the contusion and intimal injury (**C**).

- Consider an extension to median sternotomy for proximal control when injury is below the omohyoid muscle (Fig. 4.6).
- Open the carotid sheath and apply digital pressure or insert an occlusion balloon for bleeding.
- Ligate the facial vein and retract the mobile internal jugular vein laterally with the SCM.
- Dissect the common carotid artery (CCA) protecting the vagus nerve on the posterolateral surface.
- Place a Rummel tourniquet around the CCA and silastic vessel loops around the internal carotid (ICA) and external carotid arteries (ECA).
- The ECA is medial (going to face) and can be ligated without consequences.

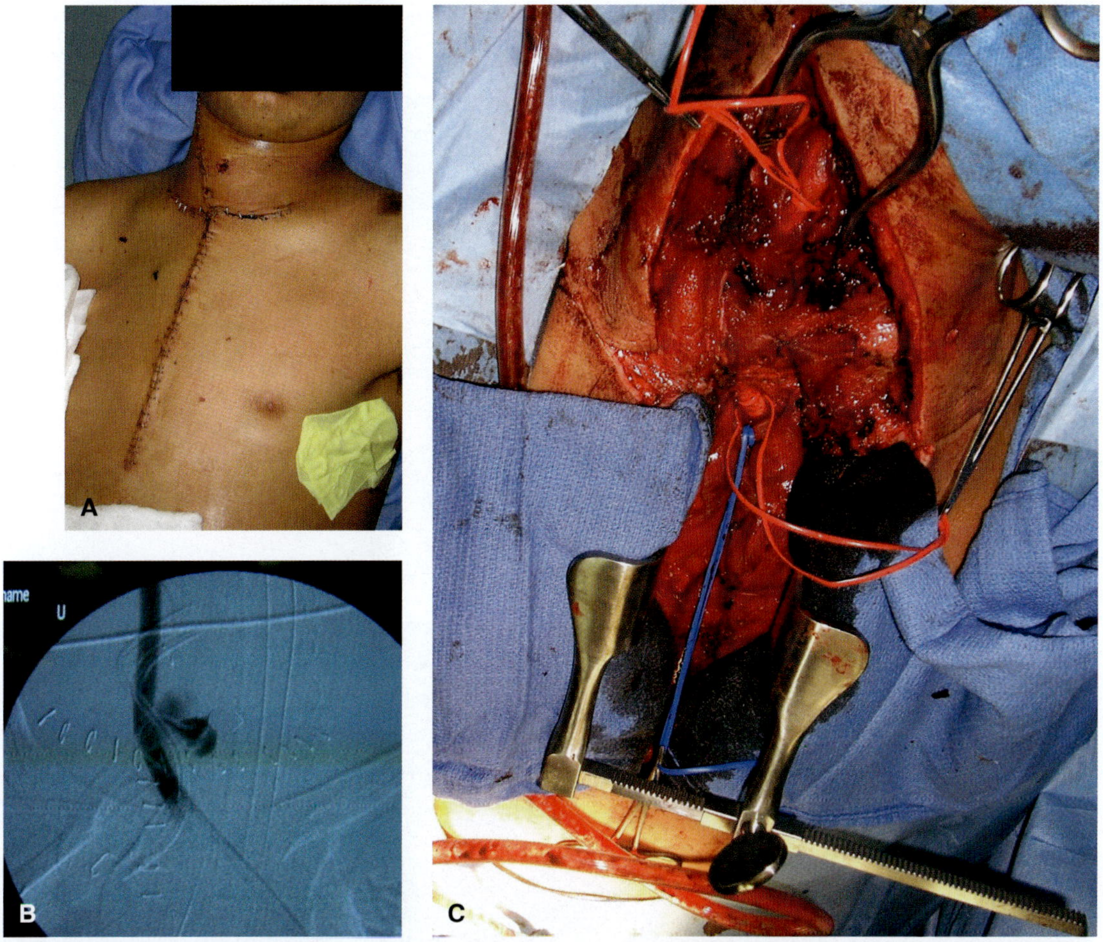

FIGURE 4.6 ▌ A patient was received following a penetrating injury to the right neck that was incompletely explored using a collar incision (**A**). The injury was located with a digital subtraction angiogram showing extravasation (**B**) and subsequently reexplored using a median sternotomy (**C**) for proximal control by placing silastic loops around the carotid bulb and the innominate artery. The injury was repaired with a reversed saphenous vein graft.

- Identify the hypoglossal nerve coursing transversely across the internal and external carotid arteries.
- The vagus nerve is seen posterolateral to the CCA.
- The ansa cervicalis courses distally on the CCA and can be divided.
- Division of the occipital artery will release the tethered hypoglossal nerve and expose more of the mid-ICA.
- Division of the posterior belly of the digastric muscle will expose the distal ICA.
- Remove the styloid process with a rongeur to reach the terminal extracranial ICA.

Thrombectomy and Shunting

TIP

Use extreme caution with the antegrade thrombectomy. Do not overinflate or pass the Fogarty thrombectomy catheter too far; intimal damage or cavernous sinus fistula can occur.

- A 2, 3, or 4 French Fogarty balloon thrombectomy catheter is passed gently and not overinflated to remove all thrombotic debris.
- Intraluminal temporary vascular shunts reestablish antegrade arterial flow.
- The Argyle shunt is easily inserted and comes in four diameters for optimal sizing.

- A Pruitt-Inahara shunt can be placed through a vein graft to perform the anastomosis without interruptions (Fig. 4.7).

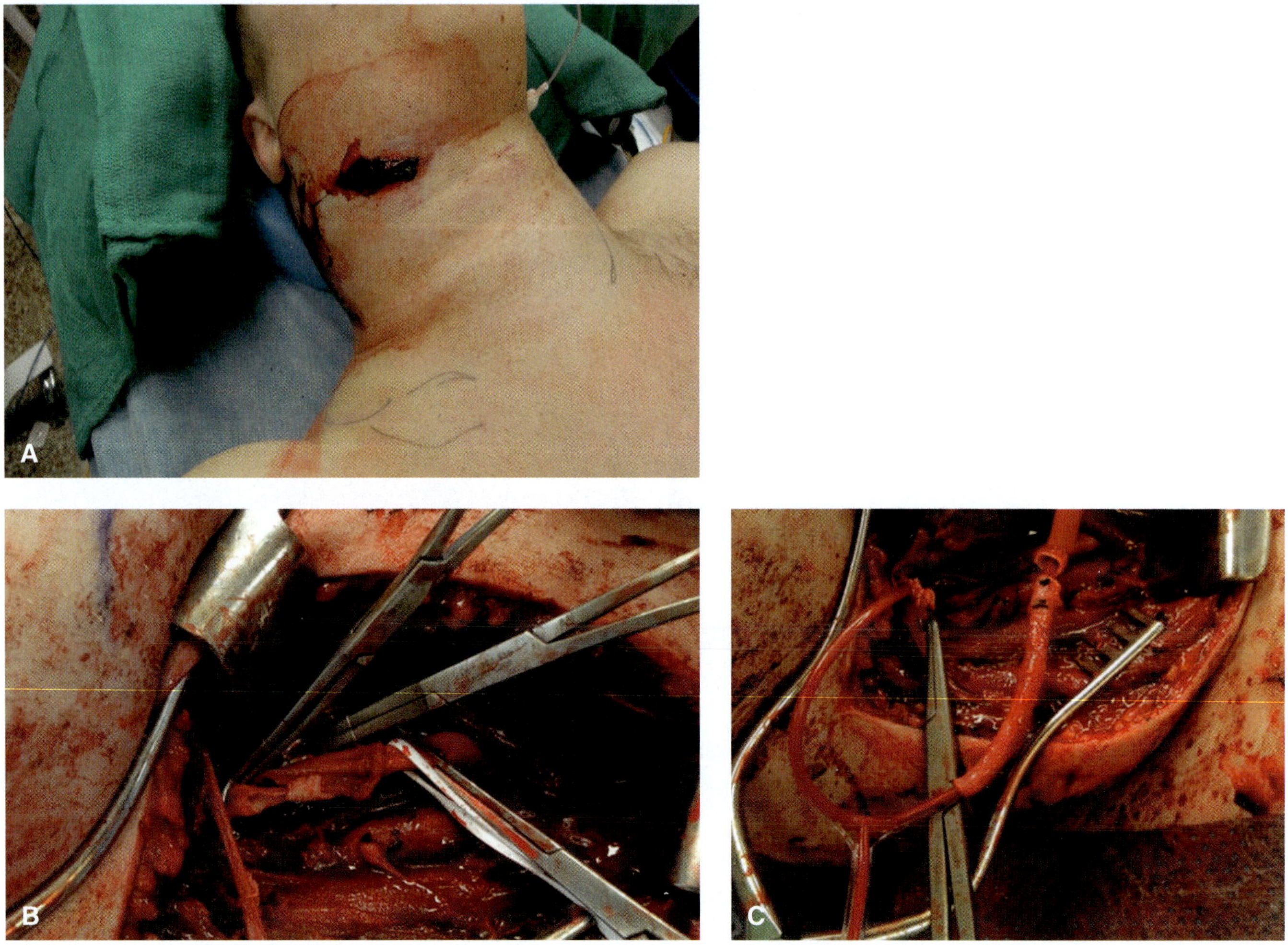

FIGURE 4.7 ▮ Penetrating right internal carotid artery injury (**A, B**) repaired with reversed saphenous vein sewn over a Pruitt-Inahara shunt (**C**).

- Robust collateral circulation via ECA to ICA excludes the need to shunt a CCA injury.
- A stump pressure (<40 mm Hg) predicts the need for shunting.
- Confirm shunt patency with Doppler, or T arm with Pruitt Inahara.
- Give intravenous heparin bolus to maintain activated clotting time >250 seconds.
- Flush vessel liberally with heparinized saline.

Carotid Reconstruction

TIP

Avoid the temptation to patch a large defect as this will result in stenosis. A prosthetic patch or vein patch is equally suitable as the neck is rarely contaminated.

- Type of repair and conduit is dictated by the degree and location of injury.
- Lacerations are sutured, and holes are patched.
- Perform a tensionless end-to-end repair for simple transections <1 to 2 cm of defect.

- Segmental defects are repaired using vein interposition grafts (contamination or ICA); however, prosthetic grafts are preferred for CCA injuries (Fig. 4.8).

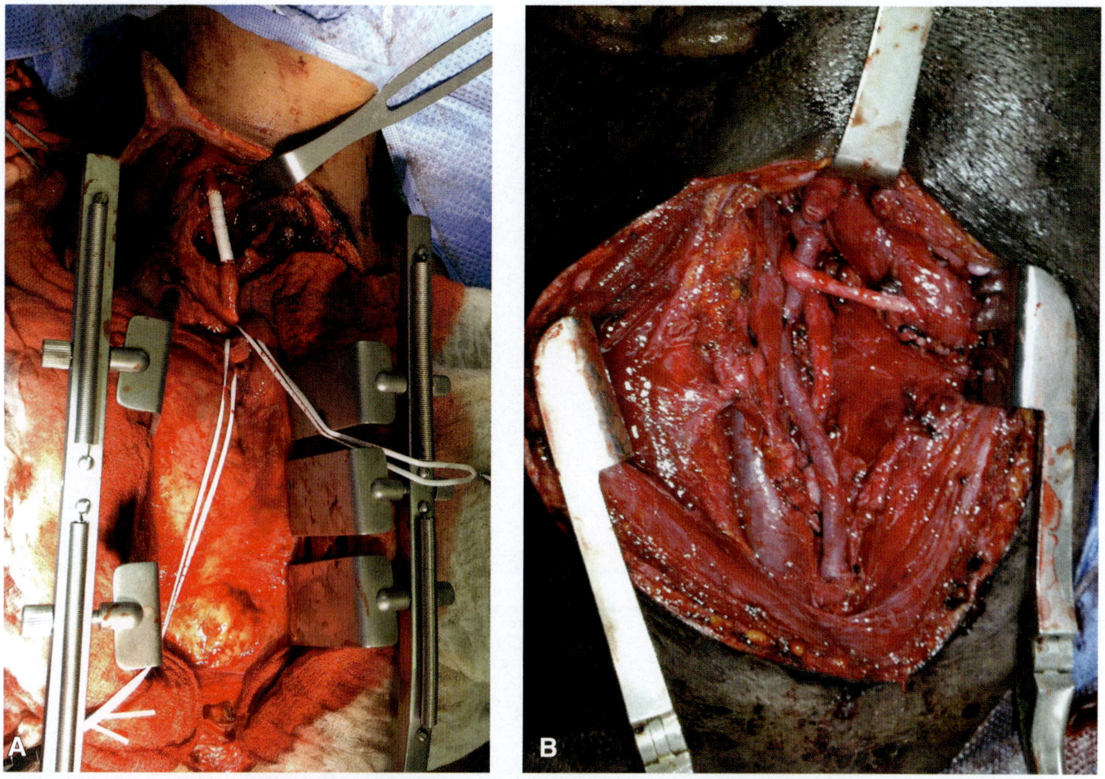

FIGURE 4.8 ▌ Oblique cervical incision with sternotomy for proximal control of a zone I injury (**A**). The CCA can be repaired with an interposition of ringed ePTFE (**A**), while the ICA is better suited for a reversed saphenous reconstruction (**B**).

- Ligation of the ICA should be avoided.
- Internal (distal) to external (proximal) carotid artery transposition is a useful autologous repair for a proximal ICA injury (Fig. 4.9).

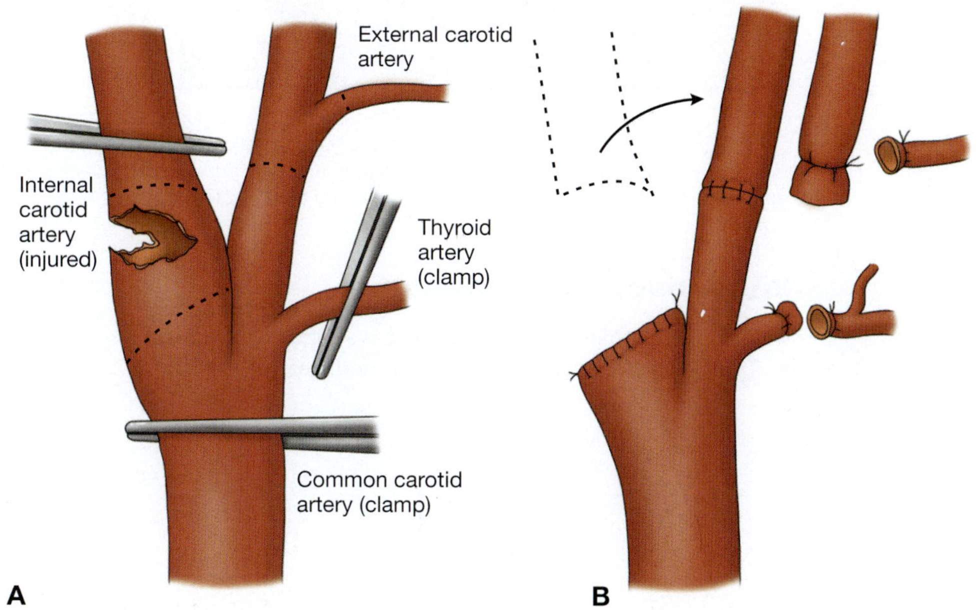

FIGURE 4.9 ▌ Transposition repair of a proximal internal carotid artery injury (**A**) to the external carotid artery is a useful autologous repair technique using a single anastomosis (**B**).

- The fresh repair is flushed first externally, then into the ECA, and finally into the ICA.
- A completion angiogram is performed with diluted hand-injected contrast arteriogram by placing a butterfly needle or angiocatheter into the CCA (Fig. 4.10).

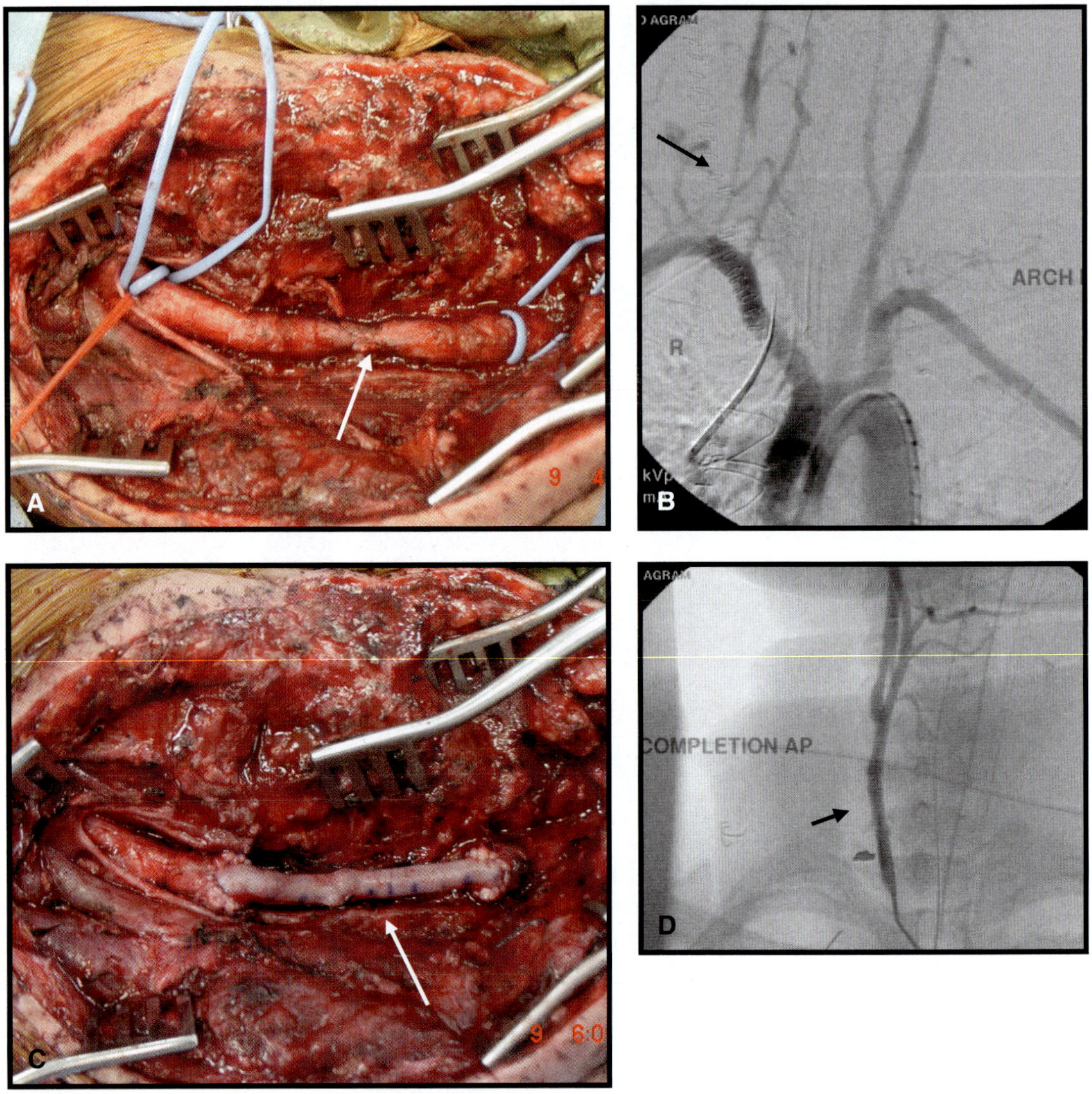

FIGURE 4.10 ▌ A right CCA fragment injury repaired with a saphenous vein patch (**A**, *white arrow*) was complicated by left hemiparesis. The angiogram shows an early thrombotic occlusion (**B**, *black arrow*) with retrograde filling of the ICA and ECA. A saphenous vein interposition graft (**C**, *white arrow*) restored antegrade circulation as shown in the completion angiogram (**D**, *black arrow*) and resolved the symptoms.

Endovascular Techniques

- Permits treatment of an injury that is surgically inaccessible.
- Typically reserved for the diagnosis and treatment of blunt cerebrovascular injuries.

- Stents are useful for tacking a dissection or sealing a transection or arteriovenous fistula (Fig. 4.11).

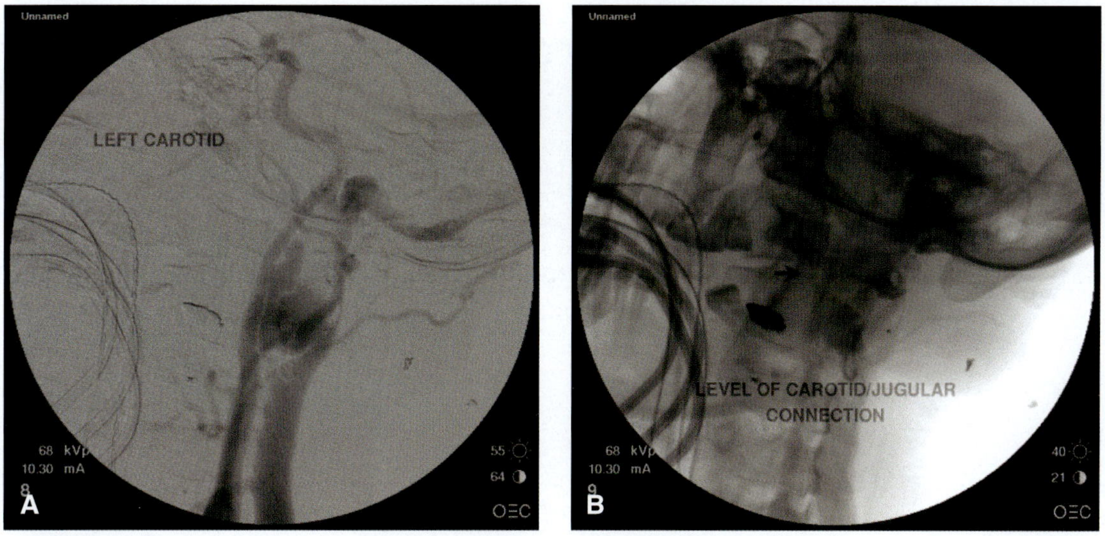

FIGURE 4.11 ▌ Left carotid artery digital subtraction angiogram discovers an occult arteriovenous fistula (**A**) characterized by early rapid jugular venous filling at the level of a metallic fragment (**B**).

- Coils are useful for occluding a branch vessel or treating some pseudoaneurysms (Fig. 4.12).

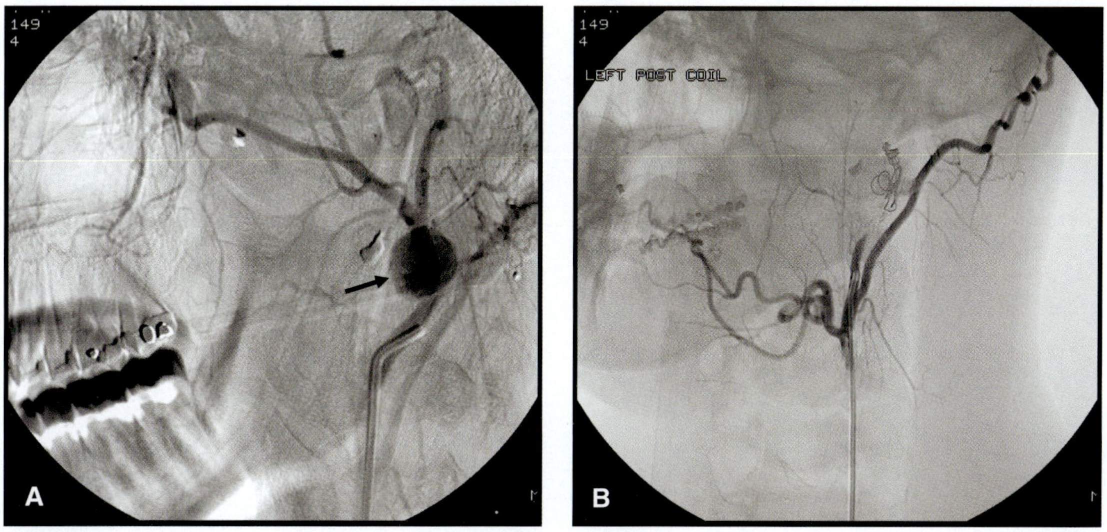

FIGURE 4.12 ▌ Left neck zone III penetrating injury with a digital subtraction angiogram showing an ECA pseudoaneurysm (**A**, *arrow*). Completion study after endovascular coiling demonstrates preservation of the occipital and lingual branches (**B**).

POSTOPERATIVE CARE

TIP

Antiplatelet therapy following carotid reconstruction is superior to systemic anticoagulation. A completion study (duplex sonography, angiography, or computed tomography angiography [CTA]) is essential to demonstrate patency of the revascularization.

- Patients with neurologic deficits should have diffusion-weighted magnetic resonance imaging.
- Initial and semiannual color flow duplex sonography is performed for 2 to 5 years to screen for the development of intimal hyperplasia.

- Indefinite single-agent antiplatelet therapy is routinely prescribed.
- Follow-up examinations and annual duplex sonography are encouraged.

Suggested Readings

Biffl WL, Cothren CC, Moore EE, et al. Western Trauma Association critical decisions in trauma: screening for and treatment of blunt cerebrovascular injuries. *J Trauma*. 2009;67(6):1150–1153.

Blitzer DN, Ottochian M, O'Connor J, et al. Penetrating injury to the carotid artery: characterizing presentation and outcomes from the national trauma data bank. *Ann Vasc Surg*. 2020;67:192–199.

Feliciano DV. Penetrating cervical trauma. "Current concepts in penetrating trauma", IATSIC Symposium, International Surgical Society, Helsinki, Finland, August 25–29, 2013. *World J Surg*. 2015;39(6):1363–1372.

Sperry JL, Moore EE, Coimbra R, et al. Western Trauma Association critical decisions in trauma: penetrating neck trauma. *J Trauma Acute Care Surg*. 2013;75(6):936–940.

Chapter 5
Vertebral Arterial Injury

CHARLES J. FOX AND ERNEST E. MOORE

PERIOPERATIVE CONSIDERATIONS

Procedure Rationale

A wide variety of presentations range from a mild blunt injury to destructive penetrating wounds that may be challenging. A decision for immediate open exploration versus imaging and delayed repair is based on the mechanism and hemodynamic stability of the patient. Blunt injuries infrequently require intervention by endovascular techniques. Penetrating vertebral artery injuries are rare but may require emergent exploration. The anatomy is complex, and the surgical exposure is difficult. The majority of patients present with active bleeding or an expanding hematoma, occasionally with airway compromise, and rarely a neurologic deficit. Computed axial tomography angiography (CTA) offers a high-resolution three-dimensional imaging that has increased the ability to detect subtle injuries of the vertebral artery. Endovascular strategies are useful therapeutic options for treating the surgically inaccessible segments.

Anatomy

The vertebral artery is divided into four anatomic segments referred to as V1–V4 (Fig. 5.1).

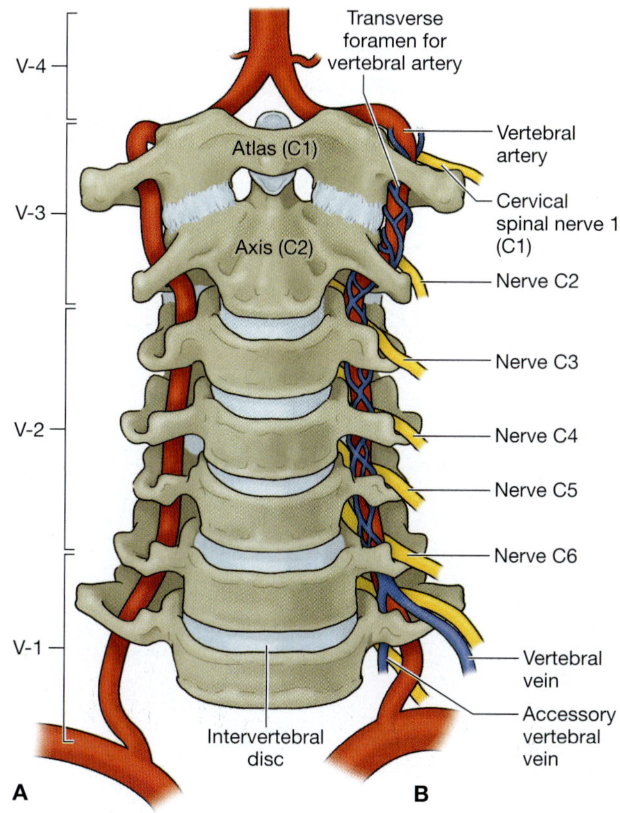

FIGURE 5.1 **A:** The four segments of the vertebral artery, (V1–V4) and the relationship between V2 and the proximal C3–C6 nerve roots (**B**).

- V1 is from the origin at the subclavian artery to the entry into the C6 transverse foramen.
- V2 (most common injury) is the interosseus segment from the C6 transverse foramen and exits the bony canal at the transverse process of C2 vertebrae.
- V3 is the extracranial segment between the transverse process of C2 and the skull base.
- V4 is the intracranial segment, terminating at the junction with the contralateral vertebral artery to form the basilar artery.
- Cervical nerve roots are in close (>4 mm) proximity to the V2 segment but in most cases, the artery remains undisturbed during anterior approaches to the cervical spine.
- Occasionally, it may be necessary to identify, expose, or mobilize the interosseus vertebral artery.
- V2 rests on the anteromedial surface of the cervical nerve roots at the level of each intertransverse space.

Essential Equipment

TIP

During the OR preparation, essential equipment must be immediately available because bleeding should be anticipated from the origin or may require a difficult bony resection to control bleeding in the interosseous region of the vertebral artery.

- Headlight
- Loupe magnification 2.5
- Self-retaining retractor
- Ryder and Castroviejo needle drivers
- Microvascular forceps
- Vessel loops
- Profunda vascular clamps (angled and straight)
- Sutures
  - 5-0 Prolene on a C1 or RB1 needle
  - 2-0 silk ties and sutures
  - 3-0 Vicryl sutures
  - 4-0 Monocryl sutures
- Heparinized saline 50 to 100 units in 1,000 mL saline
- 10-cc syringes of heparinized saline on 18-gauge IV catheter.
- Fogarty embolectomy catheters no. 2, no. 3
- Bulldog soft vascular clamps
- Linear 8- to 10-MHz Doppler probe
- Rongeur
- Bone wax

POSITIONING

TIP

Place supine in neutral cervical alignment with the arms tucked. A shoulder roll is helpful to extend the neck and will facilitate better exposure, provided that the cervical spine is not injured.

- Prep an assistant into field with temporary digital or balloon catheter occlusion (Fig. 5.2).

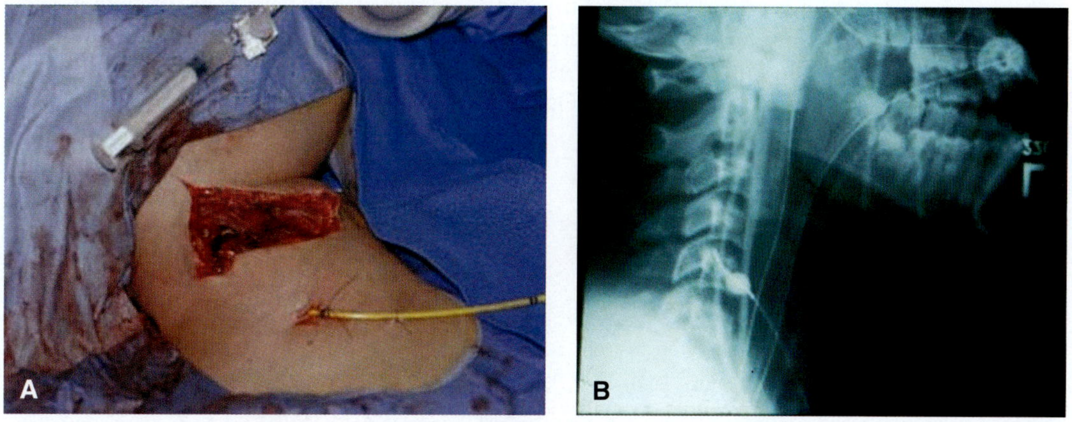

FIGURE 5.2 ▌ A penetrating injury to the right vertebral artery is controlled with digital pressure and ligation proximally with distal balloon tamponade (**A**). The lateral radiograph depicts the cervical level of the injury by filling the balloon with dilute IV contrast (**B**).

- Supine position with cervical spine maintained in neutral alignment is preferred.
- Drape from skull base to lower chest.
- A radial arterial line is recommended for continuous hemodynamic monitoring.
- A careful neurologic assessment is documented prior to induction of general anesthetic.

TECHNIQUE

Surgical Approach

TIP

Take extra time to fully dissect and mobilize all structures to completely explore the vessel and avoid iatrogenic injury. Pay particular attention to the vagus nerve and the vertebral vein. On the left side, identify, ligate, and divide the thoracic duct. A rongeur may be needed to remove the transverse foramina when dissecting a mid-distal vertebral artery injury.

Proximal Vertebral Artery (V1)

- A supraclavicular incision with wide subplatysma flaps is a good exposure for an injury isolated to the V1 segment of the vertebral artery (Fig. 5.3).

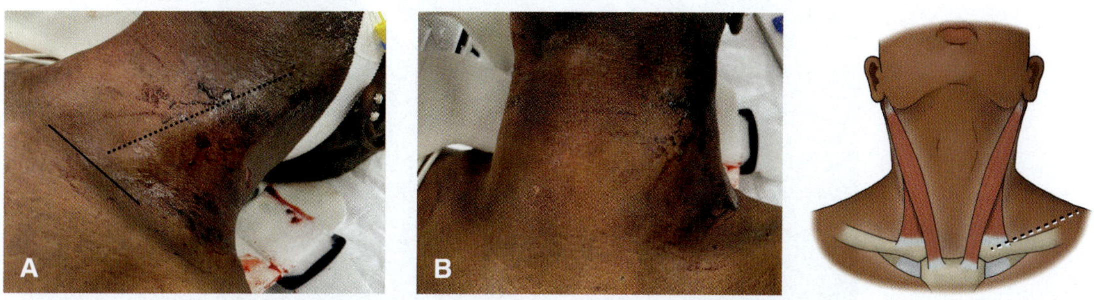

FIGURE 5.3 ▌ A left posterior cervical stab wound (**A, B**) to the vertebral artery can be exposed using a supraclavicular (*solid line*) or an oblique cervical approach (*dashed line*). **Inset:** The supraclavicular approach to the proximal vertebral artery (V1).

- The dissection is carried out between the heads of the sternocleidomastoid muscle (SCM).
- After the omohyoid muscle is divided, the jugular vein is fully mobilized and reflected laterally.
- The common carotid artery and vagus nerve are kept medial.
- The entire dissection is confined medial to the prescalene fat pad that covers the anterior scalene muscle and phrenic nerve. These structures are left unexposed lateral to the field.

- The inferior thyroid artery runs transversely across the field, which is ligated and divided.
- It is important to identify and avoid injury to the adjacent sympathetic chain.
- Caution should be exercised when isolating and controlling the vertebral artery, because it originates on the posterior aspect of the subclavian artery and deep to the vertebral vein that is ligated to improve exposure (Fig. 5.4).

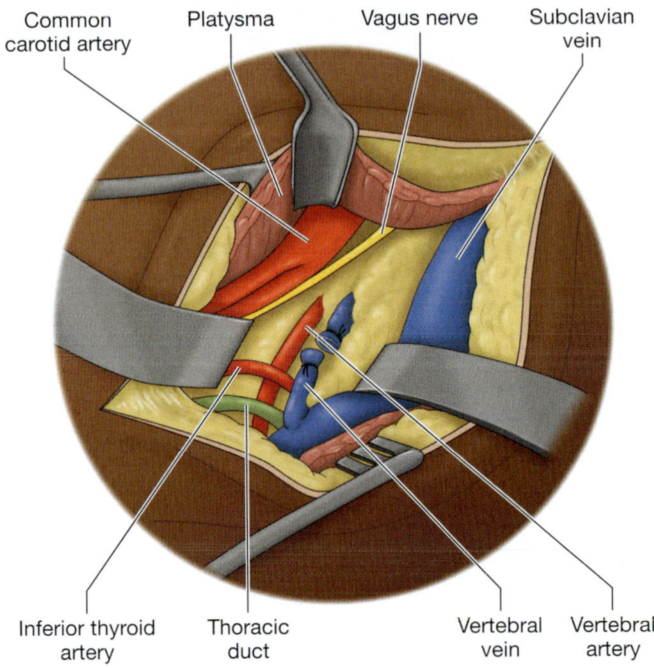

FIGURE 5.4 ❙ The carotid artery is reflected anteriorly with the vagus nerve and the subclavian vein reflected inferiorly. The vertebral vein is ligated to expose the underlying proximal vertebral artery.

- The injured vertebral artery is ligated with 5-0 Prolene and if transected, the proximal stump is further secured with a Hemoclip. Reconstruction is rarely required for a traumatic injury.
- The distal end is either ligated or the interosseus segment is packed with bone wax.

Interosseus (V2) Vertebral Artery

- Ascends within the foramina of the cervical vertebrae (Fig. 5.5).

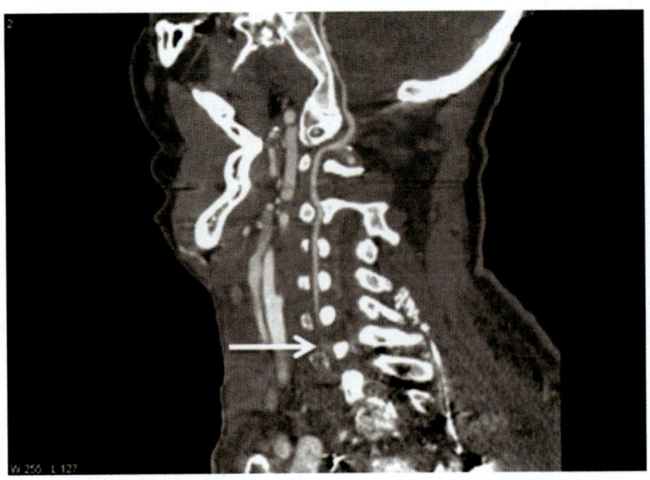

FIGURE 5.5 ❙ Sagittal CTA showing a penetrating left neck injury with retrograde filling of the vertebral artery and occlusion (*arrow*) at the interosseous segment (V2). (From Greer LT, Kuehn RB, Gillespie DL, et al. Contemporary management of combat-related vertebral artery injuries. *J Trauma Acute Care Surg*. 2013;74(3):818–824. Figure 5.2A.)

- Hemorrhage control may be easier with proximal (V1) and distal (V3) ligation.
- Direct exposure requires resection of the transverse processes.
- An oblique cervical incision is made along the SCM (Fig. 5.6).
- Surgical clips or bone wax are helpful.

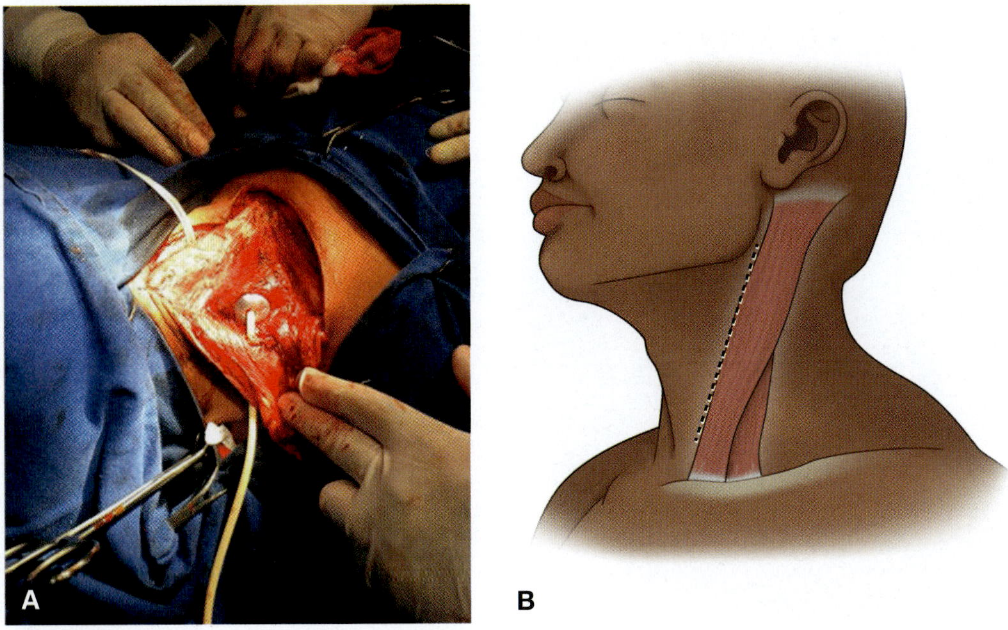

FIGURE 5.6 ‖ A: Cervical hemorrhage arising from the vertebral artery can be effectively controlled using a balloon occlusion technique with a urinary bladder catheter. (Courtesy of Adenauer Goes.) **B:** Oblique cervical incision is used to isolate the V2 and V3 segments of the vertebral artery.

V3 Exposure

- Extend an oblique cervical skin incision to just below the ear lobe.
- Dissect between the internal jugular vein and the SCM to expose the spinal accessory nerve (Fig. 5.7).

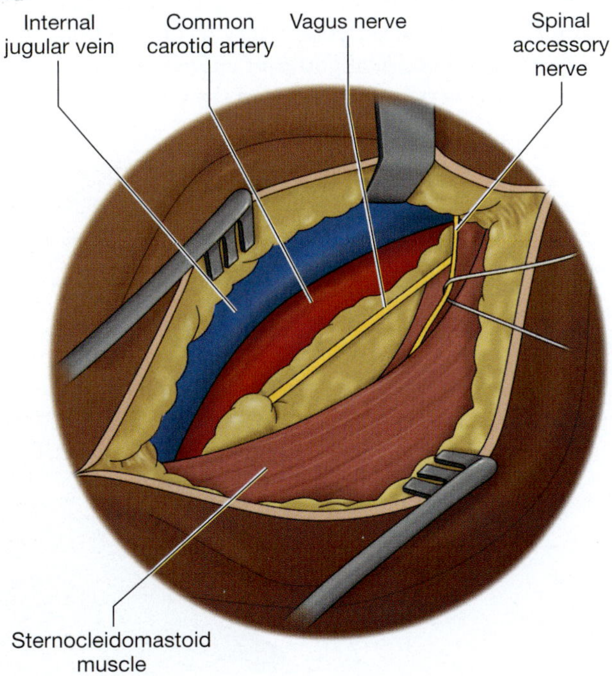

FIGURE 5.7 ‖ V3 exposure of the distal vertebral artery begins with a retrojugular dissection to identify the spinal accessory nerve.

- Follow the spinal accessory nerve as it crosses in front of the jugular vein and the easily palpated transverse process of C1.
- Divide the levator scapula muscle at the C1 transverse process (Fig. 5.8).
- Divide the anterior ramus of C2 to expose the underlying vertebral artery (Fig. 5.9).

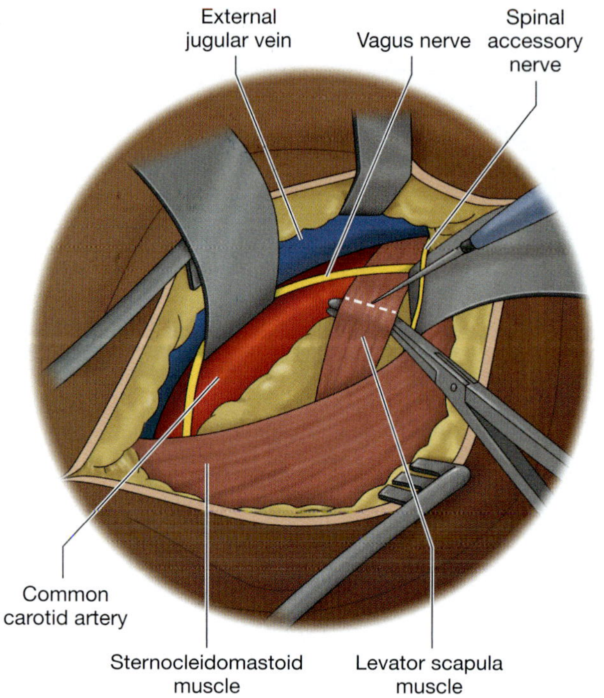

FIGURE 5.8 ❙ Expose V3 by dividing the levator scapula over the C2 ramus. The vagus nerve and internal jugular vein are anterior to the muscle.

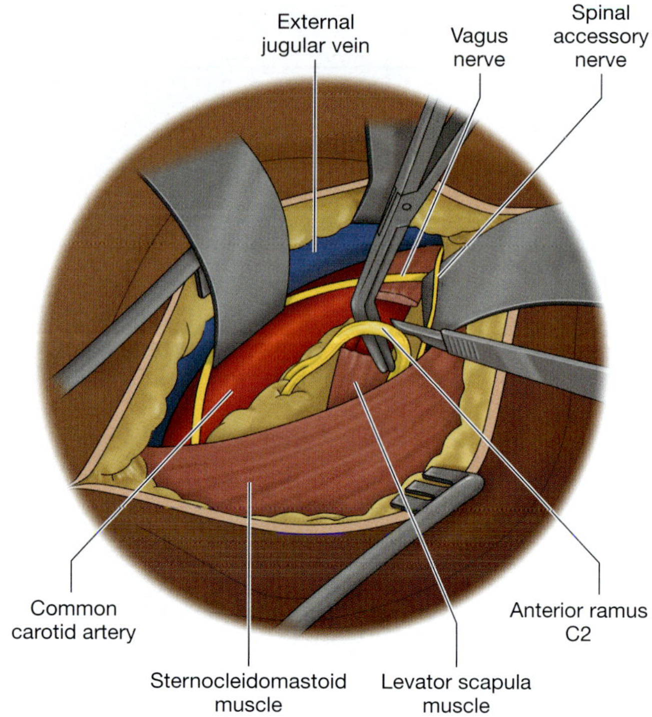

FIGURE 5.9 ❙ Divide the anterior ramus of C2 to expose the underlying vertebral artery (V3).

Distal Vertebral Artery

- Dissection above the level of C1 is technically demanding and thus very rarely performed.
- Reserved for distal vertebral artery reconstructions.
- Requires a suboccipital posterior approach (Fig. 5.10).
- Exposes the vertebral arterv from the C1 foramen to the dura mater.

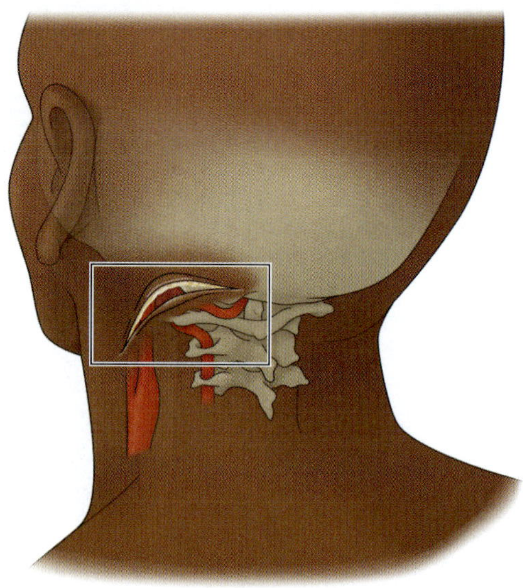

FIGURE 5.10 ❙ The suboccipital approach to the distal vertebral artery (V4).

Endovascular Techniques

- Multidetector row CTA is particularly useful for endovascular planning.
- Diagnostic confirmation with four vessel cerebrovascular digital subtraction angiography when ballistic fragment artifact renders a CTA indeterminant (Fig. 5.11).

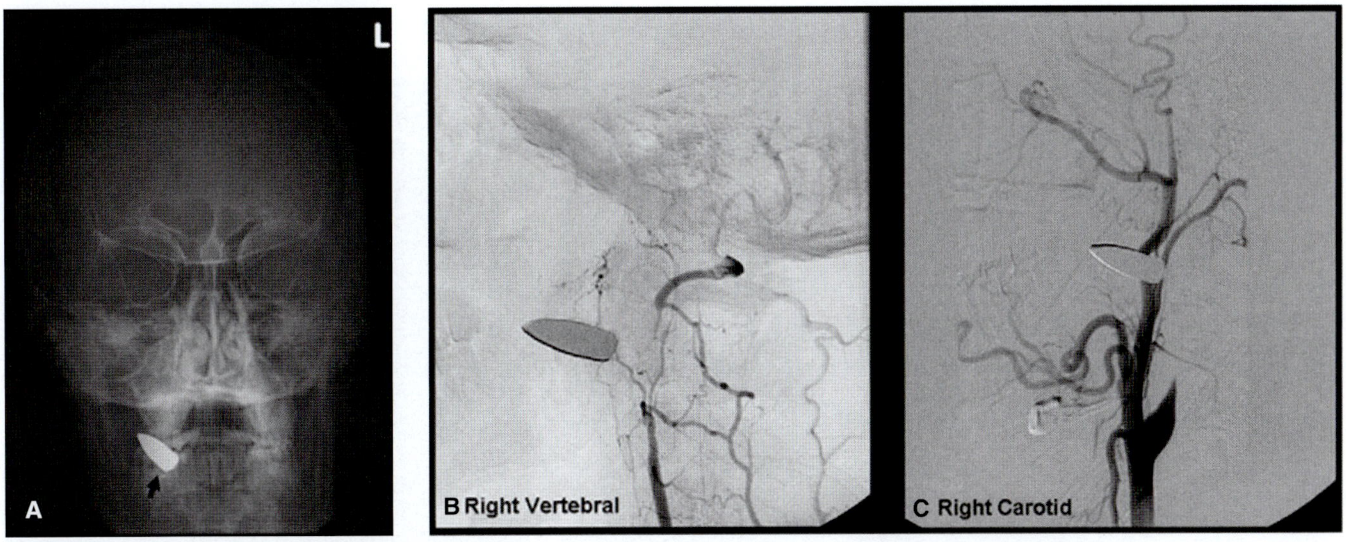

FIGURE 5.11 ▌ Plain radiographs that demonstrate retained fragments (*arrow*) will produce artifact on CTA images and limit interpretation (**A**). A contrast four vessel cerebrovascular digital subtraction arteriography is recommended when ballistic fragments are in the zone of injury as illustrated by this combined vertebral artery (**B**) and right internal carotid injury (**C**) from a cervical gunshot wound. (From Fox CJ, Gillespie DL, Weber MA, Cox MW, Hawksworth JS, Cryer CM, Rich NM, O'Donnell SD. Delayed evaluation of combat-related penetrating neck trauma. *J Vasc Surg.* 2006;44(1):86–93. Figs. 5.3 and 5.4.)

- Permits identification and treatment of a penetrating injury that is surgically inaccessible.
- Typically reserved for the treatment of high-grade blunt cerebrovascular injuries.
- Embolic coils are useful for occluding flow into a pseudoaneurysm or arteriovenous fistula (Fig. 5.12).

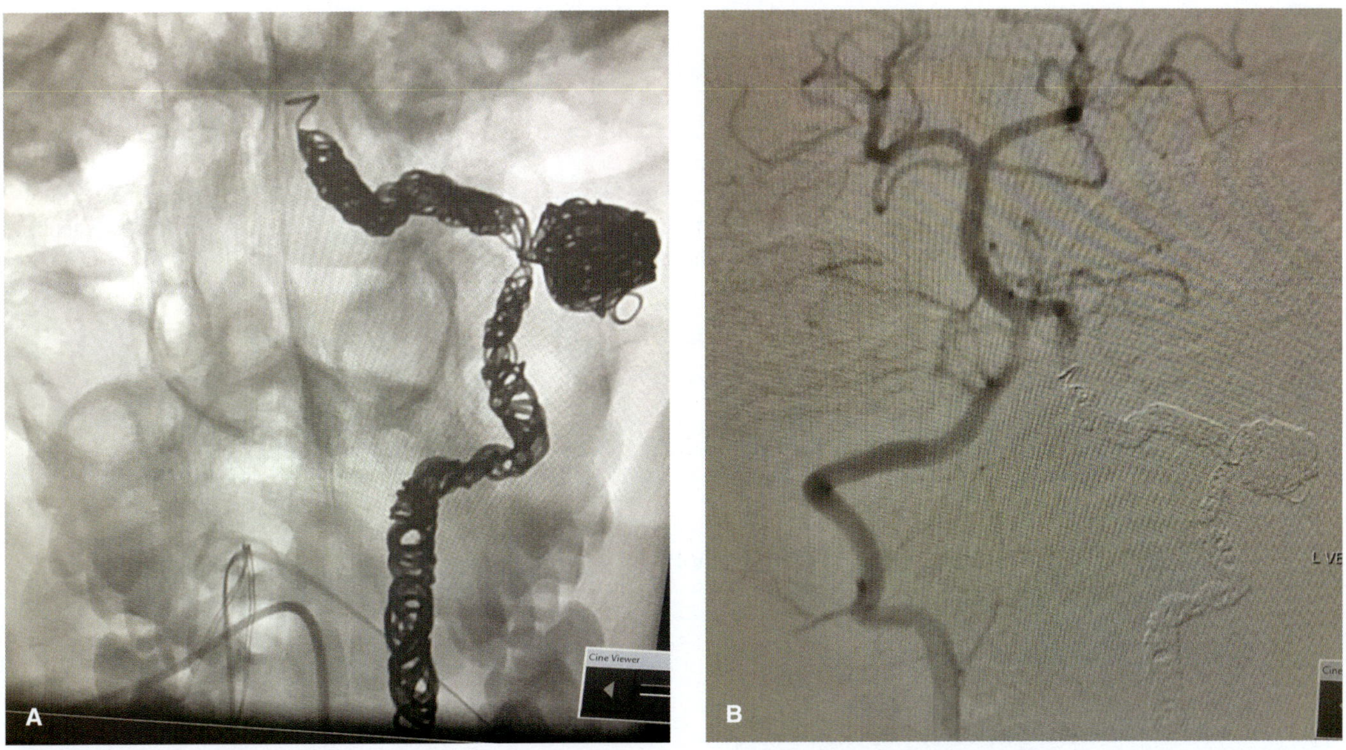

FIGURE 5.12 ▌ A left neck stab wound with a large vertebral artery pseudoaneurysm at V3 was coil embolized (**A**). Digital subtraction angiography shows successful occlusion of the artery and opacification of the distal vertebrobasilar circulation (**B**). (Courtesy of KJ Nagarsheth, MD.)

- Occasionally, stents have been used with limited success (Fig. 5.13).

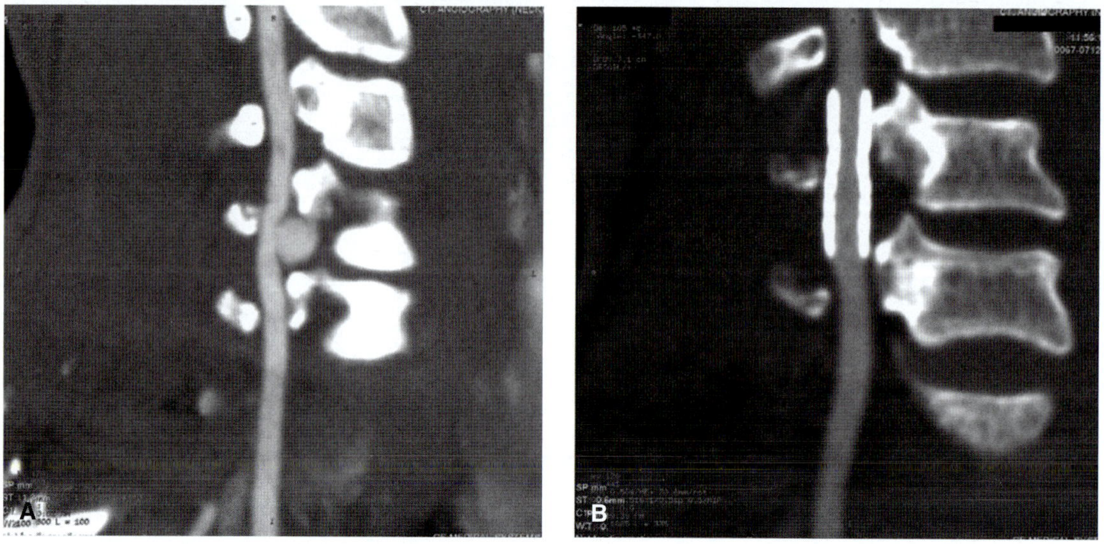

FIGURE 5.13 ▮ A vertebral artery pseudoaneurysm at C5 (**A**) before and after placement of a 5 × 22 mm balloon expandable covered stent (**B**). (From Cox MW, Whittaker DR, Martinez C, Fox CJ, Feuerstein IM, Gillespie DL. Traumatic pseudoaneurysms of the head and neck: early endovascular intervention. *J Vasc Surg*. 2007;46(6): 1227–1233. Fig. 5.4.)

POSTOPERATIVE CARE

TIP

Antiplatelet therapy following vertebral injury is recommended. A completion study (duplex sonography, angiography, or CTA) is essential to establish antegrade flow and presence of the contralateral circulation.

- Patients with neurologic deficits should have diffusion-weighted magnetic resonance imaging for evaluation of the posterior circulation.
- Follow-up examinations and surveillance imaging are mandatory for blunt cerebrovascular injury.
- A small, closed suction drain is left until after the first meal to exclude a significant chylous leak.
- Leaks that persist beyond 3 days should be reexplored.

PEARLS AND PITFALLS

Proximal Vertebral Artery Injury (V1–V2)

- Low (C7) entry to the transverse spine process
- Horner syndrome
- Vagus nerve injury
- Thoracic duct or lymph leak

Distal Vertebral Artery Injury (V3–V4)

- Spinal accessory nerve injury
- Vagus nerve injury
- Venous plexus bleeding

Suggested Readings

Asensio JA, Dabestani PJ, Wenzl FA, et al. A systematic review of penetrating extracranial vertebral artery injuries. *J Vasc Surg*. 2020;71(6):2161–2169.

Biffl WL, Moore EE, Elliott JP, et al. The devastating potential of blunt vertebral arterial injuries. *Ann Surg*. 2000;231(5):672–681.

Greer LT, Kuehn RB, Gillespie DL, et al. Contemporary management of combat-related vertebral artery injuries. *J Trauma Acute Care Surg*. 2013;74(3):818–824.

Landreneau RJ, Weigelt JA, Meier DE, et al. The anterior operative approach to the cervical vertebral artery. *J Am Coll Surg*. 1995;180(4):475–480.

Morasch MD. Technique for subclavian to carotid transposition, tips, and tricks. *J Vasc Surg*. 2009;49(1):251–254.

Chapter 6
Esophageal Injuries

DANIEL VANDERPLOEG AND FREDRIC M. PIERACCI

PERIOPERATIVE CONSIDERATIONS

Procedure Rationale

- Esophageal injuries are much more common in penetrating neck trauma than in blunt trauma. Esophageal injuries often present much more indolently but can lead to high morbidity conditions such as mediastinitis if left untreated. Furthermore, as with most trauma scenarios, injury detection requires a high index of suspicion based on injury pattern and mechanism of injury.
- Penetrating trauma is managed based on zone of injury to guide detection of at-risk structures. There is some disagreement on the zone boundaries but each trauma center has guidelines to delineate borders of zones 1 to 3 of the neck.
- Our institution defines (Fig. 6.1) zone 1 as above the angle of the mandible, zone 2 as between the manubrium and the angle of the mandible, and zone 3 as from the level of clavicles to the manubrium.

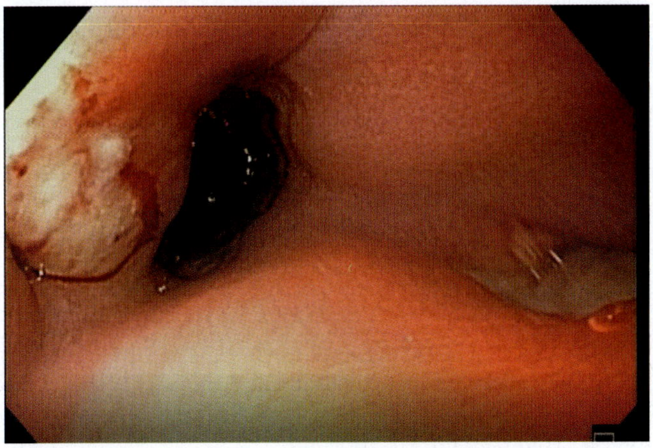

FIGURE 6.1 | Endoscopic view of mid thoracic through and through penetrating injury. The injuries are visible at 3:00 and 9:00.

TIP

Zones are important as they not only directly affect the management options available to treat injuries but also delineate the structures of the neck at risk for injury.

Zone 1 is not surgically accessible and limits treatment options. While zones 2 and 3 are surgically accessible, management is guided by patient presentation and structures injured. Zone 2 poses the highest risk of esophageal injury. Clinical signs such as dysphagia or odynophagia should raise the clinical suspicion of esophageal injury and trigger prompt investigation. Prompt detection and intervention are the key step to decreasing morbidity and mortality.

- Blunt traumatic injury to the esophagus is exceedingly rare. There are signs which should raise the suspicion of injury and prompt radiographic investigation. Neck seatbelt signs, from improperly high seatbelts, raise the risk of injury. Pharyngeal or hypopharyngeal injury is still much more common than cervical esophageal injury and management is quite different. Most pharyngeal or hypopharyngeal injuries can be managed nonoperatively with NPO, antibiotics, and proton pump inhibitors. However, cervical esophageal injuries will often require surgical or endoscopic interventions.
- Given improved outcomes with earlier detection and intervention, there have been discussions on what the diagnostic gold standard should be. Historically, double endoscopy (bronchoscopy with upper endoscopy) with or without radiographic studies was needed to evaluate for aerodigestive injuries. The advancing quality and technology of radiographic studies is able to replace this in most instances. However, there is discussion of which radiographic modality is the best. The sensitivity of fluoroscopic versus computed topography (CT) evaluation of the esophagus is often debated. There is increasing data in the radiology literature to suggest CT esophagram is as sensitive or better than traditional fluoroscopic esophagram at detecting esophageal injuries. However, a large portion of this literature is in blunt rupture after emesis and is extrapolated to trauma scenarios. Either fluoroscopic or CT evaluation of the esophagus with oral contrast is needed to rule out injury and further investigation is needed to elaborate which is the best test.
- There are two main interventional modalities for esophageal injuries. Stenting is the mainstay of endoscopic repair as primary endoscopic repair has poorer outcomes and increased likelihood of leak. Surgical approaches allow for direct primary repair but also for a wide drainage of area to decrease risk of infectious complications. Location is the primary factor behind which modality to use and where to place the incision for surgical repairs. High cervical stents are often poorly tolerated by patients given increased somatic sensation of the upper cervical esophagus. This coupled with the less morbid neck incision for exposure often pushes toward surgical repair. Thoracic esophageal injuries are ideal for stent placement. They might require stent fixation with endoscopic suturing to prevent stent migration. Distal esophageal or gastroesophageal junction injuries can be more difficult to manage endoscopically as stent migration is harder to prevent. Size or luminal extent of injury may also limit stenting options as passing a wire across the injury is necessary for successful stent deployment.

ENDOSCOPIC TREATMENT

Essential Equipment

Endoscopic Treatment

- Therapeutic gastroscope
- Stent options
- Fluoroscopy

Surgical Treatment

- Headlight
- Major abdominal and thoracic tray
  - + Bookwalter retractor or equivalent
  - + Finochietto rib spreader
  - + long needle drivers
  - 2-0 and 3-0 Vicryl sutures on SH, 36-inch thread
  - 2-0 and 3-0 PDS sutures on SH, 36-inch thread

Positioning

Endoscopic Treatment

- Preferably lateral decubitus, but often supine if in the operating room to allow for surgical access if needed.

Surgical Treatment

- Lateral decubitus is preferred if planning thoracotomy. Supine position is preferred for neck or abdominal approaches.

TECHNIQUE

Endoscopic Treatment

- The endoscope is passed through the mouth and into the esophagus under direct visualization to also rule out pharyngeal or hypopharyngeal injury. The esophagus is lightly distended with air or carbon dioxide to evaluate for injury. Once identified, injury location and extent should be evaluated. Midthoracic injuries with less than 50% of luminal disruption are most amenable to stenting. There are many different types of stents available for use but nearly all require fluoroscopic guidance for successful placement. Stents may require endoscopic suture fixation to prevent migration. Once satisfied with the deployment and coverage area, it is important to evaluate whether additional drainage procedures are indicated. For example, the pleural or mediastinum may be affected if the esophageal injury was poorly contained. Often, interventional radiology can perform such procedures but surgical washout may be indicated even if area of injury is adequately covered.

Surgical Treatment

Incision

TIP

If performing thoracotomy, it is important to preserve and harvest intercostal muscle, with and intact neurovascular pedicle, that can be used as a muscle flap if needed.

- Right posterolateral thoracotomy is preferred as the esophagus is a posterior structure; however, left posterolateral thoracotomy may be used for lower injuries near the gastroesophageal junction. The level of the thoracotomy is determined by the preoperative imaging based on the presumed level of the injury. If planning for a neck exploration, a left oblique incision, anterior and parallel to the sternocleidomastoid muscle, is preferred. Midline laparotomy can also be used for lower esophageal injuries as the distal esophagus can be mobilized from the mediastinum and brought into the abdomen if needed. Although laparotomy may not be ideal exposure for esophageal evaluation and repair, it might be a necessary approach for concomitant intra-abdominal traumatic injuries.

PEARLS AND PITFALLS

Key Steps for Repair

- Expose full extent of mucosal injury. This might require lengthening the muscle tear or injury.
- Repair in two layers. The mucosa, inner layer, is repaired with 2-0 or 3-0 PDS sutures. This can be running or interrupted based on surgeon preference. The muscularis, outer layer, is repaired with interrupted 2-0 or 3-0 Vicryl sutures.
- Wide drainage of area is vital. Leaving drains can usually prevent the infectious complications that dramatically increase morbidity in these patients. Mediastinal and pleural drains are left if a thoracotomy is performed. Jackson-Pratt drains are left if an oblique neck incision or laparotomy is performed.
- Flap coverage is optional but often performed. It is definitely encouraged in more contaminated fields or in delayed repairs as it has been associated with decreased frequency of fistula formation. Intercostal muscle flaps are ideal for reinforcing repair when a thoracotomy is performed; however, attention and flap preservation upon entry is key. Pleural or pericardial flaps are also viable options as well. Omental flaps are the most commonly used intra-abdominal reinforcement, whereas strap muscle reinforcement is used in the neck.

POSTOPERATIVE MANAGEMENT

- Timing until enteral feeds depends on chronicity of injury, surgeon preference, and concomitant injuries. Early enteral feeding is associated with improved outcomes so passing a feeding tube past your repair at the initial operation is often best. Antibiotics are usually continued 24 hours postoperatively in low contamination and 4 to 7 days in higher contamination settings.

Suggested Readings

Polireddy K, Hoff C, Kinger NP, Tran A, Maddu K. Blunt thoracic trauma: role of chest radiography and comparison with CT—findings and literature review. *Emerg Radiol.* 2022; MPID 35595942.

Sharp G, Steffens D, Koh Cherry. Evidence of negative pressure therapy for anastomotic leak: a systematic review. *ANZ J Surg.* 2021;91(4):537.

Sudarshan M, Cassivi SD. Management of traumatic esophageal injuries. *J Thorac Dis.* 2019;11(Suppl 2):S172–S176.

SECTION III Thoracic Injuries

Chapter 7
Thoracic Incisions

FREDRIC M. PIERACCI AND ERNEST E. MOORE

PERIOPERATIVE CONSIDERATIONS

Procedure Rationale

In the hemodynamically unstable trauma patient, rapid access to the thoracic cavity is essential to relieve a tension pneumothorax, prevent bronchovenous air embolization, release pericardial tamponade, or control bleeding. Access can vary from a 2-cm thoracotomy to a bilateral trans-sternal ("clamshell") thoracotomy. The quickest and most versatile thoracic incision remains the anterolateral thoracotomy with the patient in the supine position. Extension across the sternum provides exposure of virtually all major thoracic structures. By contrast, in the hemodynamically stable patient, exposure of the thoracic aorta, esophagus, or trachea is approached via a posterolateral thoracotomy. Each of these incisions described herein provides unique advantages to exposure of various intrathoracic structures.

Essential Equipment

TIP

Communicate early to the operating room staff important details including need for the thoracic set including a functioning sternal saw and Lebsche knife.

- Sternal power saw
- Sternal retractor
- Lebsche knife and mallet
- Finochietto rib spreader
- Rib cutters
- Balfour retractor
- Army–Navy retractors
- Vascular, lung, and bronchial stapling devices
- 2-0 and 3-0 silk plain and stick tie sutures
- No. 1 PDS pericostal sutures
- 2-0 PDS sutures for muscle closure
- Curved Mayo scissors
- 24-Fr chest tube for mediastinal drainage
- 28-Fr chest tube for pleural drainage
- No. 5 Ethibond sutures for chest tube
- Chest tube drainage system
- Sternal wires for closure

TECHNIQUE

Incisions

TIP

In the periarrest patient, it is quicker to perform an anterolateral thoracotomy with extension to a bilateral anterolateral thoracotomy if needed for exposure.

Anterior Finger Thoracotomy

- The patient in extremis from a tension pneumothorax should undergo a small decompressive thoracotomy in the submammary crease (fourth or fifth intercostal space) at the anterior axillary line.
- Following a skin incision, curved Mayo scissors should be used to enter the pleural space on top of the rib to avoid the neurovascular bundle (Fig. 7.1). The technical details for emergent tube thoracotomy are described in Chapter 3.

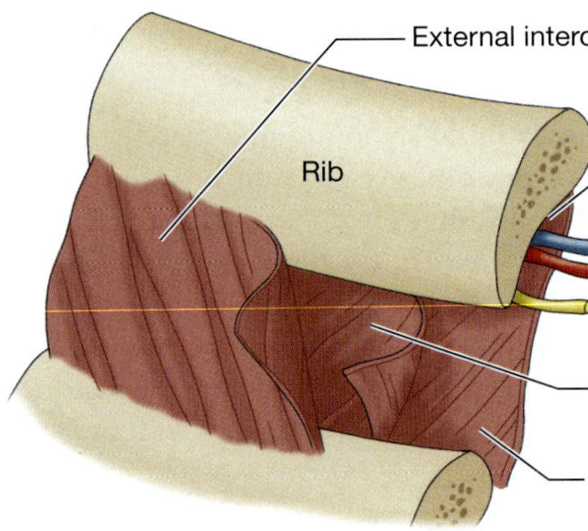

FIGURE 7.1 ▌ Anatomical considerations in performing a thoracotomy. The intercostal neurovascular bundle lies on the underside of the rib, and becomes more exposed posteriorly.

Anterolateral Thoracotomy

TIP

The anterolateral thoracotomy is the preferred access for the hemodynamically unstable patient, as shown in Chapter 1.

- In the operating room, the patient should be positioned supine with the arms extended to permit posterior extension of the incision.
- The skin incision should begin at the border of the sternum and extend posteriorly following the curvature of the ribs. The incision is continued through the chest wall musculature including the inferior fibers of the pectoralis major, anterior serratus and the anterior portion of the latissimus dorsi (Fig. 7.2). The paraspinal muscles should not be divided.
- The fifth or sixth intercostal space is optimal to enter with an unknown source of bleeding, allowing direct visualization of the pulmonary hilum and heart. Most anterior penetrating wounds to the heart can be managed from the left chest. (See Chapter 9.)

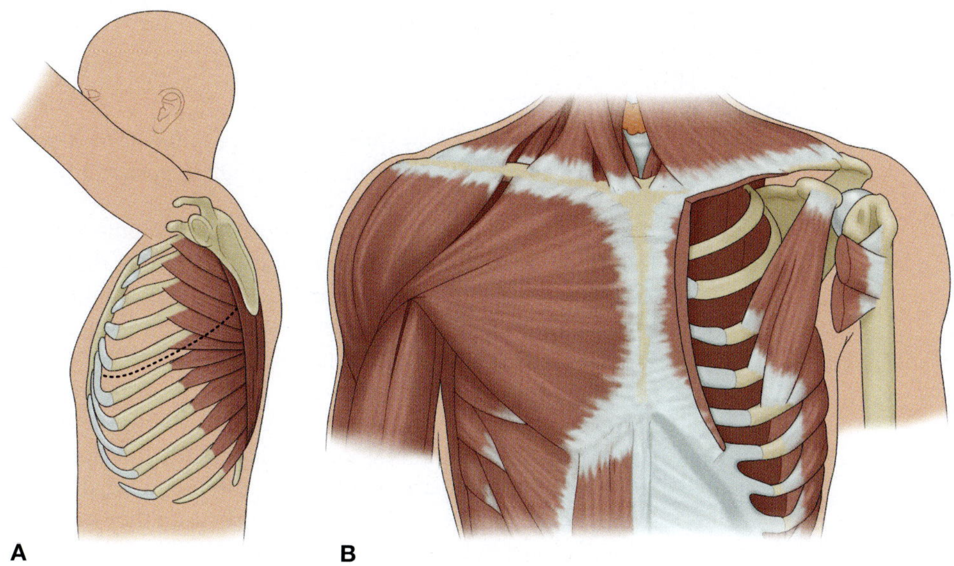

FIGURE 7.2 ❙ **A:** The anterolateral thoracotomy begins at the border of the sternum, traversing the anterior serratus and latissimus dorsi muscles. **B:** The paraspinal muscles should not be divided.

High Left Anterolateral Thoracotomy

- A distinct variant of the anterolateral thoracotomy is the high left anterolateral thoracotomy via the third or fourth intercostal space for proximal control of the left subclavian artery, described in Chapter 8.

Bilateral Trans-Sternal ("Clamshell") Anterolateral Thoracotomy

- Along the border of the sternum, an anterolateral thoracotomy across the sternum to the contralateral side greatly enhances exposure for intrathoracic structures, as shown in Chapter 1. This is clearly necessary for injuries to the opposite side but also important for posterior cardiac wounds and evaluation of the thoracic aorta or esophagus. (See Chapter 9.)
- The simplest method to cross the sternum is with the Lebsche knife. Following restoration of perfusion, the internal mammary arteries should be suture ligated proximally and distally (Fig. 7.3).

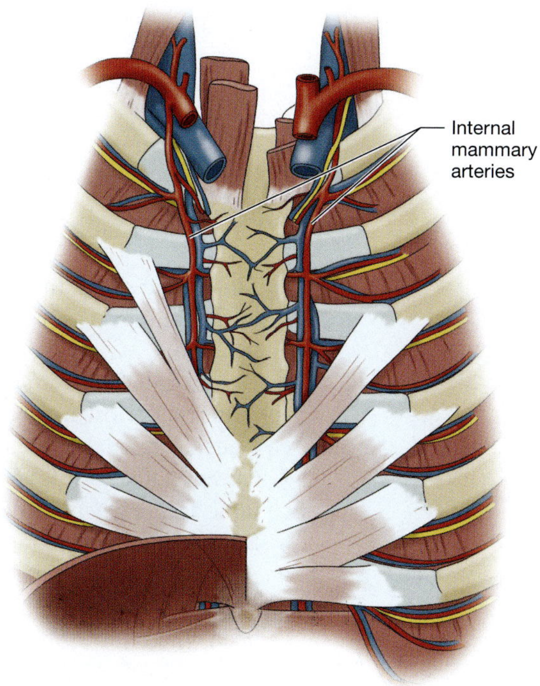

FIGURE 7.3 ❙ A transected sternum requires ligation of the internal mammary arteries coursing along the lateral border of the sternum.

Median Sternotomy

TIP

Median sternotomy provides optimal exposure of the heart and great vessels except for the left subclavian artery. It also provides limited exposure to posterior mediastinal structures.

- In the operating room, the patient is positioned supine with the arms tucked.
- A midline skin incision from the suprasternal notch to 2 cm below the tip of the xiphoid process. Carrying the incision higher is unnecessary and cosmetically unattractive.
- The incision through the periosteum of the sternum, taking care to stay in the midline.
- Use blunt dissection to clear the suprasternal notch of tissue. There is usually a transverse vein in this area measuring 3 to 4 mm, which should be ligated and divided.
- Develop the superior retrosternal space bluntly with the index finger.
- Incise the midline abdominal wall fascia directly inferior to the tip of the xiphoid, and develop the inferior retrosternal space bluntly with the index finger. Then, place one index finger in the retrosternal space superiorly and one inferiorly until they meet (Fig. 7.4). This is particularly important cephalad to separate the innominate vein.

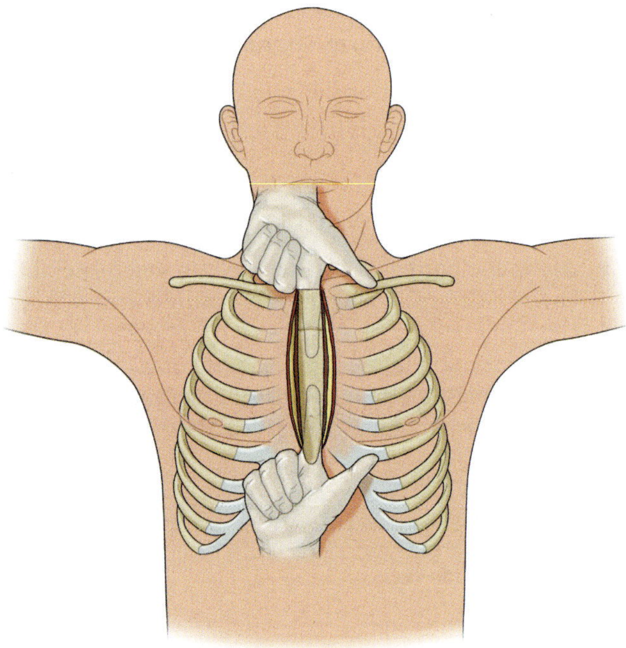

FIGURE 7.4 ❙ Prior to division of the sternum, a digital tunnel is created with finger insertion at the top and bottom of the sternum.

- The sternal saw is then introduced at either side of the sternum and its "foot" should be kept tilted toward the posterior sternal surface and held firmly against it to prevent injury to intrathoracic structures.
- Two Army–Navy retractors are then used to elevate one side of the transected sternum in order to cauterize periosteal bleeding points.
- Place the sternal retractor and gradually open the mediastinum.
- Closure after definitive surgery is preceded by careful hemostasis by means of electrocautery and topic agents when needed.
- Bone wax may be required on the sternal edges.
- A single drainage tube, sized 24 Fr, is inserted into the anterior mediastinum through a separate skin stab incision below the incision. Tubes should also be placed in either pleural space if they have been entered.

- A variety of sternal closure methods exist, including plates, zip ties, and wires. The authors prefer closure with interrupted, no. 22 steel wires, with swedged on needles, and placed 3 cm apart. The needles are driven through the sternum 2 cm lateral to the incised edge.
- Once all wires are placed, the sternum may be held approximated by one or two wires while the first wire is twisted.
- After all wires are twisted and before the ends are cut, a needle holder is used to twist each wire tightly.
- The ends of the wires are buried and the remainder of the wound closed in layers.

Median Sternotomy with Cervical Extension

- Exposure of injuries to the proximal carotid arteries and proximal right subclavian artery requires a cervical extension (Fig. 7.5).

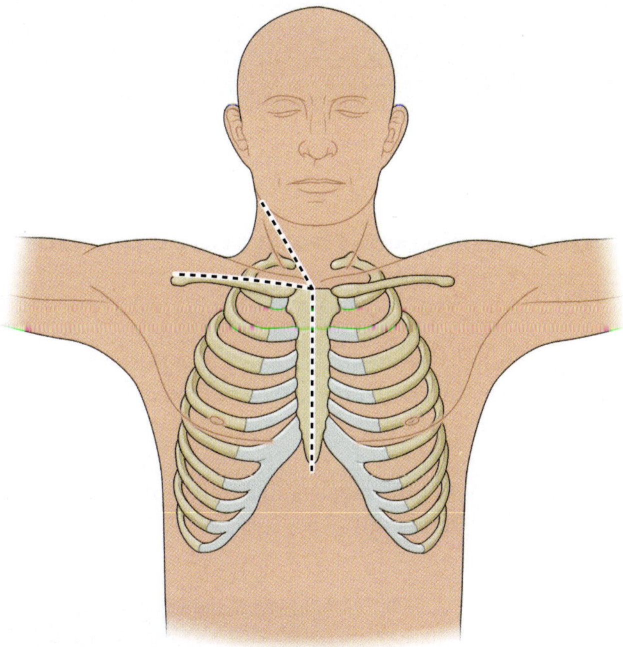

FIGURE 7.5 ❙ Exposure of injuries to the proximal carotid arteries and proximal right subclavian artery requires a cervical extension.

- Extension for carotid injuries is along the sternocleidomastoid (see Chapter 4), and supraclavicular for right subclavian artery (see Chapter 8).

Posterolateral Thoracotomy

- A posterolateral incision is employed to expose the thoracic aorta, esophagus, and trachea (see Chapter 12).
- The thoracic aorta and distal esophagus (see Chapter 6) are approached via the left thorax, whereas the proximal esophagus and trachea are accessed via the right chest.

Left Thoracoabdominal Incision

TIP

Exposure to the GE junction and the distal descending thoracic aorta can be provided via a planned left thoracoabdominal incision.

- The skin incision is initiated along the eighth rib and extended to the rectus muscle (Fig. 7.6). The diaphragm can be partially divided to enhance exposure.
- A rib plate can provide stability across the coastal margin.

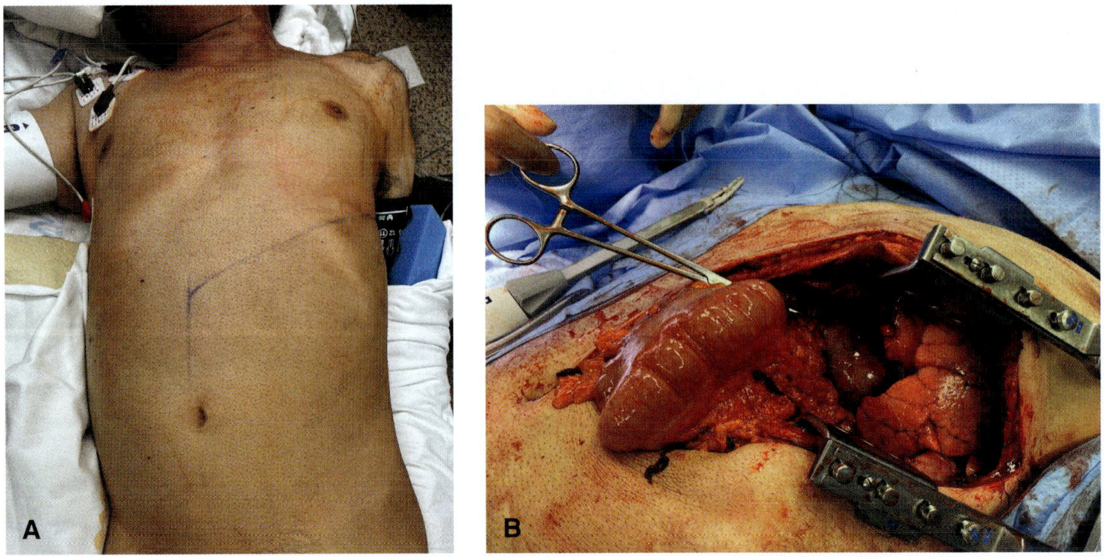

FIGURE 7.6 ❙ A, B: A left thoracoabdominal incision provides exposure of the GE junction and the distal descending thoracic aorta.

Video-Assisted Thoracoscopic Surgery

TIP

Video-assisted thoracoscopic surgery has a number of applications in trauma, including delayed hemothorax, persistent air leak, evaluation of the diaphragm, and administration of directed locoregional anesthesia.

- Standard port placement is illustrated in Figure 7.7, although optimal placement varies with the anticipated pathology.

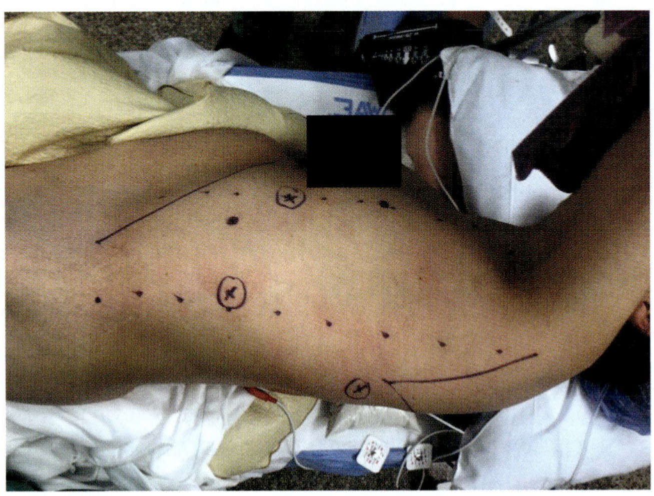

FIGURE 7.7 ❙ Standard port sites for videoscopic thoracic surgery may require adjustment depending on the anticipated pathology.

- The first incision is made in the sixth interspace along the anterior axillary line. This port can serve as the site of the chest tube placement. The second port is placed one interspace below the scapular tip. The final port is placed between the first two ports in the posterior axillary line in the eighth intercostal space. Camera placement in this port affords a comprehensive view of the thoracic cavity (Fig. 7.8).

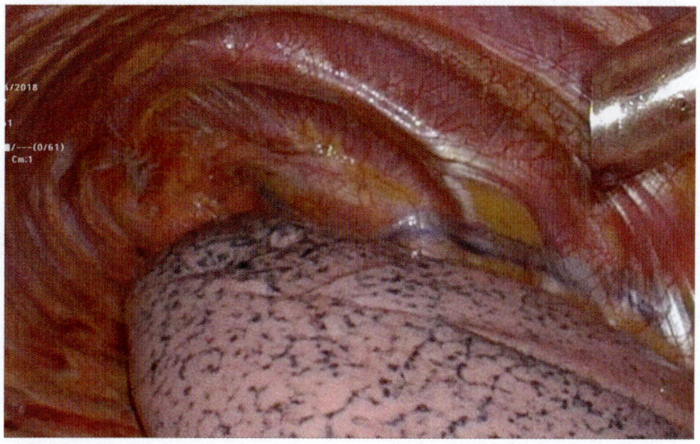

FIGURE 7.8 | Via of pleural space form posterior eighth intercostal port.

- Pleural space insufflation with CO_2 to 10 mm Hg can assist with development of space and thus exposure.
- Video-assisted thoracoscopic surgery (VATS) should not be attempted in the hemodynamic unstable patient, patients in whom one-lung ventilation is unlikely to be tolerated, or in the absence of necessary equipment or expertise.

POSTOPERATIVE CARE

- The mediastinal drain should be managed like a tube thoracostomy with pleurovac suction. The drain may be removed when there is less than 50-cc output per day.
- Routine sternal precautions (lifting, physical therapy limitations, driving, etc.) should be employed.
- Sternal infections are rare and manifest as sternal instability.

Suggested Readings

Feliciano DV, Mattox K, Moore EE. *Trauma*. 9th ed. McGraw-Hill; 2021.
Hood RM. *Techniques in General Thoracic Surgery*. Saunders; 1985.

Chapter 8
Subclavian Artery

CHARLES J. FOX AND ERNEST E. MOORE

PERIOPERATIVE CONSIDERATIONS

Procedure Rationale

Injury to the thoracic outlet vessels may appear innocuous initially may be cause unexpected or potentially catastrophic maneuvers may be needed to control bleeding. Due to extensive collateral blood flow, the majority of patients with a subclavian arterial injury will have a palpable radial pulse. On the other hand, injury to the brachial plexus should raise suspicion of a subclavian injury. In general, hard signs of injury (bleeding, expanding hematoma thrill) of injury requires immediate open operative exploration. Soft signs (proximity, brachial plexus symptoms, small hematoma, history of arterial bleeding) are best evaluated by computed tomography angiography (CTA) for preoperative planning. For the hemodynamically stable patient, there is usually time to allow for CTA to pinpoint the exact location and severity of the injury. Modern imaging technology has become increasingly relied upon in the last decade to consider endovascular options. However, persistent shock or evidence of bleeding into the thorax requires immediate operative intervention. Consequently, every on-call trauma surgeon must know the optimal exposure, how to obtain proximal control, and have the ability to place a temporary intravascular shunt or perform a vascular reconstruction. As an infrequent injury with high mortality, familiarity with the thoracic outlet area and the treatment options are essential for the best chance of survival.

Anatomy

TIP

The internal mammary artery and the thyrocervical trunk can be ligated without sequelae; doing so will allow greater mobility of the subclavian artery for a tension-free anastomosis. The phrenic nerve should be identified during the dissection to avoid injury; it is small and lies on the anterior surface of the anterior scalene muscle.

- The left subclavian artery arises from the aortic arch. The right subclavian artery arises from the innominate artery. There are rare variants in which the right subclavian artery arises directly from the ascending aorta.
- The subclavian artery is divided into three segments. The first segment is medial to the anterior scalene muscle, the second segment is posterior to the anterior scalene, and the third segment is lateral to the muscle. The subclavian continues as the axillary artery beginning at the lateral edge of the first rib.

- Important branches of the subclavian artery (sequentially the vertebral, internal mammary, and thyrocervical trunk) are in the first segment, located between the heads of the sternocleidomastoid muscle (Fig. 8.1).

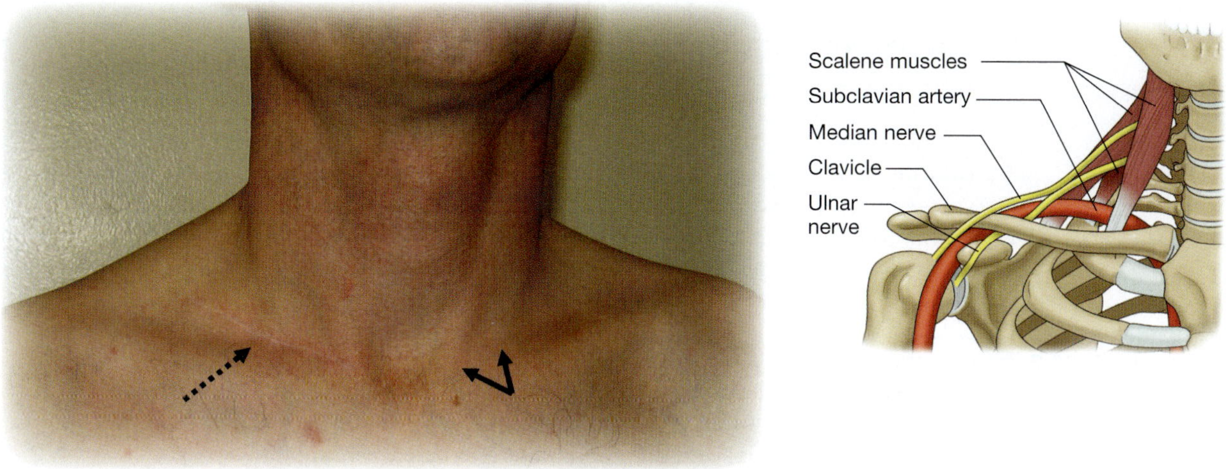

FIGURE 8.1 ▮ A supraclavicular dissection is performed between the two heads of the sternocleidomastoid muscle (*arrows*) for proximal control of the subclavian artery. The sternal head is preserved but the clavicular head can be sacrificed (*dashed arrow*) for distal exposure. The right subclavian artery was exposed after reflection of the investing lymphatic fat pad and division of the omohyoid and anterior scalene muscles (*insert*). Care must be taken to avoid injury to the phrenic nerve.

- The subclavian artery rests on the first rib and is cephalad and posterior to the subclavian vein (Fig. 8.2).

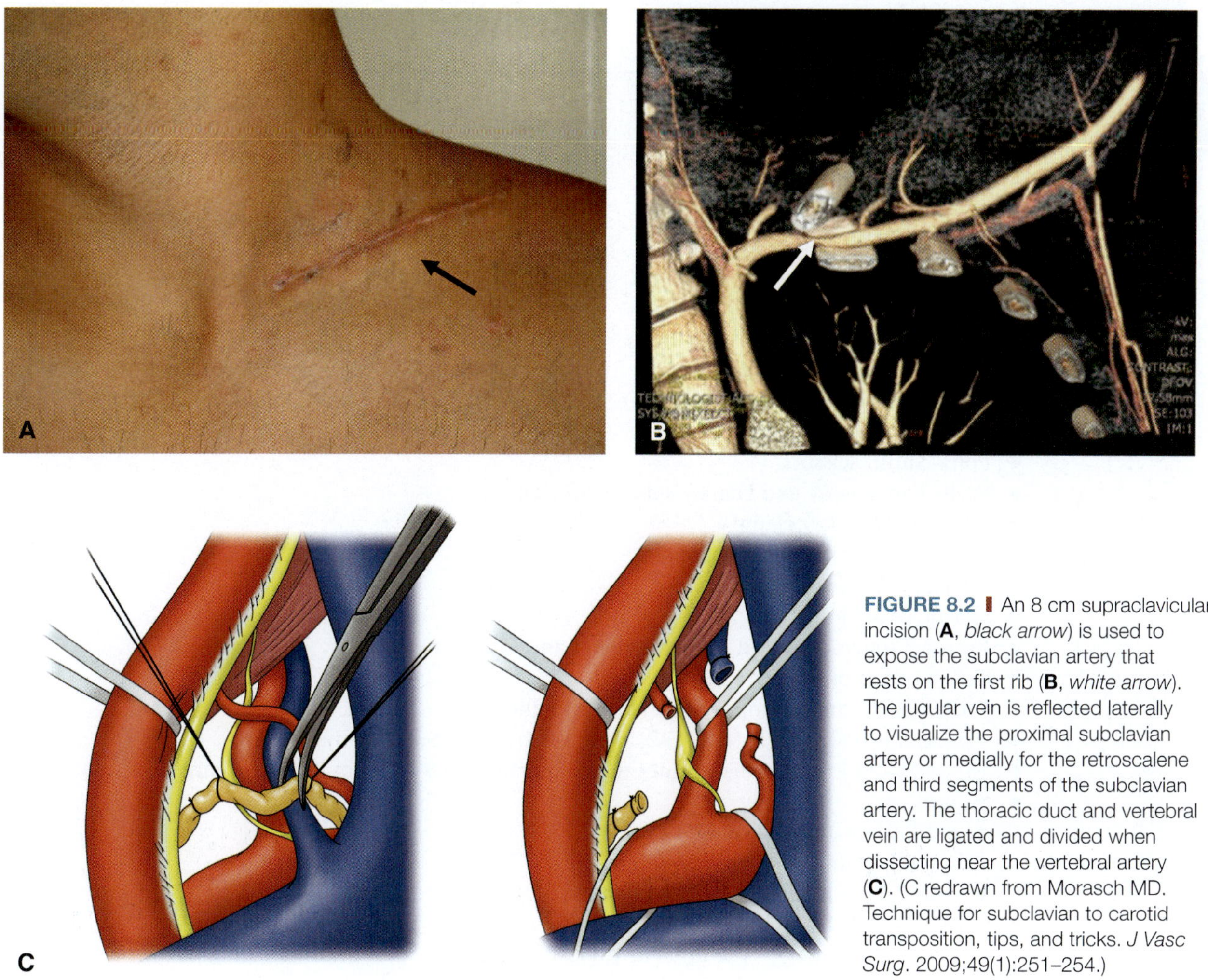

FIGURE 8.2 ▮ An 8 cm supraclavicular incision (**A**, *black arrow*) is used to expose the subclavian artery that rests on the first rib (**B**, *white arrow*). The jugular vein is reflected laterally to visualize the proximal subclavian artery or medially for the retroscalene and third segments of the subclavian artery. The thoracic duct and vertebral vein are ligated and divided when dissecting near the vertebral artery (**C**). (C redrawn from Morasch MD. Technique for subclavian to carotid transposition, tips, and tricks. *J Vasc Surg*. 2009;49(1):251–254.)

- The thoracic duct courses transversely and anterior to the subclavian artery. While the left side is larger and well known, there is typically a smaller branch entering the right subclavian vein.
- The phrenic nerve courses lateral to medial over the anterior scalene muscle.
- The brachial plexus is associated with the artery and concomitant injury is common.

Management Algorithm

TIP

Metzenbaum blunt tipped scissors and Kittners are useful tools when dissecting near the subclavian artery. Stay in a periadventitial plane close enough to see vasovasorum. The subclavian artery is very delicate vessel and easily torn. Ligate the thoracic duct on the side of injury and use extreme caution as the brachial plexus fibers are closely associated with the distal aspect of the axillo-subclavian juncture.

- Penetrating Subclavian Artery Injury
  - Wounds should not be explored digitally in the emergency department.
  - Endovascular repair of an arterial injury is reserved for stable patients when the injury can be crossed easily without sacrificing important arterial branches.
- Blunt Subclavian Artery Injury
  - Multidetector row CTA has become a fundamental diagnostic tool.
  - Obtain bilateral arm blood pressure measurements. A pulse exam is an insensitive sign of subclavian artery injury.
  - A focused neurologic exam should be completed to exclude brachial plexus injury.
  - Minor injury can be treated with antithrombotic therapy and re-imaging.

Essential Equipment

TIP

Papaverine is mixed 60 mg in 20 cc of saline. Heparin is mixed 5,000 units in 500 mL of saline. Contrast is diluted 50:50.

- Headlight
- Loupe magnification 2.5
- Adson–Beckman retractor
- Sternal and Finochietto retractors
- Sternal saw and Lebsche knife
- Castroviejo and Ryder needle driver
- Microvascular Gerald forceps
- Potts–Smith scissors
- Wylie hypogastric and Henley subclavian clamps
- Satinsky–DeBakey clamp
- Cooley pediatric vascular clamp
- DeBakey–Bahnson aortic clamp
- Silastic vessel loops
- Rummel tourniquet (red rubber catheter and umbilical tape)
- Teflon or felt pledgets
- Profunda vascular clamps (angled and straight)
- 1 pack of 6-inch Argyle (8, 10, 12, and 14 French) or Sundt shunts
- 15- or 21-cm Pruitt-Inahara shunt with T-port (9 Fr) 8–14-mm balloon diameter
- Sutures
  - 6-0 Prolene on a C1 or BV1 needle
  - 3-0 silk plain and stick ties
  - 3-0 Vicryl sutures
- Sterile 8–10-MHz Doppler probe
- Heparinized saline 50–100 units in 1,000-mL saline

- Papaverine 30 mg/mL, 10-mL vials
- Fogarty embolectomy catheters #2, #3, #4
- Bulldog soft vascular clamps
- Three-way stopcock and A-line extension tubing
- 10-, 20-cc syringes of heparin saline on 18-gauge IV catheter with blunt needle (Olive) tip
- 19- or 21-gauge butterfly needle or angiocatheter
- Contrast agent 50 mL (Omnipaque-240, GE Healthcare, Inc., Chicago, IL)
- Linear 8–10-MHz Doppler probe
- Ring reinforced 6- or 8-mm polytetrafluoroethylene (PTFE)
- Polyester or bovine pericardial patch
- Thrombin 1,000 U/mL, 20-mL vial
- Gel foam or Surgicel
- Fibrin sealant or Bioglue

Patient Positioning

TIP

Do not forget to prepare the groin for a saphenous vein harvest, but in the absence of heavy contamination an 8-mm ePTFE may be the preferred conduit due to the size discrepancy of vein for this region.

- Supine with arms out and shoulder roll; include neck and chest in the operative field.
- Anticipate the need for a saphenous vein harvest.
- Radial arterial line is placed on the opposite side of the injury.
- Anticipate blood loss and have the products with a rapid infuser in the operating room.
- Lower-body warmer.

TECHNIQUE

Exposure: Right Subclavian Artery

- Median sternotomy with a supraclavicular extension temporarily provides wide exposure. The left innominate vein should be divided temporarily for achieving proximal control when confronted with active bleeding (Fig. 8.3).

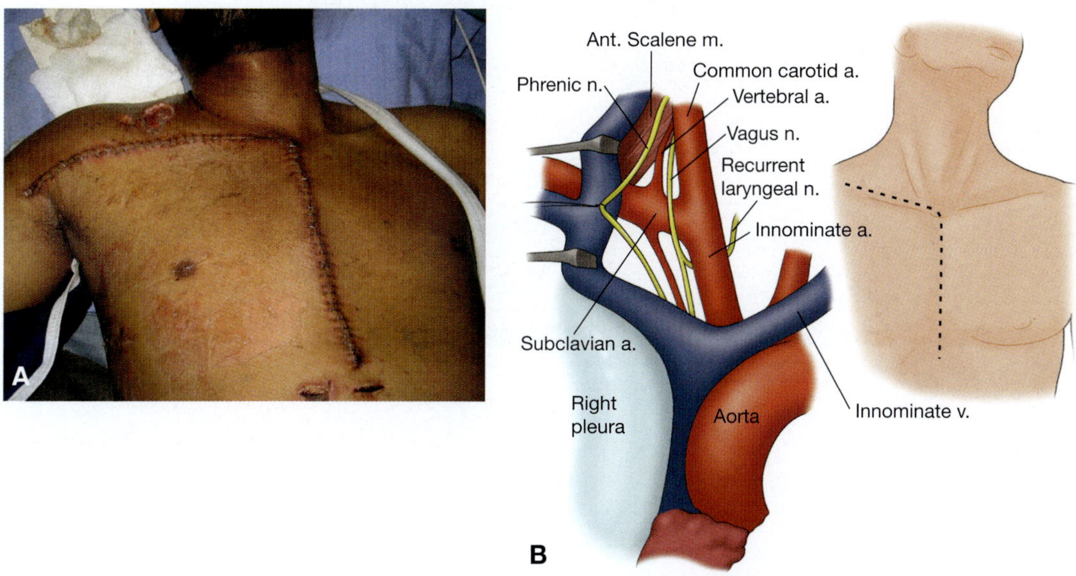

FIGURE 8.3 ▌ **A, B.** The trapdoor incision is associated with significant morbidity. Sternotomy with supraclavicular extension is the preferred approach for an unstable patient with a distal subclavian artery injury.

- Remember to ligate the right internal mammary pedicles after the sternotomy.
- A supraclavicular extension (or primary incision) for distal injury in stable patients.
- A partial clavicular resection is rapid and does not result in functional disability.
- A trapdoor approach is unnecessary and associated with many complications (Fig. 8.4).
- Apply digital pressure or insert an occlusion balloon for rapid control of bleeding.
- Avoid inadvertent venous or nerve injury during a rapid dissection with anatomy distorted by a hematoma.

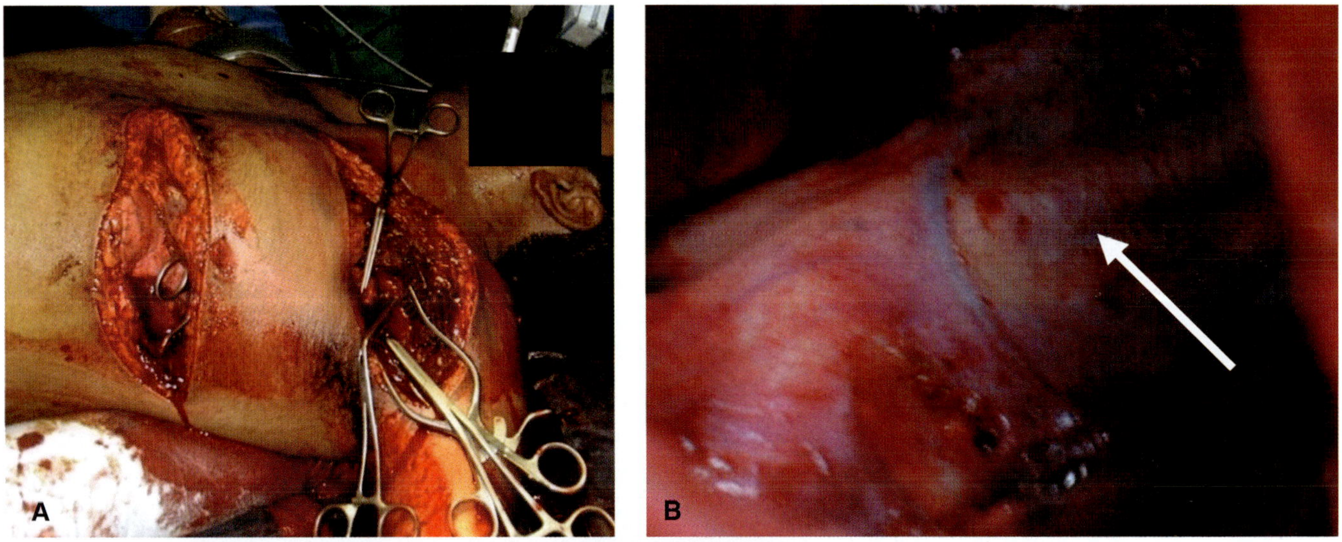

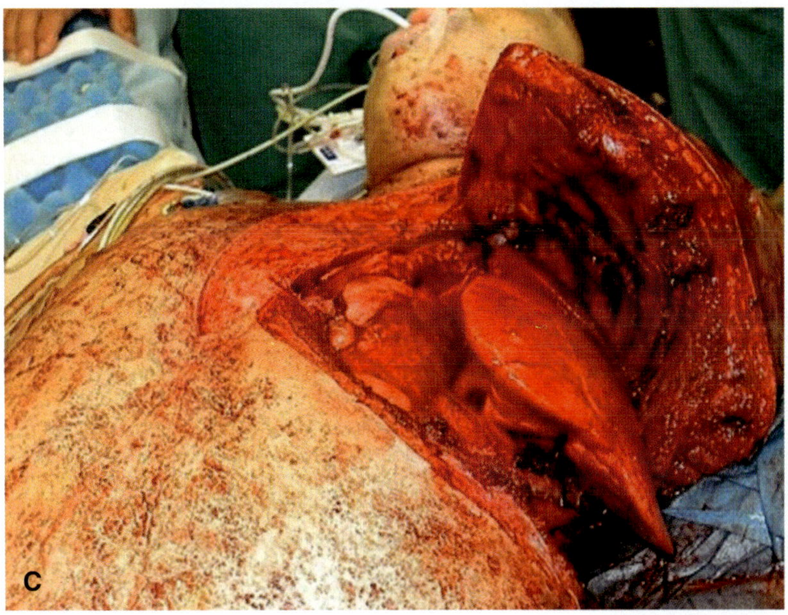

FIGURE 8.4 ▌ An unstable patient with a gunshot wound to the left shoulder was managed with anterolateral thoracotomy (**A**) and clamping of the proximal subclavian (**B**, *arrow*) artery following division of the mediastinal pleura. Next a supraclavicular incision was made to repair the transected vessel with a reversed saphenous vein graft (**C**).

Exposure: Left Subclavian Artery

TIP

Following the anterolateral thoracotomy for proximal control consider performing the reconstruction through a left supraclavicular exposure. A clavicular resection with a small oscillating bone saw is helpful for more proximal injuries.

- Third or fourth space anterolateral thoracotomy or resuscitative thoracotomy (Fig. 8.4).
- Perform a supraclavicular incision for a stable patient with non-expanding hematoma (Fig. 8.5).

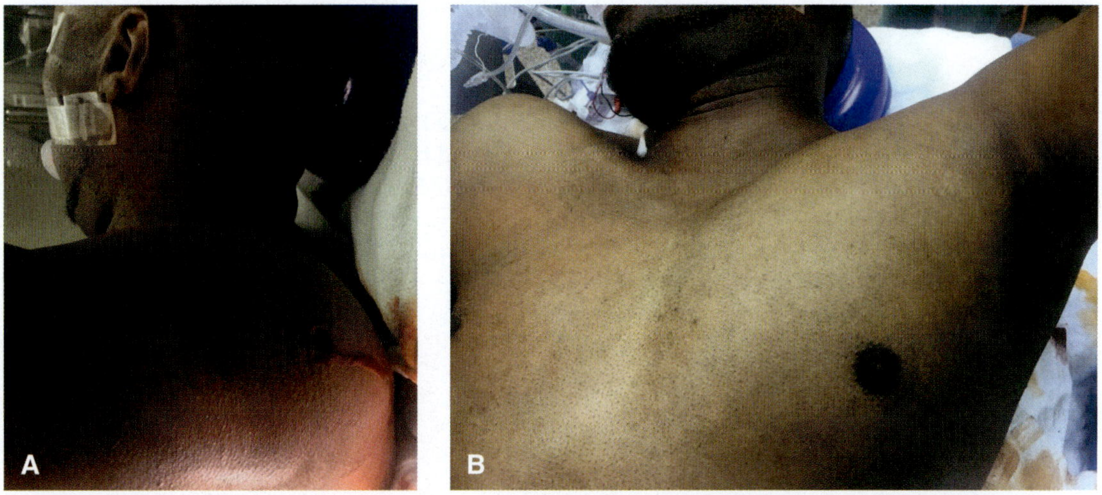

FIGURE 8.5 ▍ An isolated left posterior shoulder gunshot wound in a hemodynamically stable patient (**A**). A large nonexpanding hematoma on the left anterior chest wall challenges the supraclavicular approach (**B**).

- Apply digital pressure or insert an occlusion balloon for rapid bleeding control.
- Clavicular resection and infraclavicular extension may be needed for distal control (Fig. 8.6).

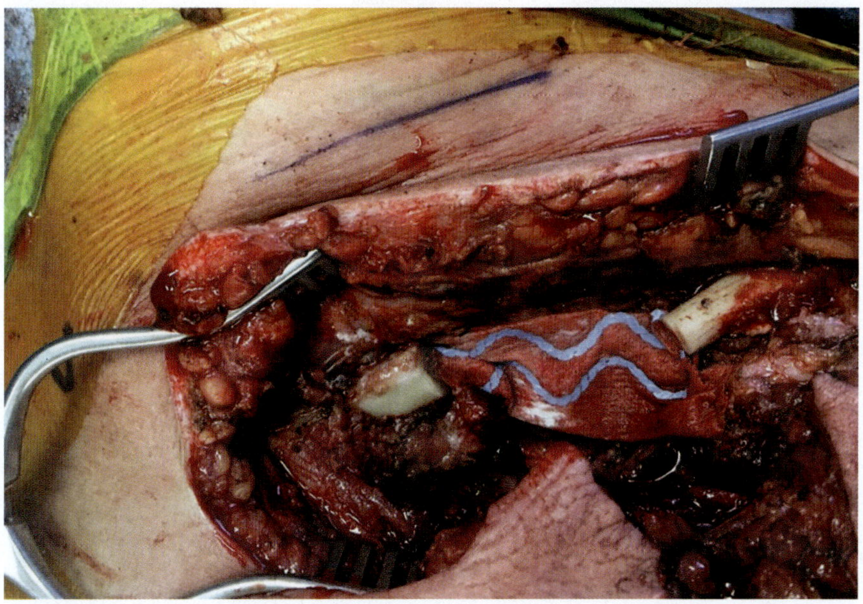

FIGURE 8.6 ▍ Iatrogenic injury to the left subclavian artery during a chemotherapy port removal necessitated a clavicular resection for proximal control.

Thrombectomy and Shunting

- A #3 or #4 Fogarty balloon thrombectomy catheter is passed gently, and not overinflated, to remove all thrombotic debris proximally and distally.
- Intraluminal temporary vascular shunts reestablish antegrade arterial flow.
- Robust collateral circulation usually prevents severe arm ischemia.
- Intravenous heparin at 50 to 75 U/kg is given to stable noncoagulopathic patients.
- Flush the artery liberally with heparinized saline.

Subclavian Artery Reconstruction

TIP

For a small child, the saphenous vein will be an acceptable and appropriately sized conduit.

- Type of repair and conduit is dictated by surgeon preference and degree of injury.
  - Suture lacerations with pledgeted bites of 4-0 Prolene using the tip of the index finger.
  - Following debridement, patch holes with vein or bovine (or patient) pericardium.
  - Perform a tensionless (nonredundant) end-to-end repair for simple transections.
  - Segmental defects are repaired with ePTFE in adults but reversed saphenous vein may be a better size match for children (Fig. 8.7).

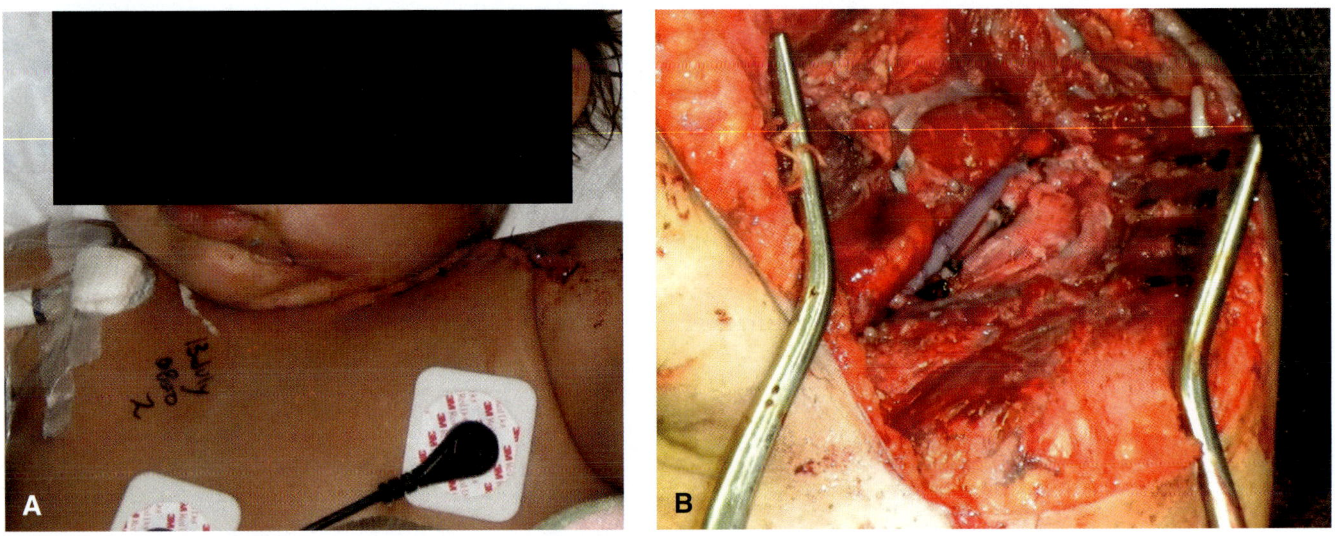

FIGURE 8.7 ▮ An 18-month-old female with a left shoulder GSW (**A**). A supraclavicular approach was used to repair the transection with a reversed saphenous vein interposition graft (**B**). She was discharged home on day 5 with a brachioplexopathy.

- Prosthetic grafts are durable. They may be better suited for large arteries or when routing under the clavicle (Fig. 8.8).

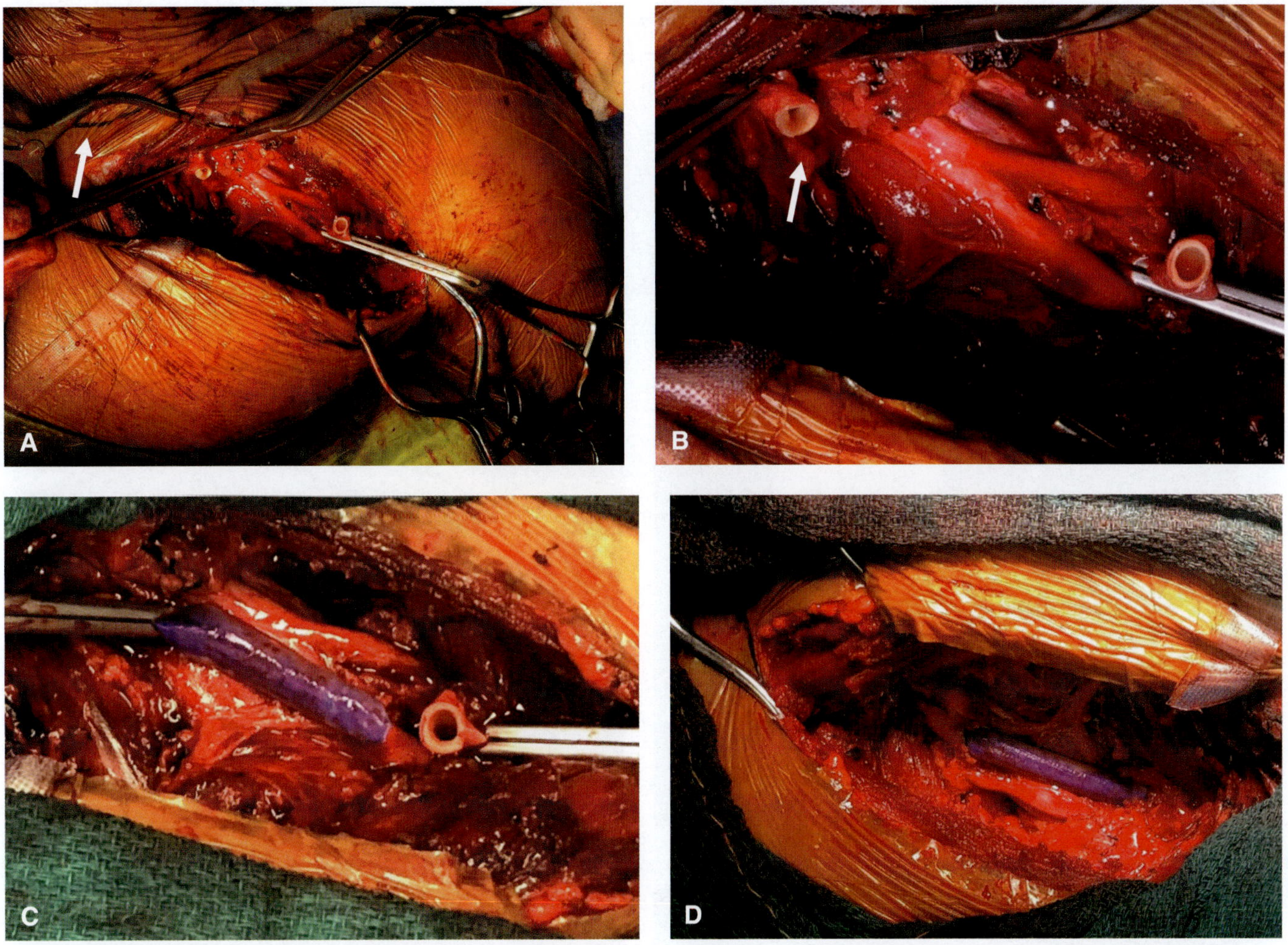

FIGURE 8.8 ❙ Left supraclavicular exposure with surgical ink on sternal notch (**A**, *arrow*). The forceps is on proximal left subclavian artery (**B**, *arrow*). The intact brachial plexus is shown with complete debridement of all thrombus and intimal injury (**B, C**). The bioengineered Human Acellular Vessel (Humacyte, Durham, NC) was an expeditious "off-the-shelf" size matching conduit (**D**). The graft was covered by the pectoralis muscles. A 10 JP was placed in the event of a thoracic duct leak.

- Ligation of the artery is often tolerated but only performed in extremis.
- Repair concomitant venous injury with lateral suture when possible; venous ligation is associated with mild to moderate swelling.
- A completion angiogram is performed with diluted, hand-injected contrast arteriogram by placing a butterfly needle or angiocatheter into the native artery.
- A Duplex ultrasound is an alternative to completion angiography.
- A drain is left in place in the event of a thoracic duct injury.
- Routine prophylactic forearm fasciotomy is not recommended.

Endovascular Techniques

TIP

An endovascular repair is best reserved for the hemodynamically stable patient with a very focal injury. Occasionally retrograde access techniques are effective when antegrade wires fail to cross the injured arterial segment.

- Allows durable treatment of an injury that is surgically challenging.
- CTA directs preoperative endovascular plans as covered stents are frequently used to treat pseudoaneurysms or arteriovenous fistulae (Fig. 8.9).

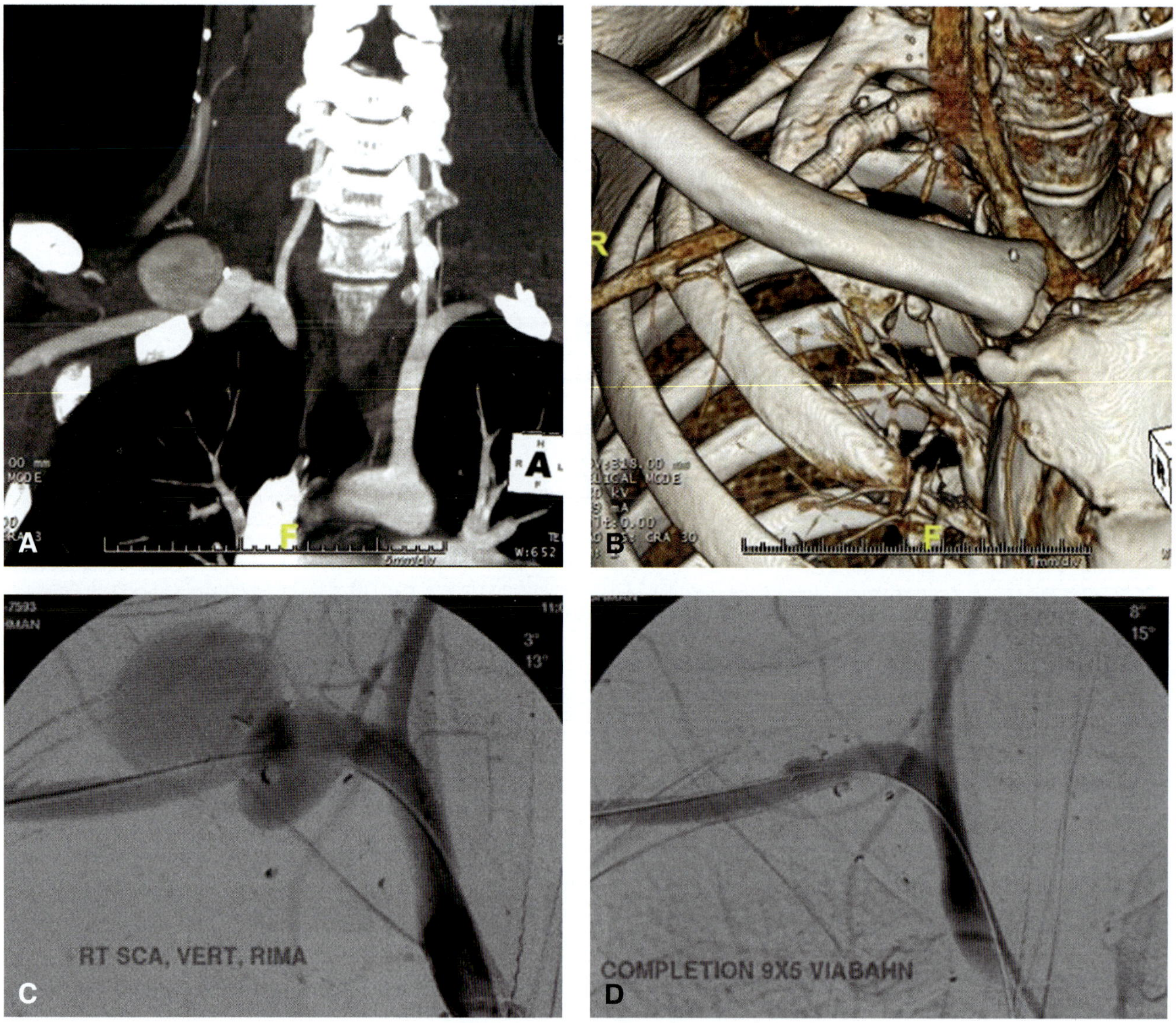

FIGURE 8.9 ▌ Multi-detector row CTA is a fundamental diagnostic tool (**A, B**). Right subclavian artery pseudoaneurysm successfully repaired with a covered stent **(C, D)**.

- In some cases, a retrograde (transbrachial) approach can revascularize a difficult transection (Fig. 8.10).

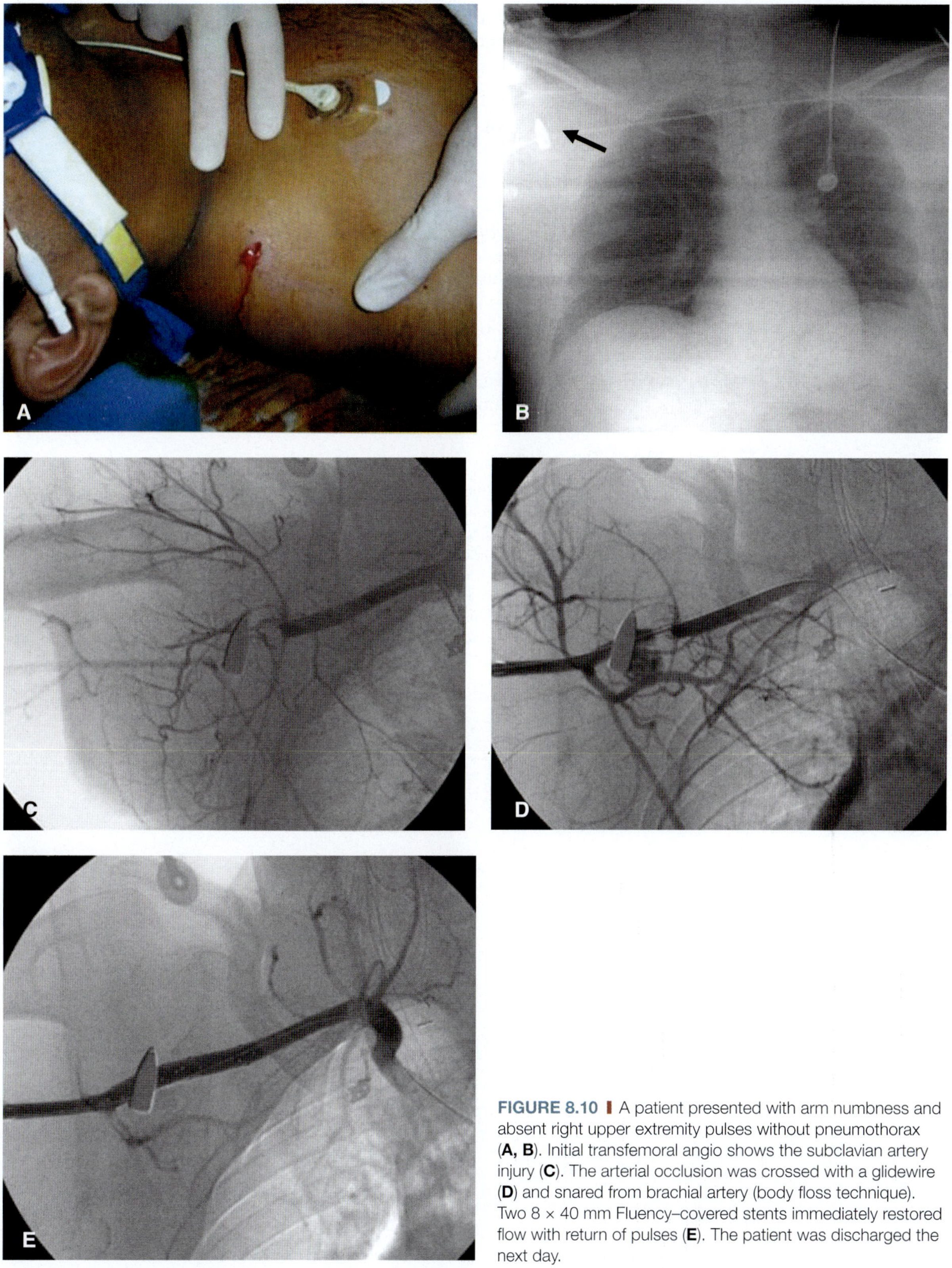

FIGURE 8.10 ▎ A patient presented with arm numbness and absent right upper extremity pulses without pneumothorax (**A, B**). Initial transfemoral angio shows the subclavian artery injury (**C**). The arterial occlusion was crossed with a glidewire (**D**) and snared from brachial artery (body floss technique). Two 8 × 40 mm Fluency–covered stents immediately restored flow with return of pulses (**E**). The patient was discharged the next day.

- Coils are useful for occluding a branch vessel or treating pseudoaneurysms.
- Percutaneous ultrasound-guided transfemoral arterial access may be useful if the patient suddenly requires balloon occlusion.

POSTOPERATIVE MANAGEMENT

TIP

Brachial plexus injuries are common and early involvement of the Hand team is recommended.

- Normal mean arterial pressure (80–100 mm Hg) should be maintained.
- Single-agent antiplatelet therapy is routinely.
- Monitor for pain and neurologic deficits that may suggest the onset of compartment syndrome and need for forearm fasciotomy.
- Persistent left-sided drainage should be evaluated for elevated triglycerides and chylomicrons consistent with thoracic duct injury.

Suggested Readings

Cox CS Jr, Allen GS, Fischer RP, et al. Blunt versus penetrating subclavian artery injury: presentation, injury pattern, and outcome. *J Trauma*. 1999;46(3):445–449.

Hajarizadeh H, Rohrer MJ, Cutler BS. Surgical exposure of the left subclavian artery by median sternotomy and left supraclavicular extension. *J Trauma*. 1996;41(1):136–139.

Shalhub S, Starnes BW, Hatsukami TS, Karmy-Jones R, Tran NT. Repair of blunt thoracic outlet arterial injuries: an evolution from open to endovascular approach. *J Trauma*. 2011;71(5):E114–E121.

Waller CJ, Cogbill TH, Kallies KJ, et al. Contemporary management of subclavian and axillary artery injuries: a Western Trauma Association multicenter review. *J Trauma Acute Care Surg*. 2017;83(6):1023–1031.

Chapter 9
Cardiac

ERNEST E. MOORE AND FREDRIC M. PIERACCI

PERIOPERATIVE CONSIDERATIONS

Procedure Rationale

- Cardiac injuries can result from diverse insults, broadly divided into penetrating and blunt. Similarly, the lesions range widely from ice pick perforations that require no operative intervention to large blunt ruptures that are technically unsalvageable. Following penetrating wounds, due to the predominance of anterior and left lateral entrance, the most common locations of injury are the right ventricle, left ventricle, and right atrium. Stab wounds (SWs) typically violate one wall of a cardiac chamber, whereas gunshot wounds (GSWs) often involve multiple chambers and may damage internal cardiac structures (Fig. 9.1).

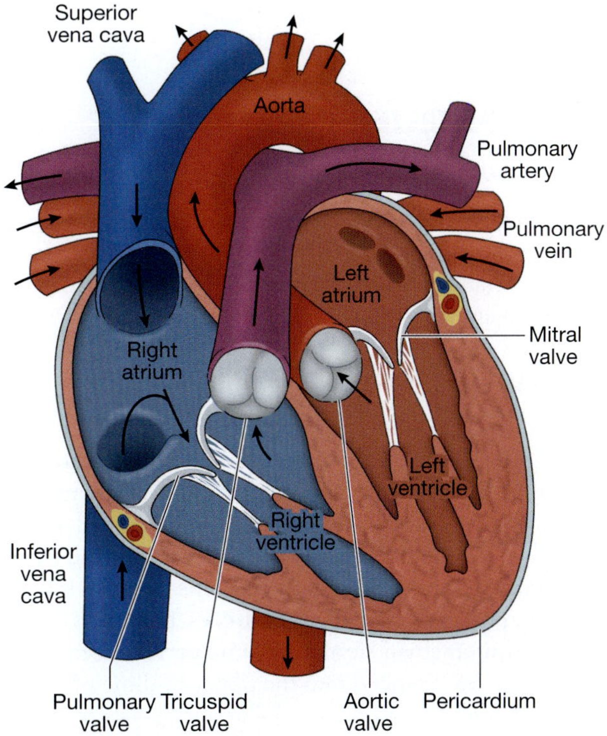

FIGURE 9.1 | Intracardiac structures are vulnerable to injury, particular with GSWs.

- The low-pressure atria are at risk for air embolism, and the left is particularly dangerous with the chance for cerebral air emboli. With blunt trauma, the frequency of injury location is related to topographic exposure to the usual anterior directed force; rupture of cardiac chambers is most frequent in the right ventricle, followed by left ventricle, right atrium, and left atrium; valvular disruption, septal defects, and coronary arterial dissections can occur. However, cardiopulmonary bypass is rarely needed for the initial management of cardiac trauma.

Essential Equipment

Emergency Department

- Betadine-soaked 4 × 4 gauze to prep the anterior chest
- 10-blade scalpel
- Curved Mayo scissors
- Finochietto chest retractor (rib spreader)
- Toothed forceps
- Satinsky vascular clamps (large and small)
- Needle holder
- Lebsche knife and mallet
- 3-0 PDS Sutures
- Teflon pledgets
- Internal defibrillator paddles

Operating Room (in Addition to the Above)

- Sternal power saw
- Sternal retractor
- Rummel tourniquets
- Army–Navy retractors
- # 1 PDS pericostal sutures
- 2-0 and 3-0 PDS sutures
- 24-Fr chest tube for mediastinal drainage
- 28-Fr chest tube for pleural drainage
- #5 Ethibond sutures for chest tube
- Chest tube drainage system
- Sternal wires for closure

TECHNIQUE

Surgical Approach

- Cardiac injuries producing hemodynamic instability are typically exposed and repaired via a resuscitative thoracotomy (RT) in the emergency department (ED) (see Chapter 1), whereas with hemodynamic stability, the heart is usually accessed with a median sternotomy in the operating room (OR) (see Chapter 9).

Pericardiotomy

- Following RT, the pericardium is opened longitudinally anterior to the left phrenic nerve (see Chapter 1). When there is a tense hemopericardium, it is difficult to grasp the pericardium with clamps for elevation and opening. In this situation, a small opening in the pericardium should be made with a knife and the incision extended with scissors. The pericardium should be opened widely to permit delivery for the heart into the left chest for inspection and repair. The left thoracotomy should be extended across the sternum into the right chest (clamshell thoracotomy) for right atrial, posterior cardiac, or multiple-chamber injuries.
- Following median sternotomy, the pericardium should be opened widely in the midline. The incision can be extended into the upper midline of the abdomen for additional exposure.

TIP

The pericardium should be grasped with Kocher clamps and mobilized into the wound for decompression. Blunt dissection will advance the pericardium into the mediastinum and make access difficult.

Subxiphoid Pericardial Window

- A subxiphoid pericardial window can be performed in the ED or OR, with local or general anesthesia depending on the indications. An upper abdominal incision is made around or through the xiphoid process. The diaphragm is grasped on both sides of the anticipated pericardiotomy with Kocher clamps, as superior as possible beneath the xiphoid process (Fig. 9.2).

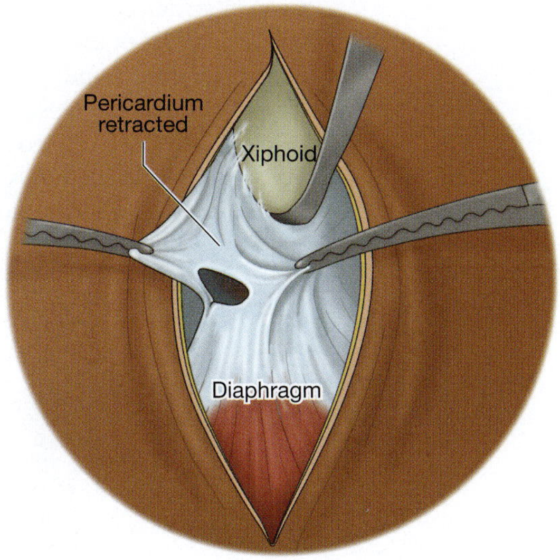

FIGURE 9.2 ▌ A subxiphiod window is made via a midline diaphragmatic incision. Kocher clamps are used on either side of the incision site to provide countertraction.

- The xiphoid can be elevated with an Army–Navy retractor or excised if large. Scissors are used to traverse the diaphragm and underlying pericardium. Ongoing bleeding from the pericardium is followed promptly with a median sternotomy to expose the heart. In the event of transient bleeding, there may be role for pericardial lavage to determine if a sternotomy is required. In this circumstance, it may be useful to leave a 10-mm Jackson–Pratt drain to identify recurrent bleeding.

TIP

Bleeding from the ventricle should be controlled with finger pressure. While a Foley is suggested, the balloon may enlarge the defect and preclude simple suture repair.

Bleeding Control and Cardiorrhaphy

- Following pericardiotomy, the blood clots should be evacuated and a rapid search done to identify bleeding sites. A finger should be placed over ventricular wounds to minimize bleeding. Atrial wounds should be controlled promptly with an appropriate-sized Satinsky clamp (Fig. 9.3).

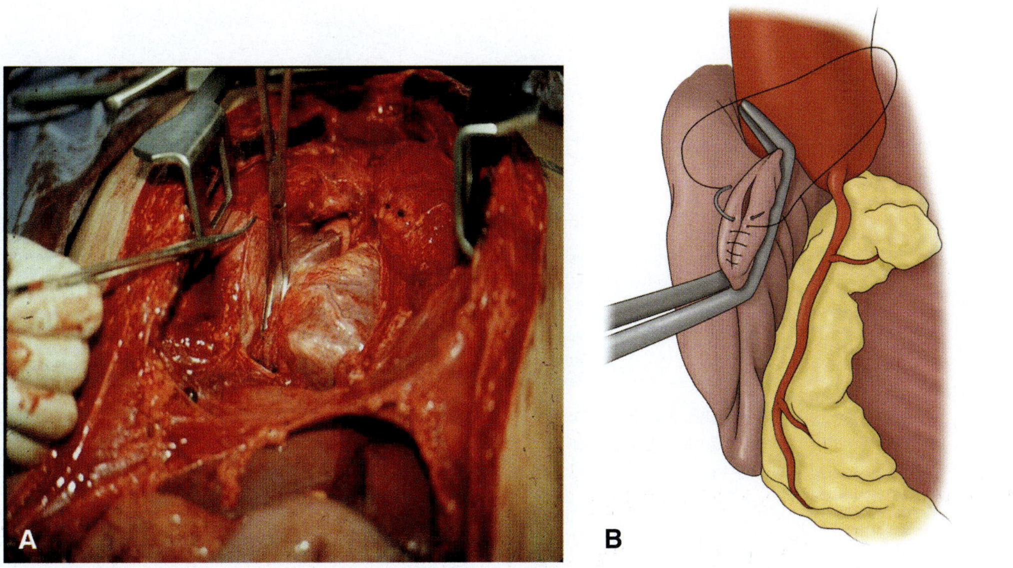

FIGURE 9.3 ▌ Bleeding from atrial wounds is controlled with a Satinsky clamp and the injured oversewn with a running 3-0 PDS suture. (**A**) Operative photograph; (**B**) schematic.

- This is particularly critical on the left atrium to minimize the risk of air embolism. Atrial wounds are repaired definitely with a running 3-0 Prolene suture.
- The management of ventricular wounds is controversial. Poor technique can result in enlarging the cardiac defect or endangering an adjacent coronary artery. There is some enthusiasm for Foley balloon control of bleeding. However, we discourage this maneuver because of the risk of enlarging the ventricular wound, particularly in the relatively thin-walled right ventricle.
- We perform suture closure of the ventricular wound with 3-0 Prolene. Interrupted 3-0 Prolene sutures with Teflon pledgets are used routinely for the relatively thin-walled right ventricle (Fig. 9.4), whereas wounds in the left ventricle are repaired with continuous 3-0 Prolene or additional interrupted sutures for more extensive wounds (Fig. 9.5).

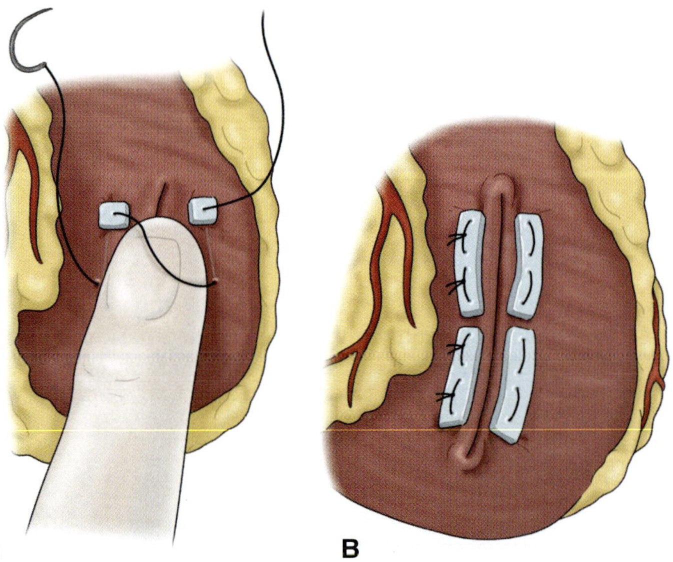

FIGURE 9.4 ▌ Right ventricular wounds are typically sutured (**A**) with Teflon pledgets (**B**) because of the relatively thin ventricular wall.

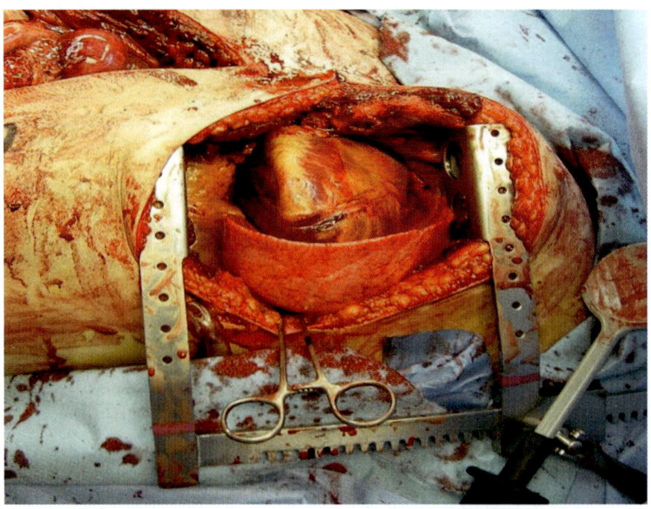

FIGURE 9.5 ▌ Left ventricular injuries are usually suture repaired without pledgets because of the thick ventricular wall. However, irregular wounds due to GSWs may warrant pledget support.

- Skin staples may be used for large ventricular wounds for rapid control of bleeding in the ED (Fig. 9.6). The staple line is usually re-enforced or replaced with interrupted sutures in the OR.

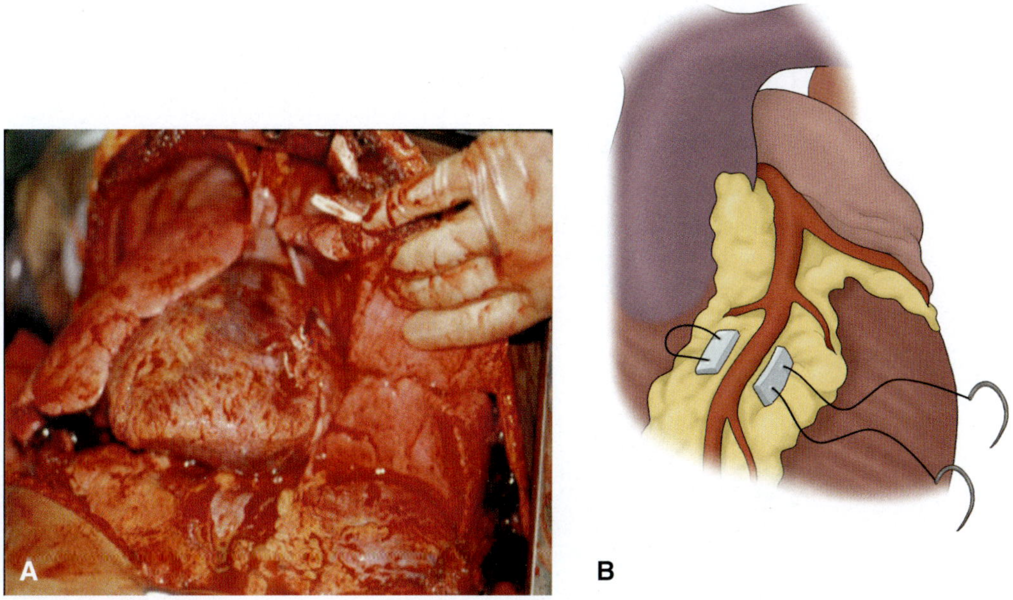

FIGURE 9.6 ▌ Ventricular injuries adjacent to the left anterior descending coronary artery are reapproximated with sutures deep to the artery, with sufficient tension to arrest bleeding without compromising coronary flow. (**A**) Operative photograph; (**B**) schematic.

- Defibrillation of a cardiac wound is delayed until the repair is completed (see Chapter 1). Similarly, calcium administration and inotropic support are withheld until the repair is deemed secure.

Coronary Artery

- When the ventricular injury is in proximity to a coronary artery, the sutures should be placed deep into the artery in a horizontal mattress fashion and tied with sufficient tension to control bleeding without compromising coronary flow (Fig. 9.7). We have used BioGlue to control residual bleeding from the loose suture line.

FIGURES 9.7 ▌ Staples are occasionally used to close large ventricular wounds, generally but require suture support or revision in the OR.

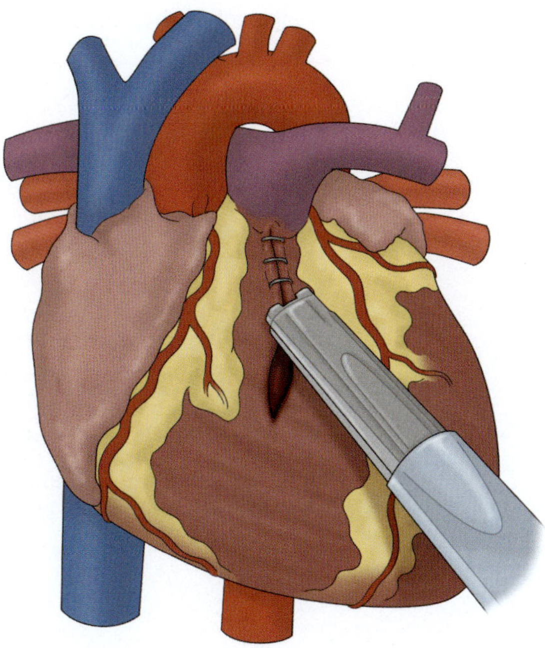

- Bleeding from a tangential injury to a coronary artery should be controlled digitally until definite repair can be attempted with magnification. Transected coronary arteries should be ligated. Coronary artery bypass is rarely required or successful.

Inflow Occlusion

- Temporary inflow occlusion may be required for complex cardiac injuries, particularly, large right ventricular ruptures due to blunt trauma. The maneuver entails limiting blood flow into the heart by occluding the superior and inferior vena cava (Fig. 9.8). The superior vena cava Rummel should include the azygous vein or the azygous can be controlled separately.

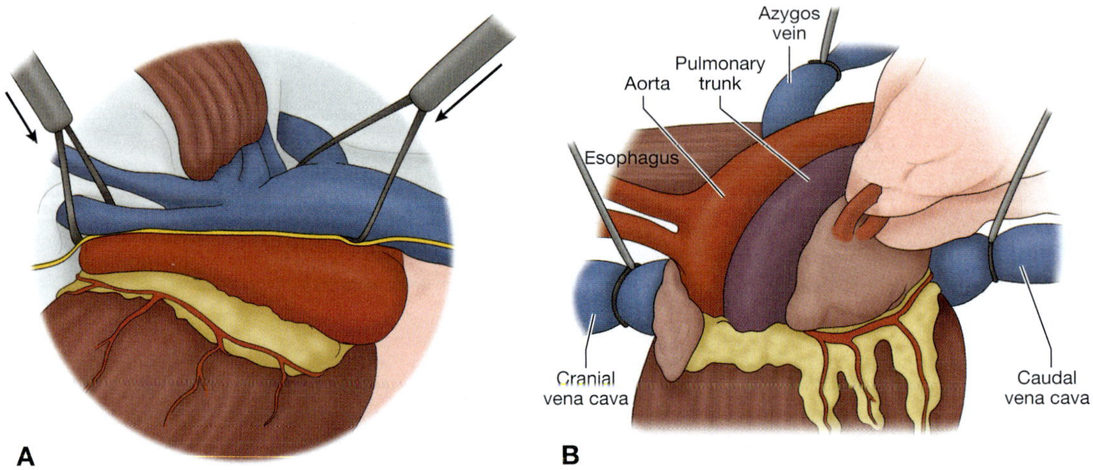

FIGURE 9.8 ▌ Temporary inflow occlusion may be required for complex cardiac injuries. The concept entails occluding the superior (**A**) and inferior vena cava (**B**).

Posterior Cardiac Wounds

- Penetrating wounds in the posterior cardiac ventricular wall should be controlled digitally until the patient's physiologic status is improved. Repair is usually feasible with sequential elevation of the apex of the heart.

TIP

Efforts to restore cardiac activity and improve contractility (epinephrine and calcium) should be withheld until the injury is repaired definitely. Vigorous cardiac activity will make the repair more difficult and may enlarge the wound with partial suturing.

Defibrillation

Defibrillation of a cardiac wound is delayed until the repair is completed (see Chapter 1). Similarly, calcium administration and inotropic support are withheld until the repair is deemed secure.

Pericardial Closure

- A large flat drain or small chest tube is placed in the pericardium, as reviewed in Chapter 1. The pericardium is closed with interrupted 2-0 PDS unless reperfusion myocardial edema obviates safe closure.

Damage Control Thoracic Closure

- Similar to visceral edema precluding physiologically tolerable abdominal wall closure, thoracic myocardial and chest wall edema may require temporary chest wall closure (Fig. 9.9)

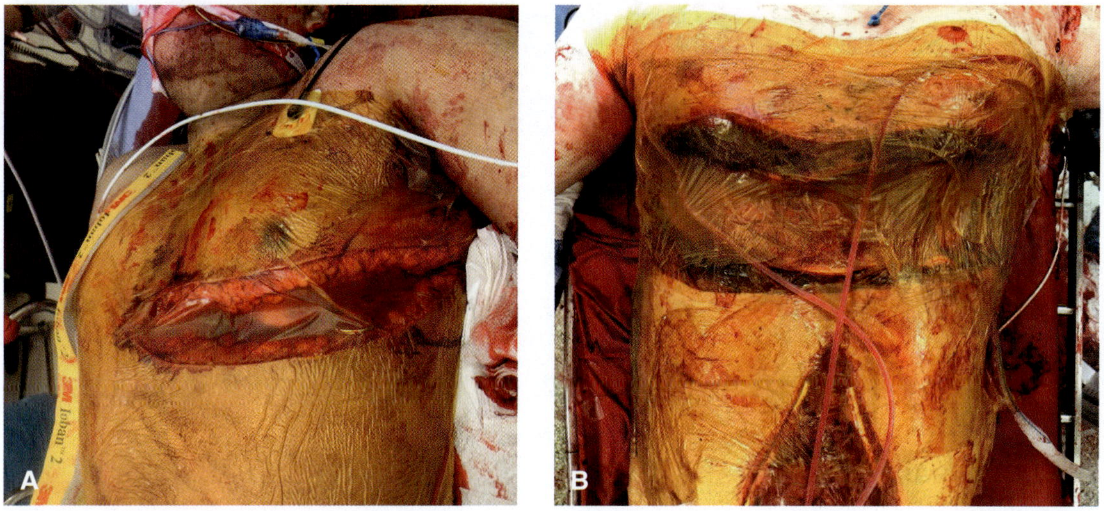

FIGURE 9.9 ▌ Damage control principles; that is, delayed incision closure, may be necessary for reperfusion edema of the heart (**A**) and chest wall (**B**).

POSTOPERATIVE CARE

Patients should undergo formal ECHO evaluation of the heart in 3 to 7 days for any lesion requiring surgical intervention.

Suggested Readings

González-Hadad A, Ordoñez CA, Parra MW, et al. Damage control in penetrating cardiac trauma. *Colomb Med (Cali)*. 2021;52(2):e4034519.

Jones EL, Burlew CC, Moore EE. BioGlue hemostasis of penetrating cardiac wounds in proximity to the left anterior descending coronary artery. *J Trauma Acute Care Surg*. 2012;72(3):796–798.

Mattox KL, Feliciano DV, Burch J, Beall AC Jr, Jordan GL Jr, De Bakey ME. Five thousand seven hundred sixty cardiovascular injuries in 4459 patients. Epidemiologic evolution 1958 to 1987. *Ann Surg*. 1989;209(6):698–705.

Moreno C, Moore EE, Majure JA, Hopeman AR. Pericardial tamponade: a critical determinant for survival following penetrating cardiac wounds. *J Trauma*. 1986;26(9):821–825.

Morse BC, Mina MJ, Carr JS, et al. Penetrating cardiac injuries: a 36-year perspective at an urban, Level I trauma center. *J Trauma Acute Care Surg*. 2016;81(4):623–631.

Chapter 10

Partial Left Heart Bypass for Thoracic Aortic Injury

ERNEST E. MOORE

PERIOPERATIVE CONSIDERATIONS

Procedure Rationale

- Modern centrifugal pumps facilitate partial left heart bypass without systemic anticoagulation, and have become the standard when open repair of the thoracic aorta is required (Fig. 10.1).

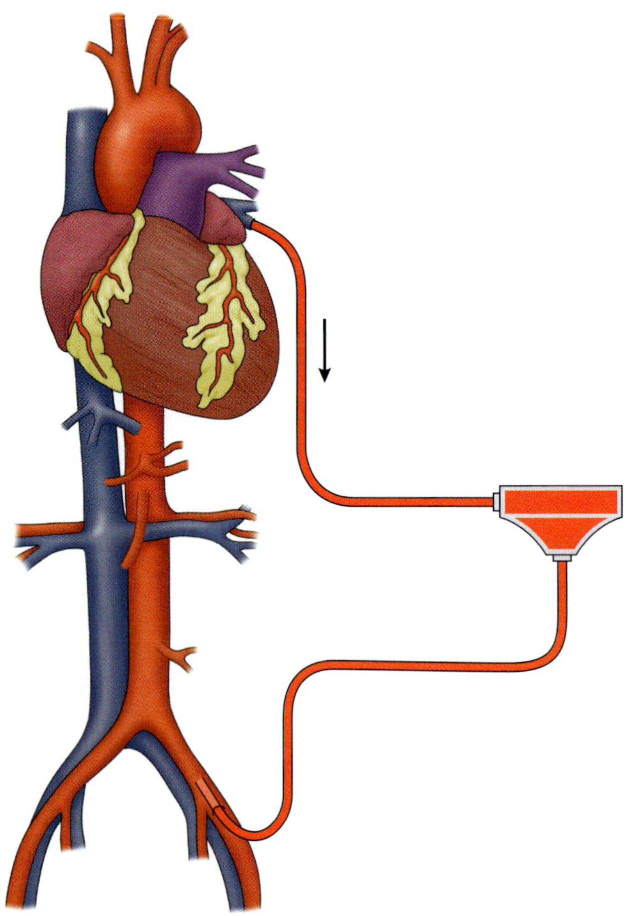

FIGURE 10.1 ▌ Partial left heart bypass is achieved by withdrawing blood from the left atrium (superior pulmonary vein) and returning it via the left common femoral artery. This perfuses the thoracic aorta distal to the cross-clamp with oxygenated blood.

- This technique virtually eliminates the risk of paraplegia associated with cross-clamping of the thoracic aorta. Previous studies have found that clamp times exceeding 30 minutes without distal aortic perfusion, or distal perfusion failing to produce a mean pressure greater than 60 Torr are significant risk factors for paraplegia. In addition, precipitous increases in left ventricular afterload following cross-clamping can contribute to myocardial dysfunction, especially in multi-injured patients with associated myocardial contusion or pre-existing cardiac disease. Partial left heart bypass prevents this physiologic stress during aorta occlusion. Finally, partial left heart bypass avoids splanchnic and lower extremity ischemia/reperfusion associated with aortic cross-clamping. These inflammatory responses have been invoked in the genesis of the adult respiratory distress syndrome (ARDS) and multiple organ failure (MOF).

Reduction of Aortic Shear Stress

- A thoracic aortic pseudoaneurysm is contained only by the pleura and endothoracic fascia. The tension in this segment of attenuated aortic wall is greater (the law of Laplace) than the adjacent normal aorta. Thus, minimizing the stress on the pseudoaneurysm is critical before definitive repair. The primary objective is to reduce the rate of rise in aortic pressure (dP/dT). This is achieved by decreasing the force of left ventricular ejection with a negative ionotropic agent (selective β_1-antagonist). Pharmacologic β-blockade is continued in the OR until the thoracic aortic tear has been isolated for proximal and distal vascular control. Esmolol is the preferred agent, and the hemodynamic targets are a heart rate <100/min and systolic blood pressure <100 mm Hg (Esmolol loading dose = 500 μg/kg with a continuous infusion begun at 50 μg/kg/min). Once the thoracic aorta is isolated for cross-clamping, it is important to remind the anesthesiologist to stop the Esmolol administration when partial left heart bypass is initiated.

Spinal Cord Protection

- In the unusual event, the patient presents with paraplegia or has aortic occlusion due to a dissection from initial disruption, an intradural catheter is placed to decompress the spinal canal for 72 hours.

Essential Equipment

TIP

The surgeon in charge should review all the essential items with the scrub nurse and pump technician before initiating the operation. A technical challenge during the procedure can be fatal if the appropriate material is not immediately available.

- Centrifugal pump with tubing, connectors, and clamps
- 28-, 30-, and 32-Fr venous cannulae; 18-, 20-, and 22-Fr arterial cannulae
- Vascular grafts: 16-, 18-, and 20-mm gel Dacron or PTFE. We prefer PTFE based on studies indicating a lower incidence of infection
- Vascular clamps: #2 Harken, medium and large Satinsky, and 2 large DeBakey aortic clamps
- Suture: 3-0 and 4-0 Prolene double-armed sutures; 0, 2-0, and 3-0 silk ties; 0 and 2-0 PDS sutures
- Teflon pledgets, precut 1 × 2 cm
- Rummel tourniquets × 6, umbilical tapes × 10
- Finochietto chest retractor
- Heparinized saline (50 U/mL)

Airway Management

- Unilateral right-lung ventilation is optimal for exposure of the descending aorta. A double-lumen endotracheal tube is typically inserted to permit selective deflation of the left lung. An alternative is a selective airway blocker, but this is operator dependent.
- A high-flow mechanical ventilator (>100 L/min flow capacity) may be required to achieve adequate single-lung ventilation. In patients with right pulmonary contusions, synchronous partial

ventilation of the left lung may be necessary to maintain adequate arterial oxygenation. This can be achieved with continuous positive airway pressure (CPAP) at a small lung volume that will not interfere with the procedure.

Hemodynamic Monitoring

- A right radial arterial catheter is placed to allow continuous monitoring of the proximal thoracic aorta during cross-clamping of the left subclavian artery.
- A right femoral arterial catheter is employed for continuous monitoring of the distal space aortic pressure during thoracic aortic cross-clamping.

Patient Positioning

- The patient is placed in a right lateral decubitus position with the left arm suspended and the thorax angled 15 degrees posteriorly.
- A large axillary roll and iliac wing pad suspend the right chest to facilitate ventilation.
- The pelvis is rotated posteriorly approximately 45 degrees to the left to facilitate access to the left common femoral artery (CFA).
- The patient is then prepped sterilely and draped to allow for simultaneous exploration of the left chest, left groin and, if necessary, the abdomen. Ioban is used to secure the drapes and isolate the skin to prevent contamination if a synthetic graft is required.
- The centrifugal pump technician is positioned at the patient's left side for a clear view of the anesthesiology monitoring equipment, including the distal aortic pressure.

TECHNIQUE

Two-Team Approach Preferred

- One trauma team performs the posterior lateral thoracotomy, places the left pulmonary venous cannula, and focuses on isolating and repairing the aortic injury (Fig. 10.2).

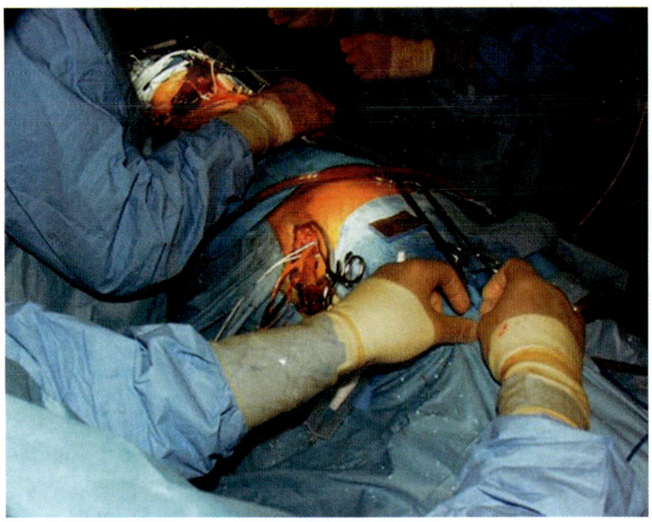

FIGURE 10.2 ▍ Repair of the torn thoracic aorta is optimally performed with two teams; one team places the left pulmonary venous cannula and focuses on repairing the aortic injury, while the second team isolates the left common femoral artery and oversees hemodynamic management during bypass.

- The second team isolates the CFA for simultaneous cannula placement and oversees hemodynamic management during partial left heart bypass.

Left Common Femoral Artery Isolation

- The left CFA and junction of the superficial femoral and profunda branches are exposed via a standard vertical groin incision (Fig. 10.3).

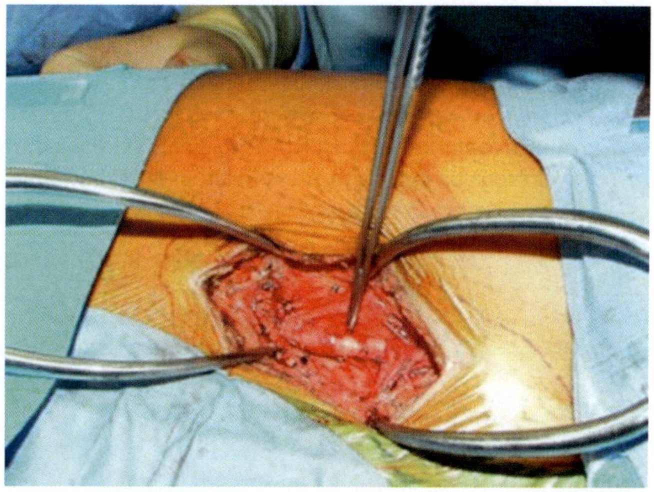

FIGURE 10.3 ▌ The left common femoral artery is cannulated to preserving collateral flow via the profunda femoris to perfuse the lower extremity.

- Although a percutaneous approach can be used, we prefer to confirm optimal position of the arterial cannula. However, the same wire-guided access technique should be used to minimize the arterial defect. Cannulation of the CFA is important to preserve collateral flow via the profunda system to maintain perfusion of the leg. The CFA is surrounded proximally and distally with umbilical tapes.
- Cannulation is delayed until pulmonary venous cannulation is initiated to minimize the risk of thromboemboli during the implementation of bypass (Fig. 10.4).

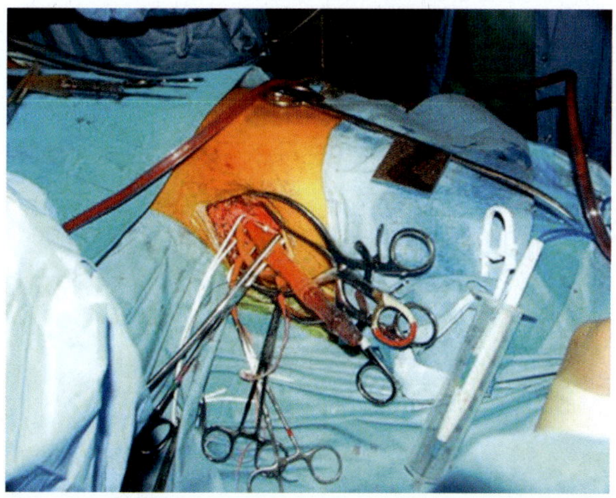

FIGURE 10.4 ▌ Left common femoral artery access is delayed until pulmonary venous cannulation is initiated to minimize the risk of femoral thromboemboli.

Left Posteriolateral Thoracotomy

TIP

The left phrenic and vagus (recurrent laryngeal) nerves are relatively small and should be isolated with vessel loops early in the mediastinal dissection to avoid nerve injury.

- The skin incision for the left posterior lateral thoracotomy begins inferior to the nipple, continued along the infrapectoral crease, proceeding cephalad 2 cm inferior to the scapula and curved parallel to the spine.
- The chest is entered through the fourth intercostal space, and the fourth rib is transected posteriorly at the level of the paraspinal muscles.

- Tolerance to left-lung deflation is ascertained at a convenient time relying on O_2 saturation recordings. The time on partial left heart bypass is minimized to avoid thromboembolic complications. Consequently, as much dissection as can be accomplished safely is done before initiating bypass.
- The left superior pulmonary vein is isolated first. Dissection of the superior pulmonary vein is begun by longitudinally incising the pleura on the anterior, superior border of the pulmonary hilum. The pulmonary vein is then encircled with two umbilical tapes using a Harken #2 clamp (Fig. 10.5).

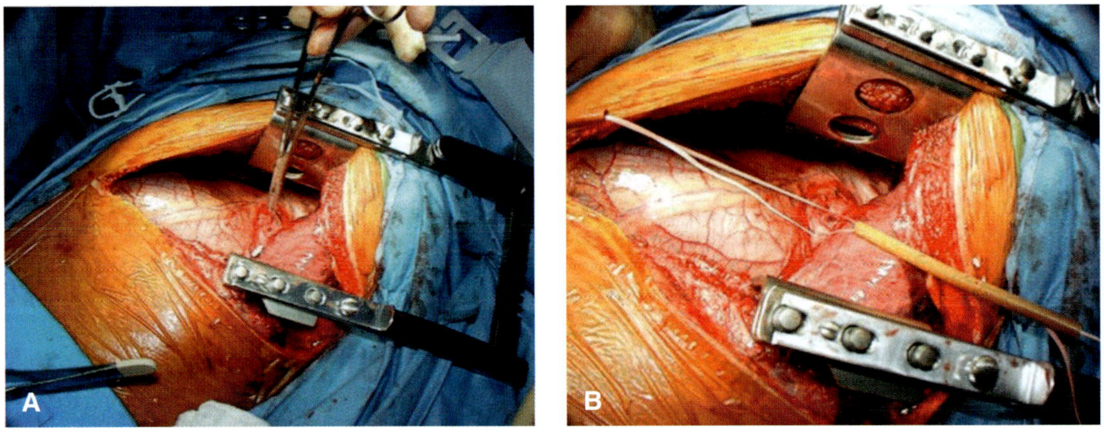

FIGURE 10.5 ❙ **A, B:** The left superior pulmonary vein is encircled with a Harkens #2 clamp for safe placement of umbilical tapes.

- The left phrenic and vagus nerves are identified (Fig. 10.6) and marked with vascular loops, and the subclavian artery is encircled with an umbilical tape (Fig. 10.7).
- It is important to control the subclavian artery proximal to the origin of the left internal mammary and vertebral arteries to avoid retrograde bleeding when the aortic injury is opened.

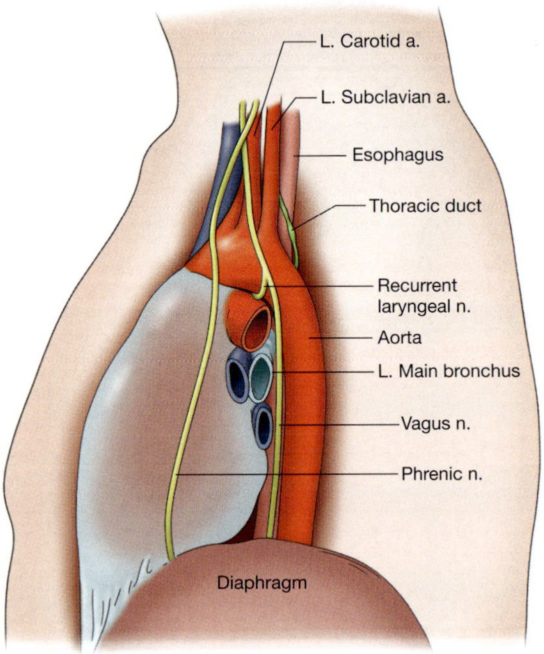

FIGURE 10.6 ❙ The left phrenic and vagus (recurrent laryngeal) nerves should be isolated with vascular loops early in the mediastinal dissection to avoid nerve injury.

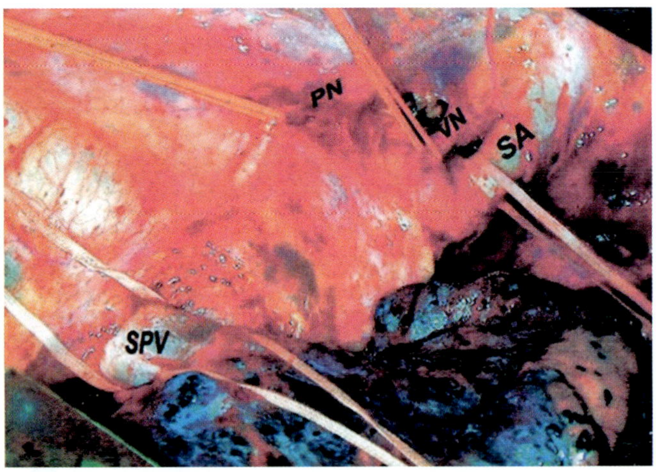

FIGURE 10.7 ❙ The first phase includes isolation of the left superior pulmonary vein (SPV) with umbilical tapes; the phrenic nerve (PN), vagus nerve (VN) with vascular loops, and the subclavian artery (SA) with a umbilical tape.

Isolation of the Aortic Injury

TIP

The decision to initiate bypass or isolate the thoracic aorta first is critical. Minimizing the time on left heart bypass is important to prevent thromboemboli, but entering the pseudoaneurysm before bypass is established may result in fatal bleeding or suboptimal clamp placement.

- The descending thoracic aorta distal to the tear is surrounded with an umbilical tape using the #2 Harken clamp, well beyond the border of the periaortic hematoma (Fig. 10.8).

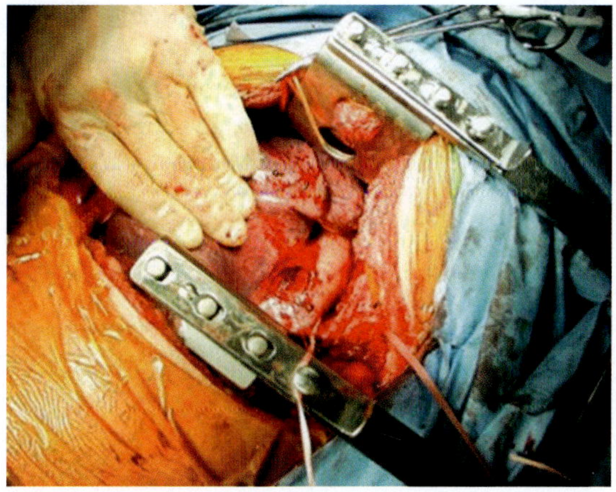

FIGURE 10.8 ▌ The descending thoracic aorta is encircled by blunt dissection, and isolated with an umbilical tape distal to the periaortic hematoma.

- Blunt dissection of the aorta should be done carefully to avoid injury to the paired posterolateral intercostal arteries.
- Dissection continues on the anterior surface of the aorta to identify the innominate, left common carotid and left subclavian arteries in the event emergent aortic cross-clamping is needed due to rupture of the pseudoaneurysm.
- Following these maneuvers, if the aortic tear is distal to the subclavian take-off and there is no hematoma surrounding the transverse arch, the thoracic aorta is mobilized between the left carotid and left subclavian arteries with an umbilical tape. However, if the aortic tear extends to the origin of the subclavian artery, bypass is initiated before isolating the transverse thoracic aorta in the event clamping must be done proximal to the left carotid artery.
- The tissue adherent to the adventitia of the inferior surface of the aorta at the level of the left common carotid artery is sharply divided to permit finger dissection under the transverse thoracic aorta. Further separation of the arch from the pulmonary artery is accomplished with blunt dissection.
- Sharp dissection is performed on the superior arch between the left common carotid and left subclavian arteries. Opposing fingers are directed around the superior and inferior borders of the aortic arch to develop a clear plane. The left vagus nerve descends between the left carotid and subclavian arteries and gives off the recurrent laryngeal nerve, which is closely adherent to the aorta in this region. A #2 Harken clamp is inserted around the aorta at this level for placement of an encircling umbilical tape (Fig. 10.9).

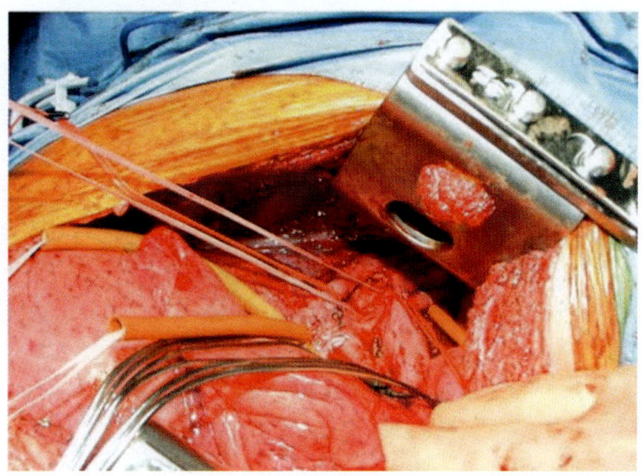

FIGURE 10.9 When the thoracic aortic tear is in the typical location, proximal aortic isolation is initiated between the subclavian artery and left common carotid artery. Encircled the aorta with an umbilical tape assists with later cross-clamping.

- Once the aortic injury has been identified, the distal aortic clamp can be moved closer to the injury to avoid unnecessary exclusion of collateral blood flow to the spine from intercostal arteries as well as to avoid back-bleeding from the intercostals when the aorta is opened.

Left Superior Pulmonary Vein-Common Femoral Artery Bypass

TIP

Cannulation of the left superior pulmonary must be done carefully to avoid air entering the left atrium, which could result in cerebral or coronary air emboli.

- The necessity for anticoagulation with centrifugal pumps remains controversial. Unless there is a clear contraindication to anticoagulation (CNS injury, unstable pelvic fracture, > grade III liver, spleen, or kidney injury), we administer systemic heparin (100 U/kg) and maintain the whole blood activated clotting time between 200 and 250 seconds. The left vertebral artery is stagnant when the left subclavian artery is occluded and a clot can produce a posterior circulation infarct.
- Before inserting the pulmonary venous cannula (28 to 32 Fr), the catheter is marked 6 cm from the tip with a 0 silk tie (Fig. 10.10) to monitor the relative position of the cannula within the left atrium during the subsequent operative course.

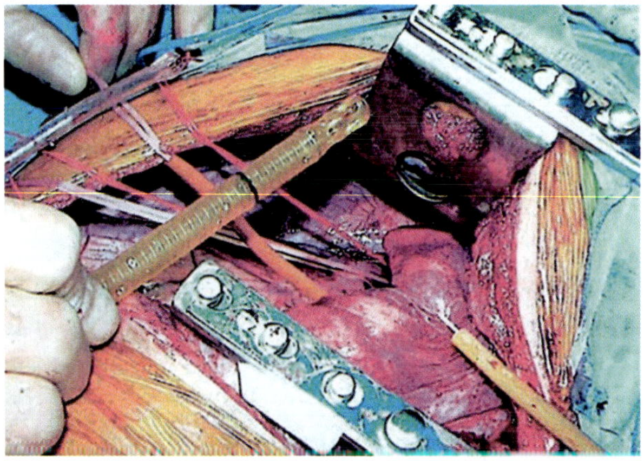

FIGURE 10.10 ■ The superior pulmonary vein cannula is marked 6 cm from the tip with a 0 silk suture to enable monitoring the position within the left atrium during bypass.

- The silk tie remains outside the pulmonary vein to monitor for inadvertent dislodgement. The cannula is filled with heparinized saline (50 U/mL), and a tubing clamp is applied to the open end of the cannula.
- The previously exposed left superior pulmonary vein is now controlled between two umbilical tape snare tourniquets. The distal snare tourniquet is cinched down, and a Satinsky clamp is placed at the juncture of the pulmonary vein and left atrium.
- A transverse venotomy is made at least 2 cm from the left atrium juncture and the clamp is released. Simultaneously, the venous cannula is advanced into the left atrium (Fig. 10.11).

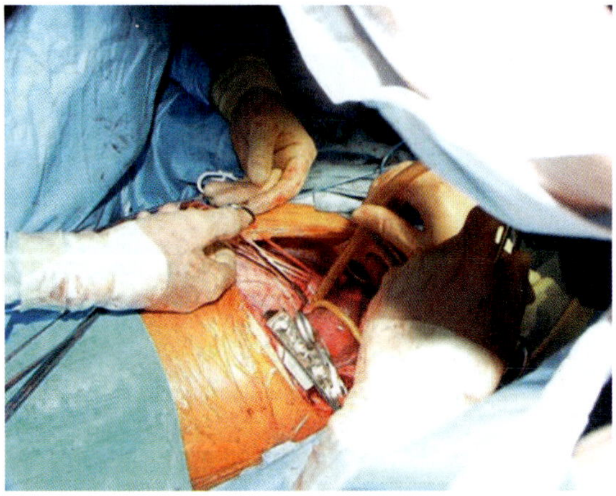

FIGURE 10.11 ■ The venous cannula (28 to 32 Fr) is advanced into the left atrium via a transverse venotomy in the left superior pulmonary vein (SPV). The SPV is encircled with a Rummel tourniquet.

- The pulmonary vein cannulation site is secured with an umbilical tape snare tourniquet. For security, both snare tourniquets are tied to the venous cannula with 0 silk sutures (Fig. 10.12).
- The clamped tubing is briefly opened to allow the cannula to back fill with blood. In connecting the venous cannula to the pump line, bubbles must be completely removed because the centrifugal pump does not eliminate air from the system (Fig. 10.13).

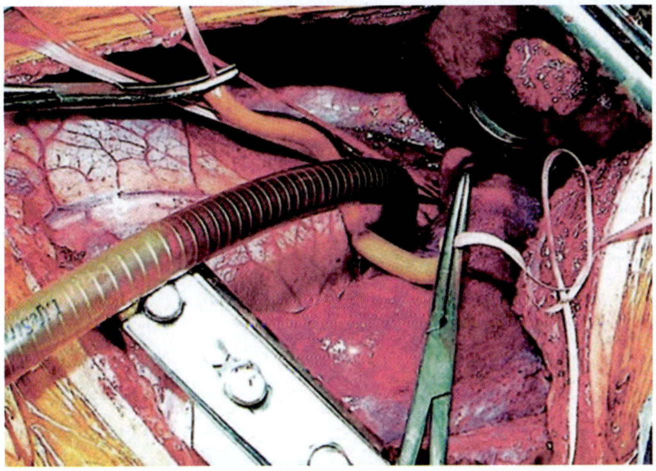

FIGURE 10.12 ▌ The left superior venous cannula is maintained in position with two umbilical tape snare tourniquets. The closure must be secure to avoid air emboli.

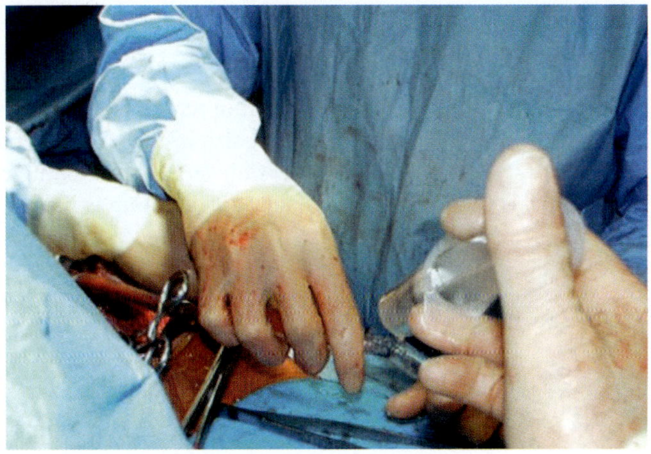

FIGURE 10.13 ▌ Air must be eliminated from the bypass system when connecting the cannulae.

- As an additional precaution to avoid accidental dislodgement of the cannula, the tubing is further secured to the patient's skin using 2-0 nylon sutures at the cannula and pump tubing connections. These sutures hold the tubing tightly to the skin and should remove all tension from the cannulae.
- Simultaneous with the superior pulmonary vein intubation, the femoral artery is cannulated. The common femoral artery is occluded by cinching the proximal snare tourniquet. A transverse arteriotomy is made and heparinized saline (50 U/mL) is flushed distally, and the distal snare tourniquet is cinched.
- An 18- to 13-Fr cannula is directed cephalad into the CFA and secured with the tourniquet. The femoral cannula is then connected to the centrifugal pump using the same precautions mentioned above to remove all air bubbles and is secured in a similar fashion (Fig. 10.14).
- The pump lines are opened with an initial flow of 1.5 L/min. Ultimately, most patients require flow rates between 3.5 and 4.5 L/min to maintain a distal aortic perfusion pressure >65 mm Hg.

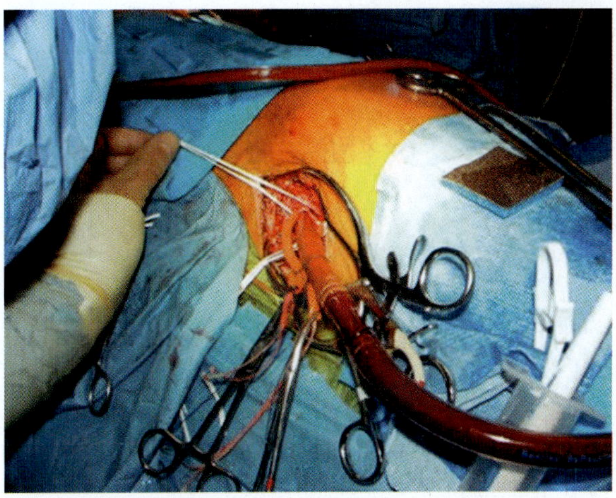

FIGURE 10.14 ▌ The left common femoral artery cannula is similarly connected to the bypass system, eliminating air and securing the cannula with 0 silk ties around the Rummel tourniquets.

Thoracic Aortic Repair

TIP

The most technically challenging part of the operation is suturing the graft to the thin posteriomedial wall of the aorta. The suture must be deep, including periaortic tissue, and the needle must follow the curve of the needle to void tearing the edge of the transected aorta.

- Every effort should be made to minimize the aortic cross-clamp time. Make certain all necessary reconstruction material is available before cross-clamping. The aorta should be assessed for appropriate graft size in the likely event primary repair cannot be achieved. If there is a question about size, select the larger graft diameter; most adult men require an 18- to 20-mm graft.
- A DeBakey aortic clamp is placed on the proximal thoracic aorta between the left carotid and subclavian arteries with gradual cross-clamping as this information is reported to the anesthesiologist and pump technician.
- The umbilical snare tourniquet is tightened on the left subclavian, and then the distal thoracic aorta is cross-clamped. For aortic tears extending proximally to the left subclavian artery, the transverse arch is clamped between the innominate and left carotid arteries.
- The mediastinal pleura is opened vertically to expose the aortic hematoma. A transverse incision should be made on the anteromedial surface of the aorta at the site of injury in the event primary aortorrhaphy can be performed.
- Aortic ruptures vary tremendously from a simple horizontal tear (repaired end to end primarily) to extensive vertical spiral dissections (repaired with an interposition graft). With more complex tears, the thoracic aorta should be divided with care to maintain sufficient aortic tissue posteriorly to provide a secure suture purchase (Fig. 10.15).
- The proximal aorta may also be freed from the recurrent laryngeal nerve to permit completion of the anastomosis proximal to the nerve. The graft is repositioned beneath the vagus nerve in preparation for the distal anastomosis.
- The level of the distal aortic cross-clamping should be moved as proximal as possible to minimize the risk of spinal cord ischemia. Intercostal arteries will require occasional ligation with 2-0 silk ligation from either within the aortic lumen or outside the aorta.
- A gel-impregnated Dacron or PTFE graft is used when segmental aortic replacement is necessary. The proximal anastomosis is performed with a continuous 3-0 double-arm Prolene suture using a parachute technique (Fig. 10.16).

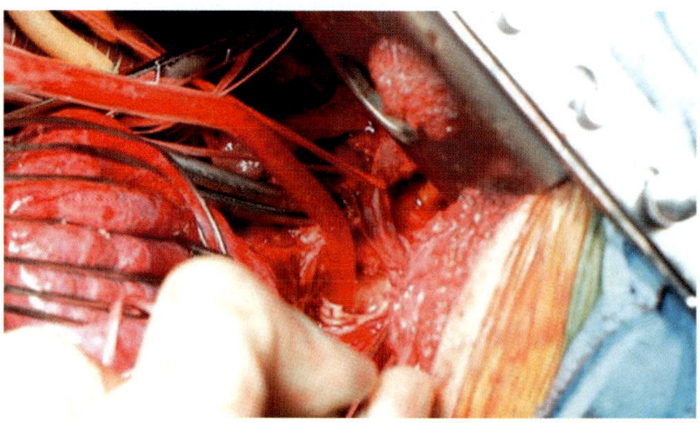

FIGURE 10.15 ❙ Aortic ruptures can be a simple horizontal tear, repaired end to end primarily, but more typically are vertical spiral dissections, requiring resection and repair with an interposition graft.

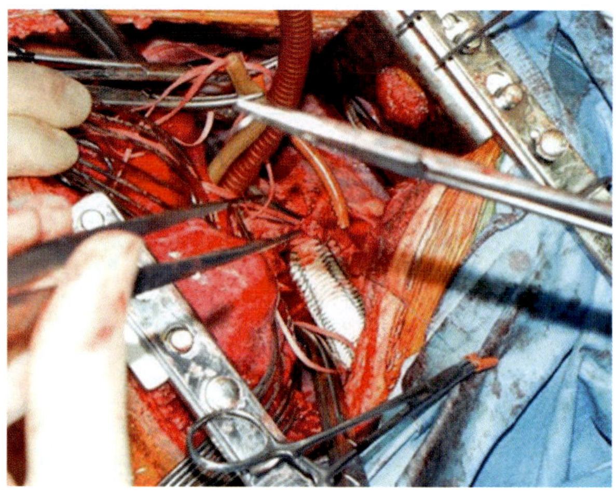

FIGURE 10.16 ❙ The proximal thoracic aortic anastomosis is done with a parachute technique to ensure adequate posterior suturing without damaging the left recurrent laryngeal nerve. The medial wall of the posterior cuff of aorta is particularly fragile, requiring deep bites incorporating periaortic tissue but avoiding the underlying esophagus.

- Suturing is initiated with a horizontal mattress outside to inside in the graft. Sutures are placed from the intimal surface through the adventia to prevent as well as repair intimal flaps. In some instances, it may be technically easier to place the proximal posterior row of sutures from outside of the aorta into the lumen; however, this method is not appropriate if the intima is loose.
- Sutures are placed deeply, incorporating periaortic tissue for added support, but taking care to avoid the underlying esophagus.
- After 3 stitches have been placed with each limb of the double-arm suture, the graft is "parachuted" down to the proximal posterior aorta. Care must be taken to remove all redundancy from these initial sutures before continuing the anastomosis.
- Tension must be maintained on the inactive limb of the suture using a rubber shod clamp and digitally on the active limb to prevent suture line hemorrhage.
- Great attention is required in the proximal suture line medially, in the region of the ligamentum arteriosum, where the aortic tissue is usually weak, thin, and easily torn. It is also important to avoid the recurrent laryngeal nerve in this region.
- Upon completion of the proximal anastomosis, the vascular clamp should be moved onto the graft to check the integrity of the proximal suture line. Leaks in the suture line are repaired using 4-0 Prolene horizontal mattress.
- When the proximal suture line is confirmed to be secure, the left subclavian tourniquet is removed to enhance collateral blood flow to the spine.
- The interior surface of the graft is irrigated with heparinized saline to remove any clot.
- The distal anastomosis is performed in a similar fashion venting air and clot out of the suture line just before releasing the distal aortic clamp (Fig. 10.17).
- The proximal aortic clamp is then released gradually while communicating with the anesthesiologist and pump technician.
- For tears extending proximal to the left subclavian artery, a short bypass graft is interposed for reconstruction (Fig. 10.18).

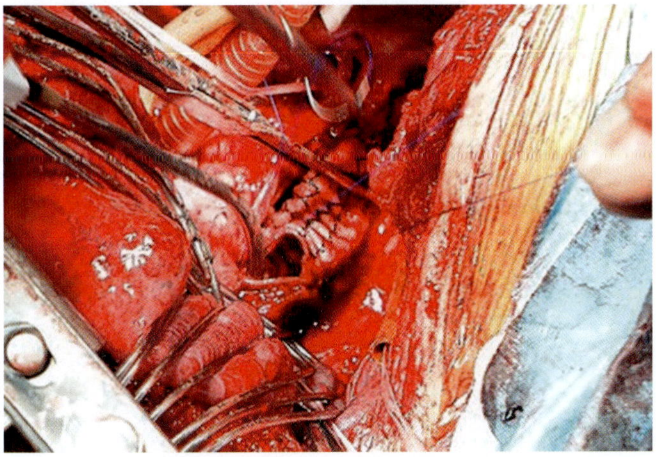

FIGURE 10.17 ▌ The distal aortic anastomosis is performed with a standard running suture, venting air out of the suture line just before releasing the distal aortic clamp.

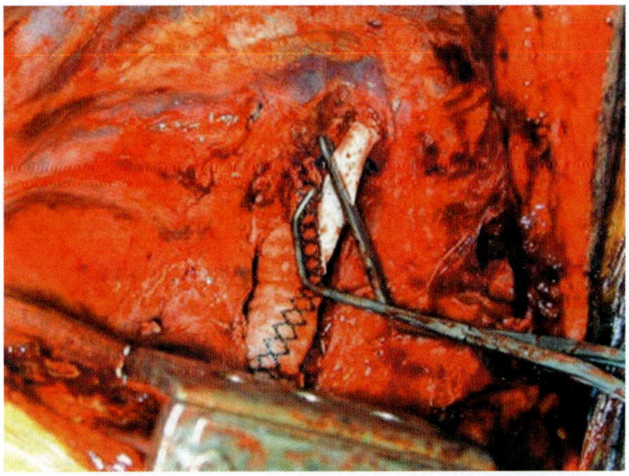

FIGURE 10.18 ▌ In the unusual setting of a tear extending proximal to the left subclavian artery, a short bypass graft from the aortic graft is placed for reconstruction.

Removal of Bypass Cannulae

- After aortic reconstruction is deemed secure, the superior pulmonary venous and femoral arterial cannulae are clamped and extracted. The respective arteriotomy and venotomy sites are closed with running 5-0 Prolene suture.
- The pulmonary venotomy must be flushed free of clot and air before removing the Satinsky clamp to avoid potentially devastating emboli from the left side of the heart.

Thoracotomy Closure

- The left chest is vented with a posterior straight 32-Fr thoracostomy tube.

- Pain control is achieved with a chest wall pain catheter or intercostal injection of mixture of short-acting and long-acting (liposomal) anesthetics is instilled into two intercostal spaces above and below the transected rib.
- The ribs are approximated with 0-PDS pericostal sutures and muscle layers closed sequentially with a continuous 2-0 running PDS suture.

Optimization of Resuscitation in the OR

- The patient's left lower and left upper extremity vascular integrity are confirmed with Duplex peak systolic pressures and flow measurements before leaving the OR.
- If heparin has been administered, we usually reverse with protamine (heparin T [1/2] = 90 minutes; 1 mg of protamine for 100 U of residual heparin).
- Hemodynamic and pulmonary stability are confirmed before transport to the surgical intensive care unit (SICU), including ABGs and lactate levels.

POSTOPERATIVE CARE

- Coagulation status, preferably a viscoelastic assay, should be obtained before leaving the operating room and repeated at the arrival time in the SICU, avoiding unnecessary blood products.
- Early transient hypertension is common. The systolic blood pressure should be maintained <140 mm Hg with Esmolol for the first 72 hours to avoid suture line stress. Calcium supplementation should be guided by ionized calcium levels, and administered slowly.
- Vascular integrity of the extremity undergoing CFA cannulation (usually left) should be ascertained every 4 hours for the first 24 hours postoperatively.
- Patients with a torn thoracic aorta usually sustain multiple injuries, including high dissections of the carotid and vertebral arteries and, thus, a systematic tertiary survey should be done in the SICU and appropriate imaging completed as soon as feasible.

Suggested Readings

Kim FJ, Moore EE, Moore FA, Read RA, Burch JM. Trauma surgeons can render definitive surgical care for major thoracic injuries. *J Trauma*. 1994;36(6):871–876.

Moore EE, Burch JM, Moore JB. Repair of the torn descending thoracic aorta using the centrifugal pump for partial left heart bypass. *Ann Surg*. 2004;240(1):38–43.

Szwerc MF, Benckart DH, Lin JC, et al. Recent clinical experience with left heart bypass using a centrifugal pump for repair of traumatic aortic transection. *Ann Surg*. 1999;230(4):484–490.

Verdant A. Contemporary results of standard open repair of acute traumatic rupture of the thoracic aorta. *J Vasc Surg*. 2010; 51(2):294–298.

Chapter 11
Pulmonary Injuries

FREDRIC M. PIERACCI

PERIOPERATIVE CONSIDERATIONS

Procedure Rationale

- The majority of pulmonary injuries can be managed nonoperatively. Approximately 15% of patients require operative intervention, predominantly for either hemorrhage or air leak. Patients suffering from penetrating trauma are more likely to have defined pulmonary injuries that are amenable to surgical repair or resection.
- Conversely, blunt injury is typically more diffuse, with uncertain margins between healthy and injured tissue. Pulmonary contusion and pneumatocele are the two most common blunt injuries and usually resolve with nonoperative management.
- Pulmonary parenchymal, vascular, and bronchial lacerations however, can occur following blunt trauma.

TIP

Patients with either hemorrhagic shock or uncontrolled air leak require emergent thoracotomy. Stable patients with either ongoing bleeding or air leak, on the other hand, are able to undergo additional diagnostic testing (e.g., CTA, flexible bronchoscopy) and may be considered for less invasive treatment modalities (e.g., angioembolization, endobronchial valve placement).

Essential Equipment

- Flexible bronchoscope
- Major thoracotomy tray
  - Finochietto rib spreader
  - Rib cutters
  - Lung, vascular, and bronchial clamps (Fig. 11.1)

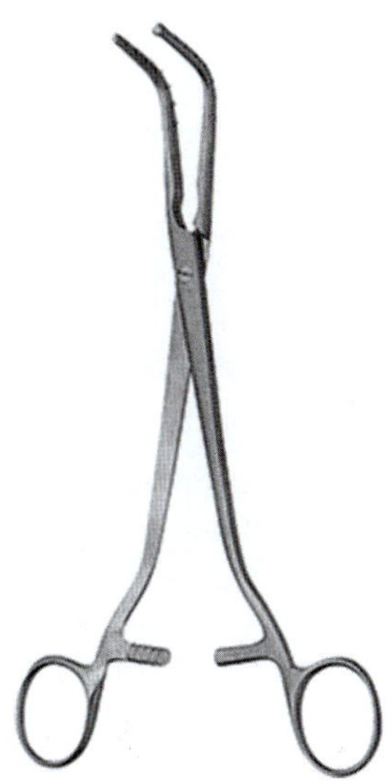

FIGURE 11.1 | Sarot bronchus clamp.

- Topical hemostatic agents
- Linear staplers—A staple height of 0.5 to 1.5 mm is typically used for pulmonary segmental or lobar vessels, 1 to 2 mm for lung parenchyma, and 2 to 3 mm for bronchi. All staple heights refer to after firing.
- “Peanut” gauze dissectors

Positioning and Preparation

- In the unstable patient, or when the source of hemorrhage is uncertain (e.g., thoracic vs. abdominal), the patient is positioned supine.
  - A “bump” with either a sheet or a roll may be placed to facilitate exposure.
  - Thoracic hemorrhage from an intra-abdominal source (e.g., liver laceration bleeding into the right chest via a diaphragm rupture [Fig. 11.2]) is possible and the supine position affords the best opportunity to address this scenario.

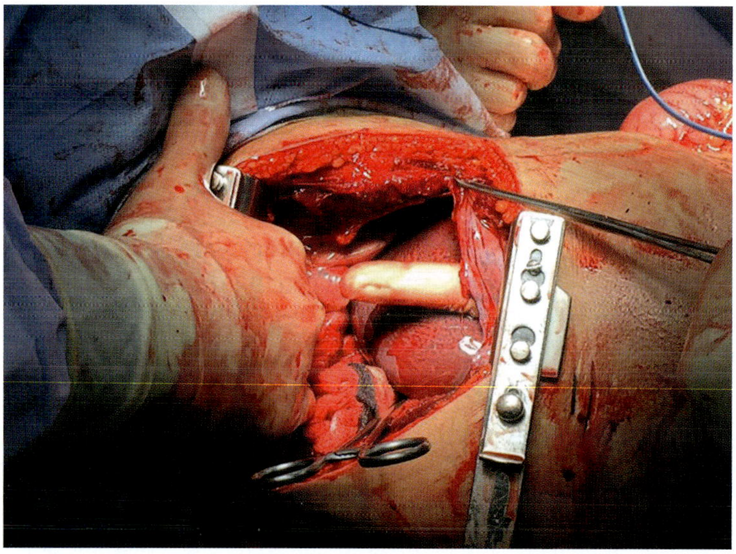

FIGURE 11.2 ▌ Coexisting hepatic laceration and right hemidiaphragm rupture presenting as massive right hemothorax. A gloved finger is traversing the diaphragm rupture via the midline laparotomy incision.

- In a stable patient in which other injuries have been excluded, the lateral decubitus position affords the best exposure to the pulmonary hilum and posterior mediastinum.
  - This position should be employed over the supine position only when the patient is stable and the source of hemorrhage/injury has already been identified by imaging.
- Pulmonary repair or resection (including lobectomy) is readily accomplished on double-lung ventilation.
- Ventilation of the patient’s entire lung capacity facilitates resuscitation.
- Active ventilation of the injured lung parenchyma allows air leaks to be identified more easily.
- For these reasons, in the trauma/emergent setting, double-lung ventilation is preferred.
- In rare cases of patient stability and isolated injury, single-lung isolation may be considered, and can be accomplished via a variety of means, including advancement of the endotracheal tube into the left main stem bronchus, bronchial blockers, and double-lumen endotracheal tubes.

Indications for Surgery

- Hemodynamic instability with suspected thoracic source of hemorrhage
- Tube thoracostomy drainage
  - Blunt trauma
    - Initial drainage of ≥1,500 mL of blood
    - Subsequent drainage of ≥250 mL of blood per hour for at least 2 hours
  - Penetrating trauma
    - Initial drainage of ≥1,000 mL of blood
    - Subsequent drainage of ≥200 mL of blood per hour for at least 2 hours

- Air leak with ≥1 of the following:
  - *Inability to ventilate:* This typically occurs when >33% of the inspired tidal volume (V_T) is lost via the injury. In an intubated patient, the percentage leak may be calculated as the expired V_T divided by the inspired (delivered) $V_T \times 100$
  - *Worsening pneumothorax or subcutaneous emphysema despite functional, well-positioned chest tube(s):* Control of an air leak may be conceptualized as the ratio of two parameters. The first is flow of air from the trachea–bronchial tree, through the parenchymal or bronchial injury, and into the pleural space. The second is flow of air out of the pleural space and into the chest tube(s). If the first parameter is greater than the second, air will continue to accumulate. Flow of air, in turn, is most dependent upon the radius of the vessel. Practically, this concept often means that one or more large-bore chest tubes will be required to adequately control an air leak, as opposed to smaller (e.g., 14-Fr) percutaneous catheters. Thus, the first step in addressing a persistent or worsening pneumothorax from a lung injury is often to upsize or add an additional chest tube. Subcutaneous emphysema from an uncontrolled air leak can be both extensive and alarming (Fig. 11.3), but is almost always able to be either temporized or definitively managed with the placement of additional, large-bore chest tubes

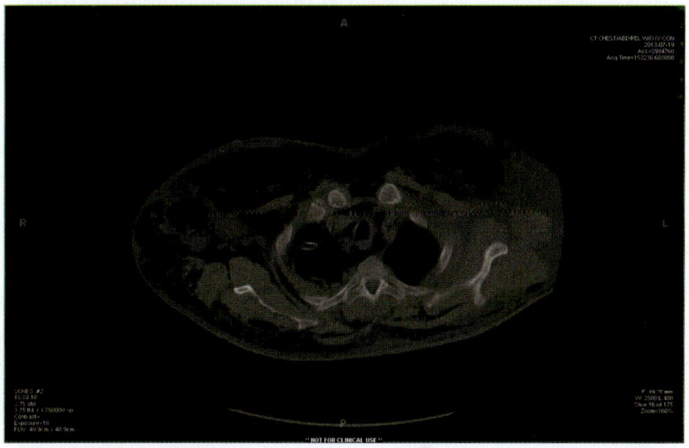

FIGURE 11.3 ▮ Extensive subcutaneous emphysema secondary to a right upper lobe parenchymal laceration due to a rib fracture.

  - *Persistent air leak:* Persistent air leak is typically defined as >7 days postinjury. Closure of a lung parenchymal injury is most dependent upon two parameters, and these two parameters should be optimized whenever possible before labeling an air leak as persistent
    - Apposition of the parietal and visceral pleura (i.e., resolution of the pneumothorax)
    - Minimization of positive airway pressure
- In stable patients, and where there is institutional expertise, endobronchial valves may be considered for management of air leaks

Anatomic Considerations

- Lung parenchyma is thin and friable, and usual hemostatic maneuvers such as suturing and clipping often only worsen the degree of injury. Accordingly, either topical hemostatic maneuvers (e.g., pressure with hemostatic gauze) or wedge resection via stapling are usually more effective.
- Pulmonary arteries differ from systemic arteries in that they are thin walled and tear easily. This is due to the relatively low pressure of the pulmonary arterial system (normal pulmonary arterial pressure is <12 mm Hg). Thus, great care must be exercised when dissecting around pulmonary arteries. Furthermore, when bleeding from a pulmonary artery occurs (including the main pulmonary artery), initial control via direct pressure with a finger or "peanut" gauze is almost always effective. This initial maneuver allows time to obtain proximal and distal control.

TIP

When bleeding from a pulmonary artery occurs, apply digital pressure for at least 1 minute as the initial maneuver. Attempting to immediately repair the vessel with suture or clips usually results in worsening of the injury.

- The lung is comprised of unique bronchopulmonary segments. Although anatomic variations are common, the following general principles are relatively preserved:
  - The pulmonary veins are the most anterior structures, followed by the pulmonary arteries and, finally, by the bronchi, which are the most posterior structures.
  - There is a superior and inferior pulmonary vein. In rare cases, a common venous trunk is present, and the existence of two veins should be confirmed prior to transecting either the superior or inferior pulmonary vein.
  - Pulmonary arteries, in general, follow bronchi, with lymph nodes typically present at bifurcation points.
  - Although both the left and right pulmonary arteries have superior and inferior divisions, the blood supply to the upper lobes arises from both the superior and inferior divisions. Thus, when performing a lobectomy, each segmental pulmonary artery branch must be identified and individually ligated. The superior divisions of the pulmonary arteries are found at the apex of the hilum. The inferior divisions are most easily found at the base of the fissures.
  - Regarding the right lung:
    - The upper and middle lobe typically both drain into the superior pulmonary vein. Thus, each segmental tributary must be identified and ligated separately when performing either an upper or middle lobectomy.
    - The superior segmental bronchus (lower lobe) and middle lobe bronchus arise in opposite directions but very close to each other (Fig. 11.4). For this reason, when performing a lower

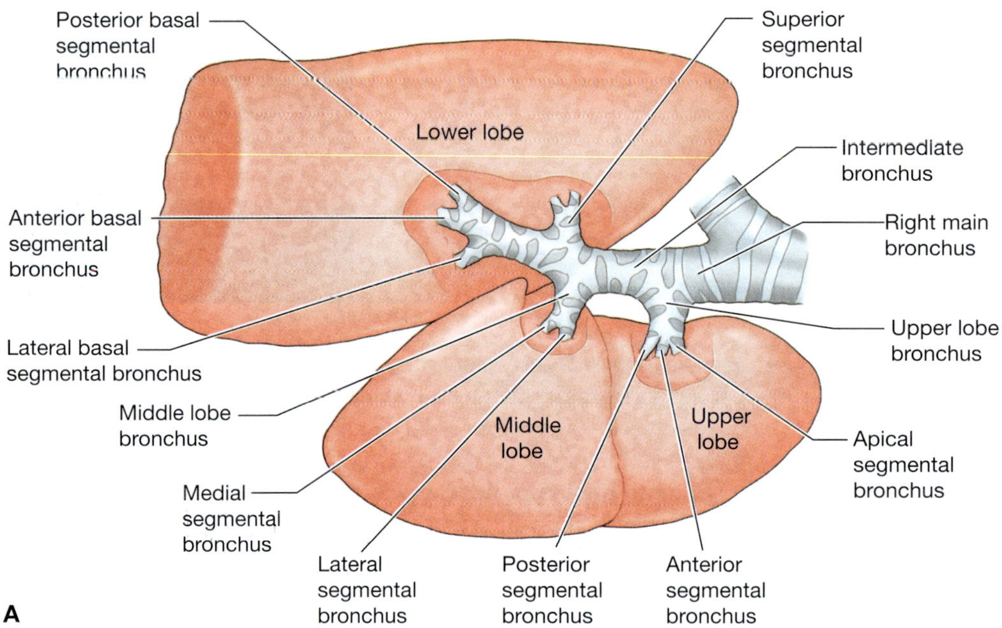

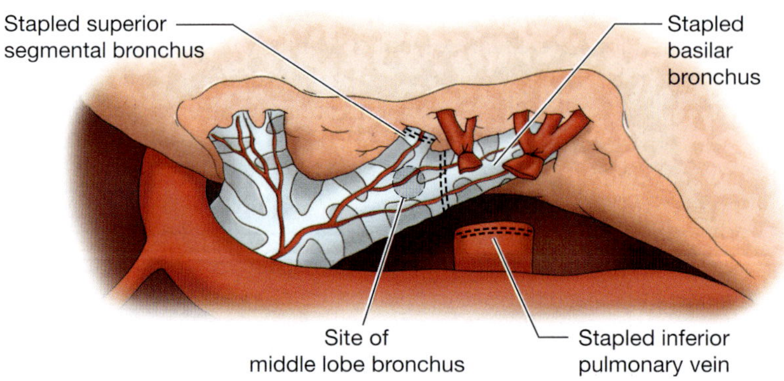

FIGURE 11.4 ❙ Right lung bronchial anatomy, shown both overall (**A**) and during RLL lobectomy (**B**). Note the relationship of the superior segmental bronchus to the middle lobe bronchus.

lobectomy, the superior and basilar segmental bronchi should be taken separately so as not to impinge on the middle lobe bronchus.
- Regarding the left lung:
  - The left main stem bronchus is longer and arises from the carina at a less acute angle than the right main stem bronchus. This makes lung isolation via bronchial blocker easier on the left side.
  - The left recurrent laryngeal nerve is at risk when dissecting out the superior hilum. Stay close to the hilum at this point.
  - The upper lobe arterial branches are highly variable and may number from 3 to 8.

TECHNIQUE

- The techniques for both anterolateral and posterolateral thoracotomies are described in Chapter 7.
- Exploration of the chest should occur in a standardized fashion, akin to a trauma laparotomy, and include specific assessment of the following structures:
  - Lung
  - Hilum
  - Pericardium
  - Diaphragm
  - Mediastinum, including the esophagus. An oro- or nasogastric tube placed intraoperatively will assist in both identification and assessment of the esophagus.
  - Ribs, intercostal vessels, and chest wall muscles
- After pulmonary injury has been identified, the degree of injury is assessed. Injuries may be grouped into one of the following seven categories:
  - Superficial laceration, not actively bleeding or leaking air—no intervention required.
  - Superficial laceration, active bleeding, and or air leak—topical hemostatic maneuvers +/− wedge resection via stapling +/− suture repair.
  - Deep laceration involving one segmental vessel or bronchus—suture ligation of the effected structure.
  - Deep laceration involving ≥2 segmental vessels or bronchi—lobectomy.
  - "Through-and-through" laceration from penetrating injury, not actively bleeding or leaking air—no intervention required.
  - "Through-and-through" laceration from penetrating injury, active bleeding, or air leak—pulmonary tractotomy.
  - Injury to main (right or left) pulmonary artery, or otherwise devastating hilar injury—pneumonectomy.
  - Diffuse, blunt injury to multiple lobes with parenchymal oozing and coagulopathy—damage control thoracotomy.

Specific Pulmonary Procedures

- *Wedge resection:* A pulmonary wedge resection is employed when a relatively peripheral portion of the lung is devascularized, bleeding, or leaking air. A wedge resection is accomplished by closing the jaws of a linear stapler across healthy parenchyma below the injured portion and firing the stapler to remove the damaged portion of the lung (Fig. 11.5).
- In certain cases, multiple stapler fires will be needed, and multiple wedge resections of a single lobe, or multiple lobes, may be performed. When a tear in the peripheral lung has already detached a portion of parenchyma, the trajectory of the linear stapler for the wedge resection should extend below the tear.

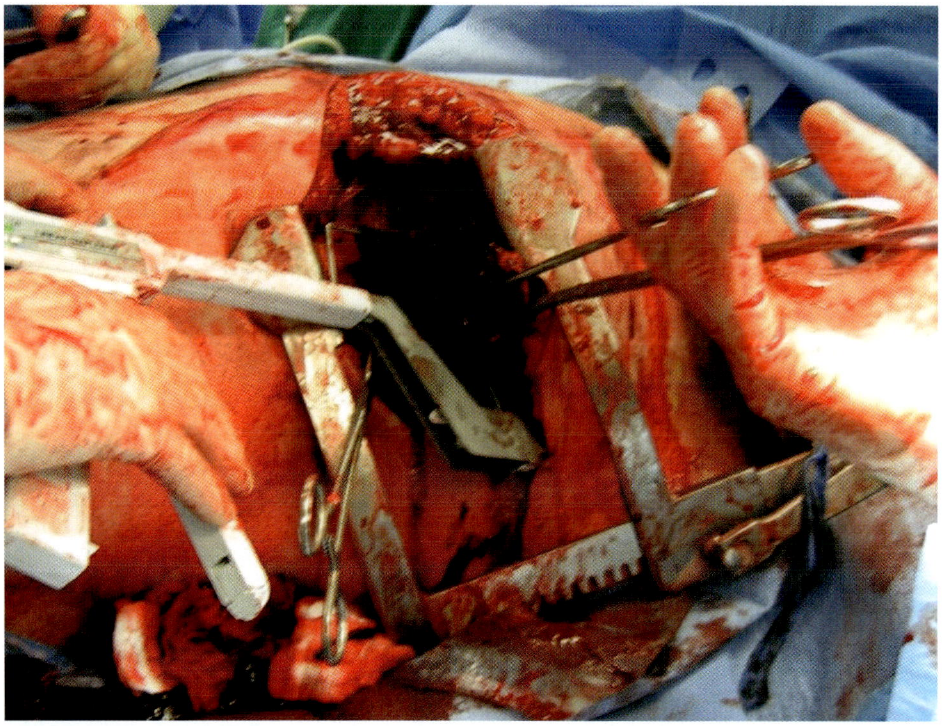

FIGURE 11.5 ▌ Pulmonary wedge resection. Note the relatively peripheral location of the parenchymal laceration.

- *Tractotomy:* Pulmonary tractotomy is employed in cases of "through-and-through" penetrating injuries to the lung. The area of parenchymal injury is circumferentially "filleted" open in order to delineate and definitively address vascular or bronchial injuries (Fig. 11.6).

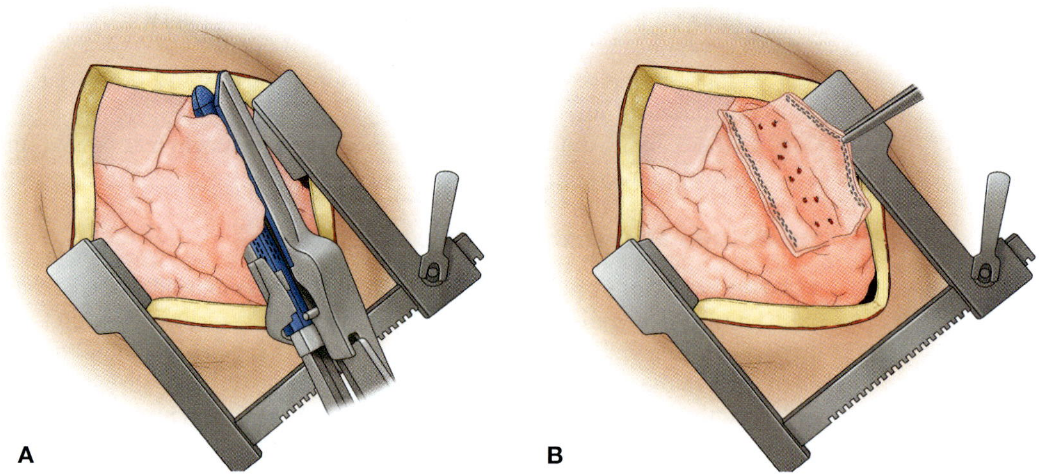

FIGURE 11.6 ▌ Illustration of pulmonary tractotomy. **A:** A linear stapler is fired through the tract, exposing its base. **B:** Areas of hemorrhage and air leak are sutured.

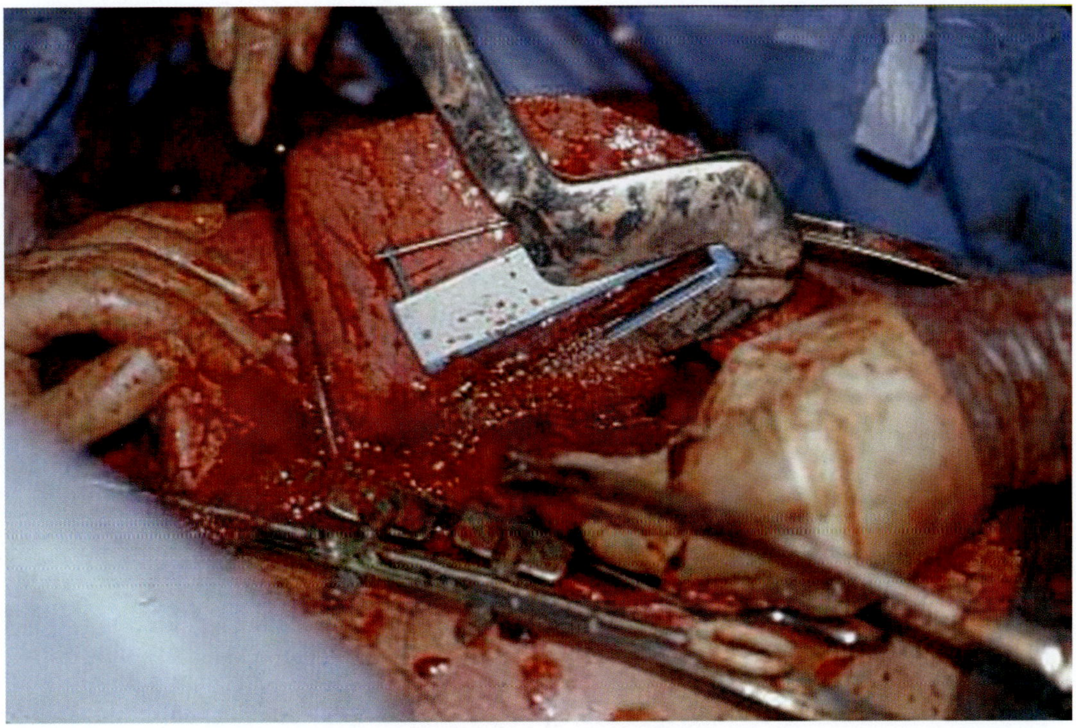

FIGURE 11.7 ▌ Pulmonary tractotomy. A linear stapler is advanced into the tract. After the stapler has been fired, the base of the tract is examined, and areas of bleeding and air leak are repaired.

- The bottom lip of a linear stapler, typically 60–90 mm in length with a 1.5–2.5-mm staple height, is introduced into the parenchymal hole, such that the tip of it is visible coming out the other end (Fig. 11.7).
- The stapler is closed and fired, opening up the area of injury in its entirety.
  - At this point, several options are considered depending upon the degree of injury that range from application of topical hemostatic agents to suture ligation, to conversion to lobectomy in the case that the tractotomy reveals persistent, deep bleeding from one or more segmental vessels (Fig. 11.8).
- *Lobectomy:* Lobectomy is reserved for cases in which there is ongoing, major bleeding from ≥2 segmental bronchi, a main trunk of the pulmonary artery, or such extensive parenchymal damage to a lobe that salvage is not possible. In the case of pulmonary artery injury, bleeding is often brisk and massive. As this is a low-pressure system, digital occlusion is almost always an effective initial maneuver to establish control.

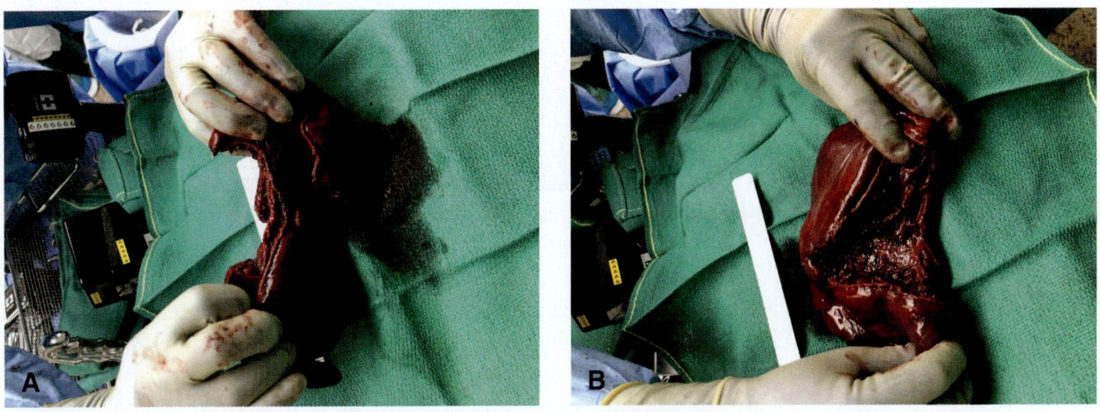

FIGURE 11.8 ▌ Left lower lobe pulmonary tractotomy (**A**) converted to lobectomy (**B**). Note the multiple staple lines extending down to the pulmonary hilum, at which level several segmental pulmonary arteries were injured.

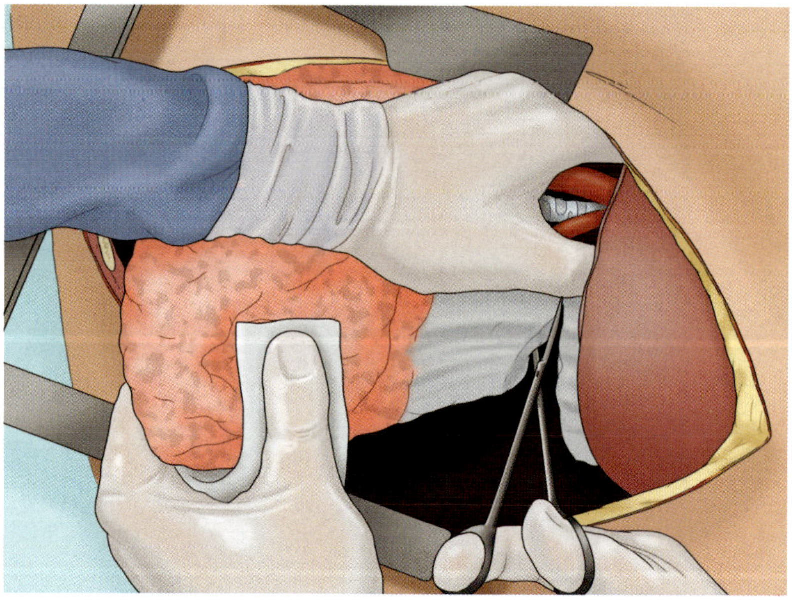

FIGURE 11.9 ▌Holding hilum between thumb and index finger.

- The surgeon, standing on the patient's ipsilateral side, places their left hand under the lung and pinches the hilum between their thumb and index finger (Fig. 11.9).
- In rare cases of massive hilar injury, proximal control may be accomplished via pericardiotomy and intrapericardial dissection of the main pulmonary artery or vein. Clamping of these vessels will allow for temporary hemorrhage control, but should be used judiciously as extended clamp times invariably result in hemodynamic embarrassment.
- Open lobectomy is typically begun by identifying the pulmonary arterial branches in the fissures, ligating these branches, and then proceeding to ligate the vein (Fig. 11.10).

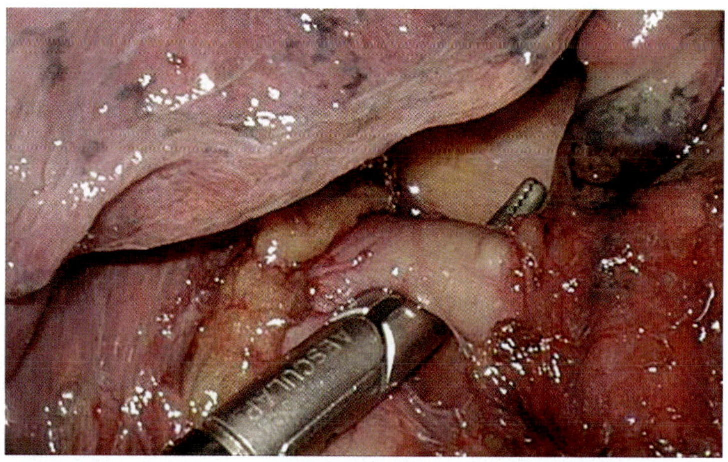

FIGURE 11.10 ▌Identification of pulmonary artery branches in the fissure prior to a left lower lobectomy.

- The fissures are completed.
- The bronchus is then ligated.
  - Linear staplers may be used to ligate the pulmonary arteries, veins, fissures, and bronchi, and are a rapid, effective means of progressing through the operation.
  - Prior to firing the stapler to transect the bronchus, confirmation that the other lobes are still ventilating is made, indicating that impingement on them has not occurred.
- In cases of lobectomy for acute bleeding or air leak, tissue coverage of the bronchial stump is not required.

TIP

A detailed description of each of the five anatomic pulmonary lobectomies is provided in the suggested readings.

- *Pneumonectomy:* Trauma pneumonectomy is a nearly universally fatal operation due to acute right heart failure. Accordingly, it should be undertaken only as a last resort and, when available, in conjunction with cardiopulmonary bypass to offload the right heart (see Chapter 13). After closure of the chest following pneumonectomy, a chest radiograph is obtained in the operating room to assess the position of the mediastinum. Air is then either instilled into or removed from the ipsilateral side to adjust the mediastinum to the midline. Placement of a chest tube is not routinely necessary following pneumonectomy.
- *Damage control thoracotomy:* Damage control thoracotomy is considered in cases of extensive, multilobar pulmonary parenchymal damage (Fig. 11.11), usually seen in blunt trauma, and in conjunction with hemodynamic instability, acidosis, and coagulopathy.

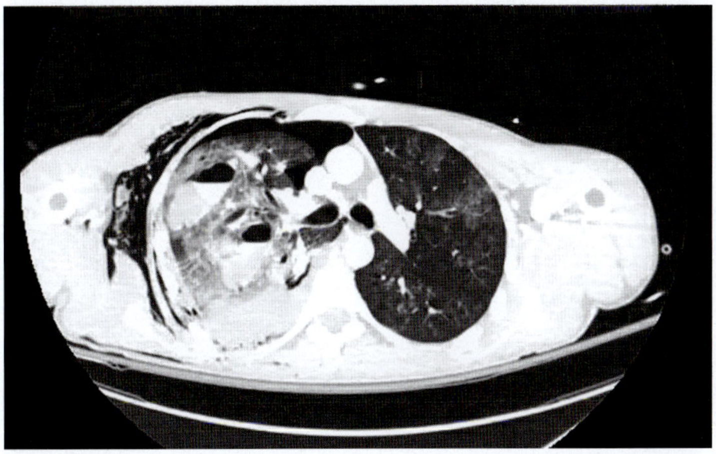

FIGURE 11.11 ❙ Extensive, multilobar parenchymal damage, including pneumatoceles, in a patient who underwent right damage control thoracotomy.

In this scenario, the lung parenchyma is packed with gauze (+/− hemostatic agents) and the skin of the thoracotomy incision is stitched closed over chest tubes. Alternatively, the skin may be left open and covered with an air-tight, translucent adhesive (Fig. 11.12). The patient is then transported to the intensive care unit for resuscitation, with a plan for a second look in 12 to 36 hours.

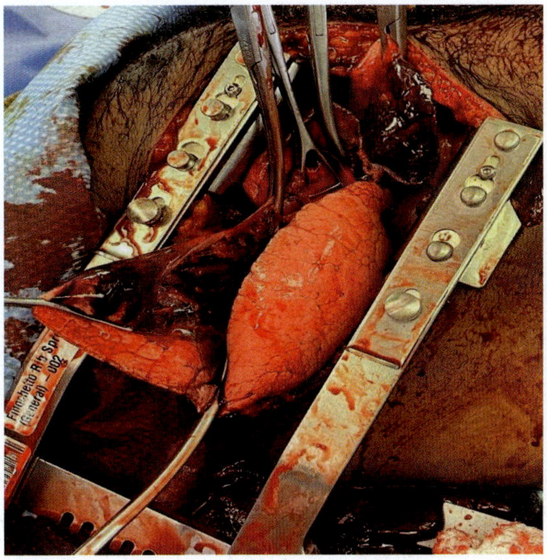

FIGURE 11.12 ❙ Open chest after damage control thoracotomy.

POSTOPERATIVE CARE

- Chest tubes are placed to water seal and monitored for both quantity and quality of drainage.
- Positive pressure ventilation is eliminated as soon as possible.
- Patients who undergo lobectomy or greater are at increased risk for cardiac arrhythmia. Although chemical prophylaxis has been shown to be effective in the elective thoracic literature, this benefit has not been evaluated in trauma patients.
- Patients who undergo lobectomy or greater have an acute increase in their pulmonary vascular resistance, and are at risk for pulmonary hypertension and its sequelae. Volume resuscitation should be employed judiciously in this situation.

Suggested Readings

Amar D, Roistacher N, Rusch VW, et al. Effects of diltiazem prophylaxis on the incidence and clinical outcome of atrial arrhythmias after thoracic surgery. *J Thorac Cardiovasc Surg*. 2000;120(4):790–798.

Cothren C, Moore EE, Biffl WL, Franciose RJ, Offner PJ, Burch JM. Lung-sparing techniques are associated with improved outcome compared with anatomic resection for severe lung injuries. *J Trauma*. 2002;53(3):483–487.

Hood RM. *Techniques in General Thoracic Surgery*. Saunders; 1985;245.

Chapter 12
Thoracic Trachea and Bronchi

FREDRIC M. PIERACCI

PERIOPERATIVE CONSIDERATIONS

Procedure Rationale

- Thoracic tracheal and bronchial injuries, whether arising from penetrating or blunt trauma, are infrequent. The extent of injury ranges widely, from minor tears (<10% of the airway circumference) (Fig. 12.1) to complex through-and-through lacerations from missiles (Fig. 12.2).

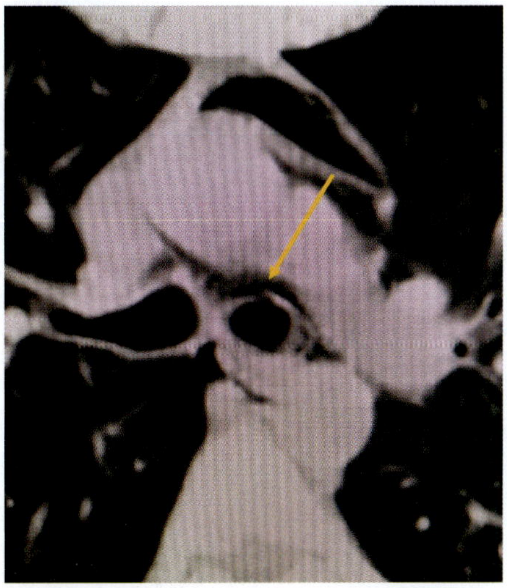

FIGURE 12.1 ▌ Small, less than 10% of airway circumference tear (*arrow*) of the left main stem bronchus from blunt trauma.

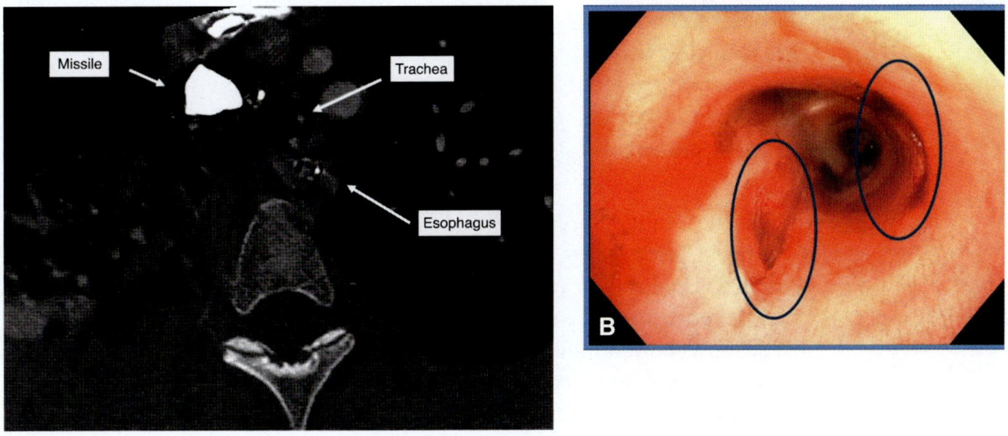

FIGURE 12.2 ▌ Through-and-through injury to the distal trachea from a bullet. **A:** CT image of the missile lodged in the posterior mediastinum. **B:** Bronchoscopic view of the through-and-through injury.

- Most injuries that involve less than 1/3 of the circumference of the airway will heal spontaneously.
- Patients who present with tracheobronchial injuries typically fall into one of three clinical categories:
  - Uncontrolled air leak with massive pneumothorax, subcutaneous air, and inability to ventilate—these patients require emergent thoracotomy.
  - Stable patient with injury recognized on CT imaging—these patients are stable enough to undergo additional diagnostic maneuvers such as bronchoscopy and can be considered for nonoperative, bronchoscopic, or operative management based upon the size and location of the injury.
  - Patients in whom the injury was not recognized during the initial presentation - these patients present weeks to months later with complete healing, stricture, post obstructive atelectasis, and recurrent pulmonary infections.
- For stable patients (i.e., group 2), operative intervention is most often performed for a tracheal or bronchial injury that is >2/3 of the circumference of the airway. Additional scenarios in which operative repair may be considered include a tracheal or bronchial injury that is 1/ to 2/3 of the circumference of the airway with prolonged (>7 days) air leak not amenable to bronchoscopic maneuvers (e.g., stenting).

Essential Equipment

- Headlight
- Flexible bronchoscope
- Major thoracotomy tray
  - Finochietto rib spreader
  - Rib cutters
  - Lung and bronchial clamps
- 2-0 and 3-0 vicryl sutures on SH needle 36-inch thread
- Nerve hook for retraction of the bronchus and bronchial injuries
- Chest tubes (24 to 32 Fr) and chest tube drainage system
- Tracheal jet ventilation apparatus
- 6.0 to 8.0 endotracheal tubes (ETTs) with a sufficient ventilator tube to achieve in-field, transtracheal ventilation

Patient Postioning

- In a stable patient, flexible bronchoscopy is performed in the supine position as an initial maneuver to characterize further the location and extent of the injury. The airways are examined to the level of the segmental bronchi. An adult bronchoscope (minimum 2.0-mm diameter) should be used to improve visualization and ability to suction and irrigate. Accordingly, intubation should occur with at least an 8.0 ETT when possible.

TIP

In order to evaluate the laryngo-tracheo-bronchial tree completely, consider performing an awake bronchoscopy under conscious sedation in the stable patient prior to induction of general anesthesia. Alternatively, pull the ETT back under bronchoscopic vision in order to visualize the maximum length of the trachea. This maneuver will minimize the risk of a missed proximal tracheal injury. Unstable patients should not under bronchoscopy prior to thoracotomy.

- The chest tube, if present, should not be clamped but can be left to water seal.
- Lung isolation is best achieved by advancing the ETT into the unaffected mainstem bronchus under direct visualization and palpation once the thoracotomy has been performed. This means that the initial portion of the operation will be performed using two lung ventilation.
- Although both double lumen tubes and bronchial blockers also provide lung isolation, each is a time consuming maneuver in the face of an uncontrolled leak.
- Transtracheal jet ventilation, when available, is a method of achieving exposure of the injury without lung isolation.

- Unless the injury is known to be on the left and is more than 2 cm distal to the carina, the injury is approached through a right posterolateral thoracotomy. When the injury is greater than 2 cm from the carina, then the injury is approached through a left posterolateral thoracotomy.
  - Lateral decubitus position is appropriate.
  - Flexing the operating table will increase the distance between rib spaces thereby improving exposure and minimizing the likelihood of inadvertent rib fracture when engaging the rib spreader.

TECHNIQUE

- Begin with a right posterolateral thoracotomy. Enter the chest through the 5th intercostal space. The respiratory status of the patient may be critical, and it may be necessary to make the chest incision rapidly.
- Open the mediastinal pleura over the trachea (if not already open), identify the injury, and temporarily control the leak with a finger to improve ventilation (Fig. 12.3).

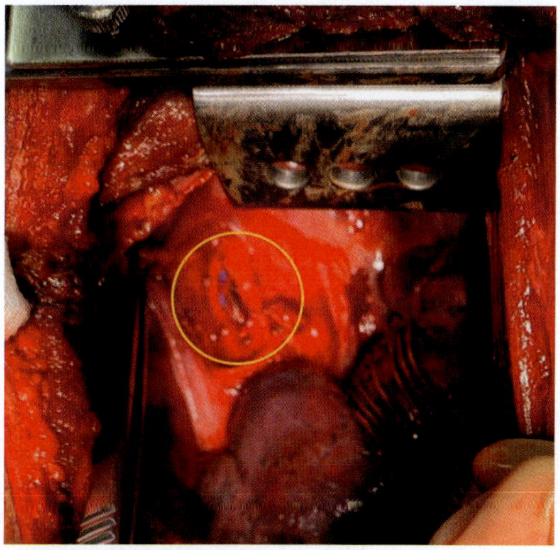

FIGURE 12.3 ▌ Endotracheal tube visible through a longitudinal injury to the trachea after the mediastinal pleura has been opened.

- Dissect out the surrounding pleura and assess the margins of the injury. Then, digitally occlude the injury and under direct visualization and palpation, advance the ETT into the uninjured bronchus (or left mainstem bronchus in the case of a tracheal injury) and inflate the cuff. This should provide adequate ventilation during the repair.

TIP

Concurrent esophageal injury is possible and should be ruled out routinely. Intraoperative esophagoscopy with leak bubble test under saline may facilitate this. However, minimize dissection in the trachea–esophageal groove in order to avoid injury to the recurrent laryngeal nerve. Coincident vascular injury, except for bronchial vessels, is rare.

- Options for repair depend upon the location, directionality, and extent of the injury.
  - Transverse injuries to either the trachea, main stem bronchus, or bronchus intermedius that are <85% of the diameter may be repaired primarily.
  - Repair of transverse injuries >85% of the tracheal diameter is usually facilitated by completing the transection and performing an end-to-end anastomosis (Fig. 12.4**A**).
  - Repair of longitudinal injuries are usually repaired primarily (Fig. 12.4**B**).
  - Repair of extensive injuries to lobar bronchi are best managed with lobectomy in the emergent situation. When these injuries present in a delayed fashion, the injury is debrided back to healthy tissue and an end-to-end anastomosis is created.

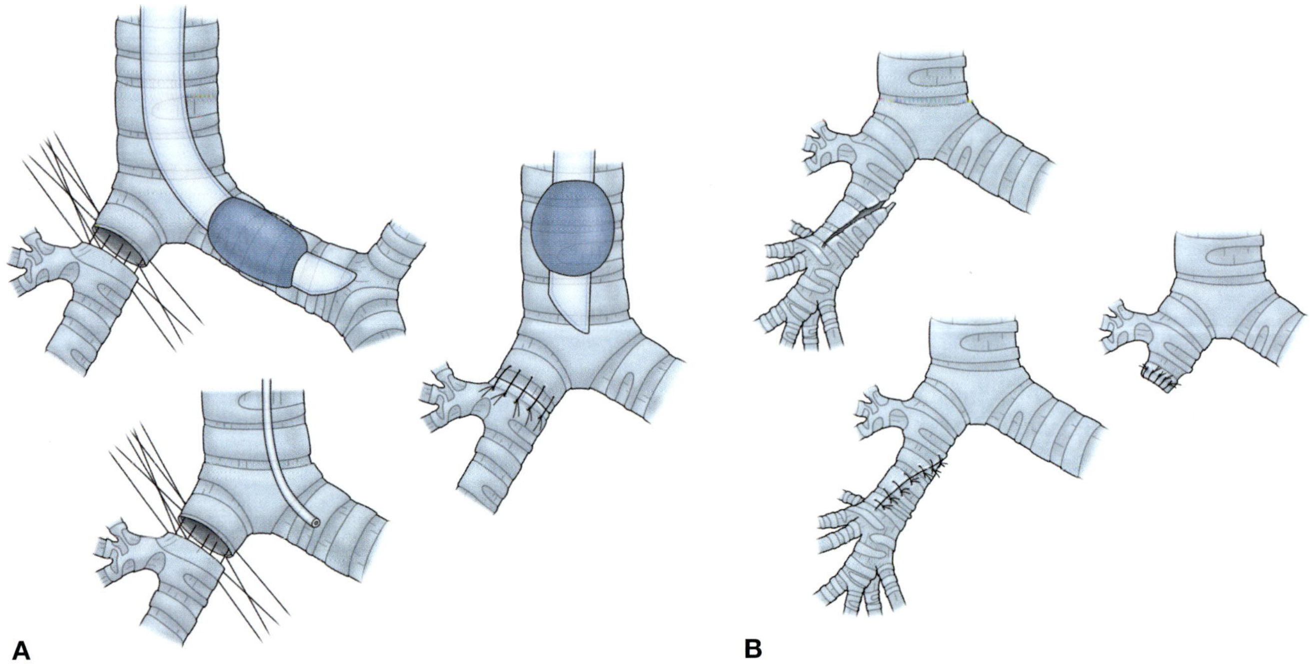

FIGURE 12.4 ▮ **A:** Repair of right main stem bronchus injury facilitated by completion of the near transection, and end-to-end anastomosis. Note that the endotracheal tube has been advanced into the left main stem bronchus. **B:** Options for management of a longitudinal injury to the bronchus intermedius include primary repair versus right middle and lower (bilobe) lobectomy.

- In general, repairs are fashioned with interrupted 3-0 or 4-0, braided, absorbable sutures placed approximately 2 to 3 mm from the edge of the injury and 2 to 3 mm apart (Fig. 12.5). Although many advocate for placing all of the knots externally, this is probably unnecessary, and placing the posterior row of knots internally will facilitate tying.

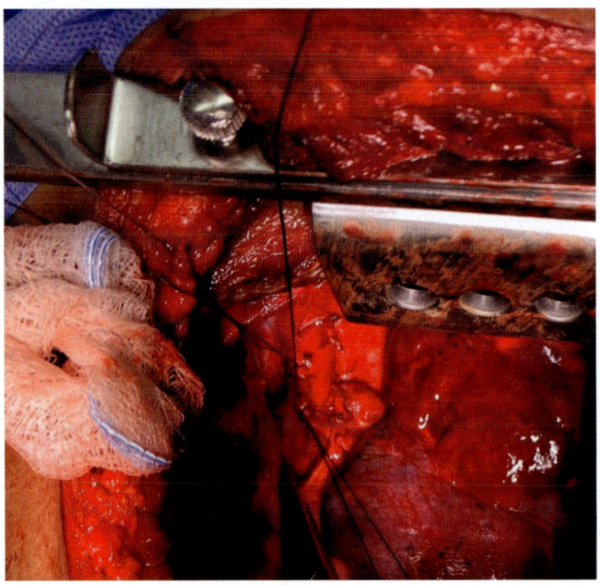

FIGURE 12.5 ▮ Primary suture repair of longitudinal injury to distal trachea with interrupted, 4-0 vicryl sutures.

TIP

Particular care must be exercised when taking bites through the membranous portion of either the trachea or bronchi as they will tear through if not taken at a right angle and following the curvature of the needle.

TIP

It is better to place the posterior row of sutures before they are tied so that each may be placed accurately.

- Once the repair is complete, it is:
  - Submerged under saline
  - The endotracheal tube is retracted to the proximal trachea
  - The airway pressures are elevated to 35 cm H_2O
  - Inspect for bubbles
- Tissue coverage of the repair is debated but we prefer to add this. Options include an intercostal muscle (Fig. 12.6), pleural, pericardial, and omental flaps.

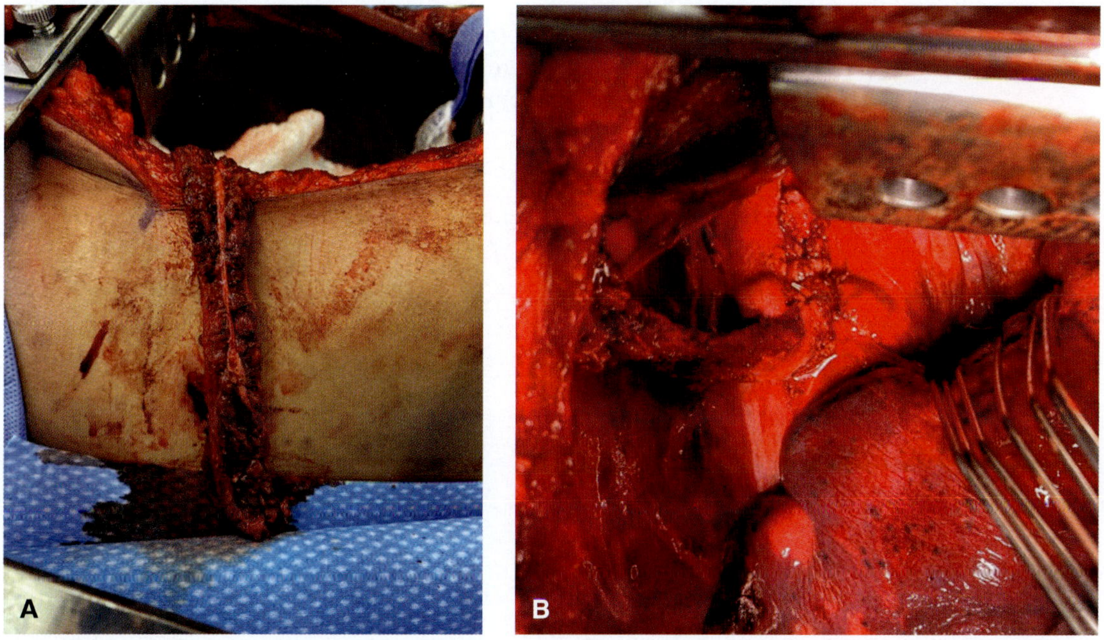

FIGURE 12.6 ▌ Intercostal muscle flap harvested during the initial thoracotomy (**A**) and sutured over a primary repair of the trachea (**B**).

TIP

When tissue coverage of a trachea-bronchial repair is being considered, harvest an intercostal muscle flap during the opening of the thoracotomy so that (1) it will not be damaged by the rib spreader and (2) there will be a period of time to assess its viability prior to using it.

- Place a single chest tube posteriorly and positioned toward the apex near the level of the repair.
- Placement of a proximal tracheostomy is controversial but probably unnecessary. Advantages include easy access for suction clearance and monitoring of the repair but there is a clear disadvantage of additional trauma to the trachea, risk of blind suctioning by personnel unaware of the anatomy, and overuse of positive pressure ventilation.

POSTOPERATIVE CARE

- Positive pressure is minimized by prompt extubation and, when extubation is not possible, low-pressure ventilation.
- Adequate analgesia is imperative to facilitate clearance of pulmonary secretions via coughing. Locoregional modalities are particularly effective in this regard.
- Blind suctioning (e.g., nasotracheal suctioning) is not recommended as it may disrupt a tracheal or bronchial repair. Rather, frequent awake bronchoscopy, with direct visualization of the repair and secretion clearance, may be necessary for several days following the operation.

TIP

Place an order in the patient's medical record and a sign over the patient's bed that blind suctioning is to be avoided.

- Suction applied to the chest tube drainage system should be avoided as it may prolong air leak through the repair. Unless there is a worsening pneumothorax, the chest tube(s) should immediately be placed to water seal and remain there until removed.

Suggested Readings

Ferreira D, Lima R, Oliveira A, et al. Bronchial fracture: bronchoscopy management with bronchial stent and balloon bronchoplasty. *Rev Port Pneumol.* 2008;14(3):409–414.

Hood RM. *Techniques in General Thoracic Surgery*. Saunders; 1985:245.

Chapter 13
Peripheral Cannulation for Extracorporeal Life Support

RYAN A. LAWLESS, NICOLE L. WERNER, AND MICHAEL HINES

PERIOPERATIVE CONSIDERATIONS

- The management of adult patients on extracorporeal life support (ECLS) can be extremely challenging, and potentially out of the scope of practice for a surgeon covering trauma. However, trauma surgeons routinely gain access to major blood vessels, and thus this knowledge and experience make trauma surgeons ideal to perform peripheral cannulation for ECLS.

Procedural Rationale

- ECLS, better known as extracorporeal membrane oxygenation (ECMO), has multiple configurations, based on the routes by which blood is drained and returned to corporeal circulation. Venovenous (VV) refers to venous drainage and venous reinfusion and is indicated for pulmonary support, whereas venoarterial (VA) is configured to reinfuse blood into an artery and provides both pulmonary and cardiac support (Fig. 13.1).

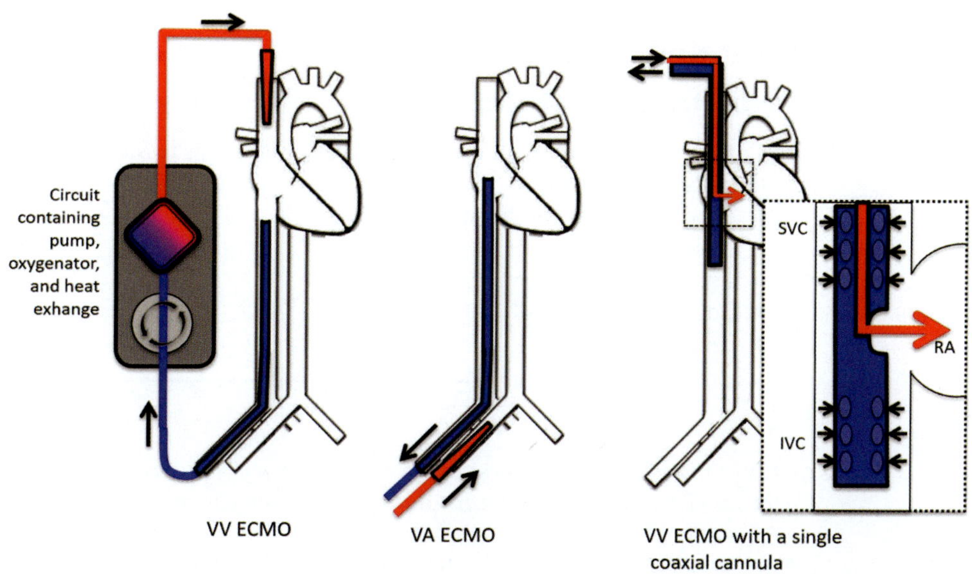

FIGURE 13.1 ❙ Configurations of extracorporeal membrane oxygenation. VV, venovenous; VA, venoarterial.

- The majority of adult patients requiring VV ECMO are suffering from acute respiratory distress syndrome (ARDS) secondary to severe pneumonitis or severe pneumonia. ARDS can be a rapidly progressing syndrome; however, ECMO cannulation in this circumstance is often nonemergent and can be planned. Patients suffering from cardiogenic shock, heart failure, or cardiac arrest secondary to hypothermia or malignant arrhythmia may benefit from VA ECMO. Cannulation in this population is typically emergent and, at times, performed during active cardiopulmonary resuscitation with chest compressions (ECPR).

Essential Equipment

- Sterile drapes
- Ultrasound (US) for percutaneous peripheral access
- Scalpel: #11 blade for percutaneous access, #10 or #15 blade for open peripheral access
- Percutaneous kit with appropriate long guidewire and sequential dilators
- Cannula:
  - Single-lumen "arterial" cannula for inflow to the patient
  - Single-lumen venous cannula (used for two-site configurations, both VV and VA ECMO), for drainage to the circuit
  - Dual-lumen cannula for single-site cannulation (VV ECMO only)
- Heparinized saline
- 0 or #1 Ethibond or Silk sutures
- Fluoroscopy (recommended for dual-lumen cannula, optional for other cannulation)
- Transesophageal endoscope (optional)
- Open small vessel tray: self-retaining retractors
- Device to measure the activated clotting time (ACT) in real time in the operating room, ICU or interventional suite
- Heparin bolus and when indicated bolus of antifibrinolytic

Patient Positioning

VV ECMO

- Supine with upper extremities tucked to the sides and head turned as indicated.

VA ECMO

- Extremis or active CPR: supine with bilateral upper extremities out as needed
- More hemodynamically stable: supine with upper extremities tucked at the sides

TECHNIQUE

Prior to Cannulation

- Consider placement of all indicated lines and tubes as feasible and required for continued resuscitation and management
  - New central venous catheters
  - Nasogastric tube
  - Fecal management system
  - Tube thoracostomies
  - Tracheostomy

TIP

Given that bleeding complications are frequently encountered during ECMO support, minimizing the number of procedures needed during ECMO support may decrease bleeding complications.

- Appropriate sedation and/or neuromuscular blockade
- Confirm with US the vessels planned for cannulation are patent and patient is appropriate positioned for access
- Equipment must be ready and draped in a sterile fashion:
  - Linear probe of the transcutaneous ultrasound
  - C-arm (strongly recommended for dual-lumen cannula placement; otherwise optional)
  - Cardiac probe of transcutaneous ultrasound or transesophageal endoscope (optional)

- Anticoagulation:
  - Goal: achieve ACT >200 seconds for initiation of support
  - Heparin dosage: 70 U/kg (max 7,000 units) initial bolus

TIP

We typically administer 100 U/kg, although some centers say 50–100 U/kg—however, subsequent doses are frequently necessary. Heparin pharmacology (ATIII levels, acute phase reactant binding, factor VIII levels, etc.) is complicated in these patients, as is the risk of bleeding, particularly ongoing bleeding at the time of initiation of support.

Cannula Selection

- The cannula inner (functional) diameters should be large enough to achieve 70% of the patient's cardiac output (60 mL/kg/min).
- Each manufacturer has flow tables for their particular cannula.
- Venous (drainage) cannula size contributes to the maximum achievable blood flow through the ECMO circuit.

VV ECMO

TIP

In VV ECMO, blood is drained from the venous circulation and returned back to the venous circulation either through (1) a single double-lumen cannula placed the right internal jugular (IJ) vein or (2) a two-cannula system, with a "venous" (a.k.a "drainage") cannula inserted in a femoral vein and "arterial" (a.k.a. "return") cannula usually placed in the right IJ.

- Right internal jugular (IJ) vein access (Fig. 13.2):

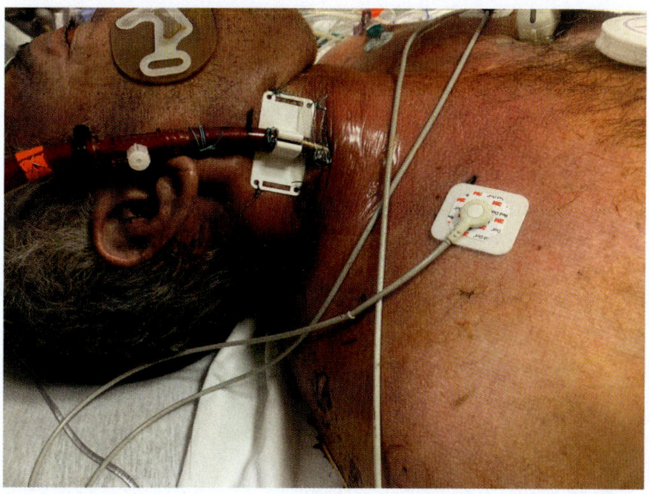

FIGURE 13.2 ▌ Right IJ cannulation for VV ECMO. This is the arterial, or return, cannula.

- Prep and drape the patient with ability to identify all necessary landmarks.
  - Right clavicle
  - Right sternocleidomastoid muscle
  - Identify the IJ vein and carotid artery with US: the vein should be compressible without appreciable clot prior to access

- Access the right IJ vein with a needle using ultrasound guidance.
- Insert the guidewire into the superior vena cava then to the inferior vena cava (under fluoroscopic imaging if available). Transthoracic or transesophageal cardiac ultrasound can also be used in the place of fluoroscopy. In urgent circumstances with unstable patients in the OR or ICU, when fluoroscopy is not available, the inflow cannula can be quickly and safely placed in the upper venous system without fluoroscopy, similar to placing a central line or dialysis catheter.

- Femoral vein access (Fig. 13.3):

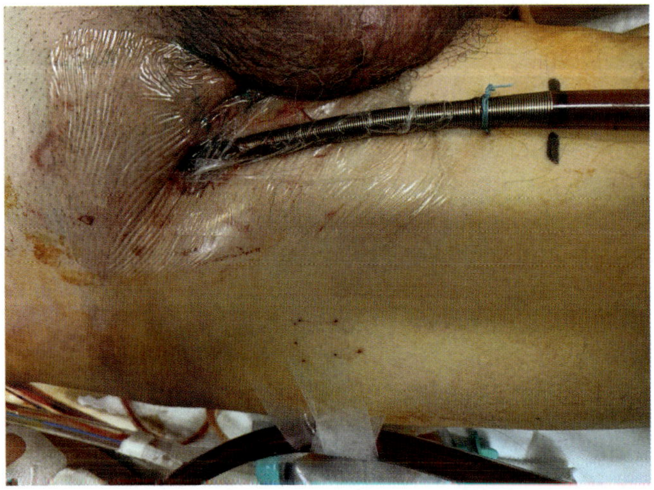

FIGURE 13.3 ▌ Right femoral vein cannulation. This is the venous, or drainage, cannula.

TIP

The right femoral vein is most commonly used for cannulation due to the gentle sloping angle compared to the left as well as the ease for right-handed surgeons. The left femoral vein can also be fairly easily accessed for cannulation.

- Prep and drape the patient with ability to identify all necessary landmarks.
  - Anterior superior iliac spine
  - Pubic tubercle
  - Inguinal ligament
  - Xiphoid and costal margin (by palpation under the drapes)
- Identify the common femoral vein, superficial femoral vein, deep femoral vein, and saphenofemoral junction
- Access the common femoral vein with a needle using ultrasound guidance

TIP

Be very careful not to stick through the inguinal ligament, as it is extremely difficult to dilate a tract sufficiently to place the large-sized ECMO venous cannulas.

- Insert the guidewire into the inferior vena cava through up into the right atrium (RA) or superior vena cava (under fluoroscopic guidance if available).
  - Transthoracic or transesophageal cardiac ultrasound can be used in the place of fluoroscopy.
  - In urgent cases the femoral cannulas can also be placed without fluoroscopy or US as long as the operator is confident with the ease of the wire access high into the IVC.

- For maximum drainage, the femoral venous cannula should have its tip positioned in the mid to high intrahepatic IVC where it cannot collapse down around the cannula under the high negative pressures that the constrained vortex of the centrifugal pump can generate. Venous femoral cannulas placed below the liver in the mid abdominal IVC are extremely prone to have difficulty draining, particularly at high flows, because of the laxity of the vein and ease with which it collapses around the cannula (in addition to the influence of any increased abdominal pressure seen in trauma patients).

TIP

In circumstances where fluoroscopy is not available, before inserting the femoral cannula, lie it on the abdomen and estimate the desired length, noting the level of the xiphoid and costal margin, and note the cm mark on the cannula. Remember, it is very easy to pull the cannula back 3 or 4 cm if there is recirculation, but it is problematic and risky to try to advance a cannula that is too low in the IVC and continuously collapsing.

- Alternate sites and two cannula configurations when the right IJ (RIJ) is not available.
  - Left subclavian vein is an acceptable access site for VV inflow and can accept the same-sized cannula as the RIJ.
  - Left IJ (LIJ) can be used but does require some manipulation of the cannula with fluoroscopic guidance.
  - Fem-Fem VV ECMO: This configuration is possible in situations where upper access is not feasible due to injury, thrombosis, etc. In order to provide sufficient venous drainage and minimize recirculation, two long "venous" cannulas must be used as properly placed using fluoroscopy (Fig. 13.4).

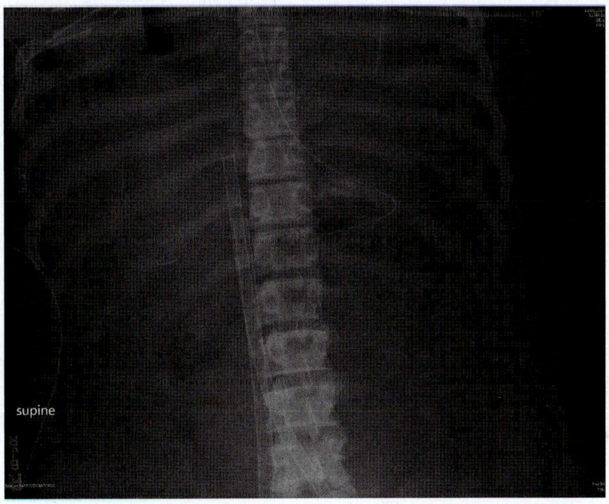

FIGURE 13.4 | Radiograph of ideal placement for femoral–femoral VV ECMO cannulation.

    - The venous drainage cannula should be placed in the usual intrahepatic IVC position, with the tip of the "arterial" inflow cannula being placed in the RA or SVC. These long cannulas have multiple holes as they are designed for venous drainage.
    - "Arterial" cannulas are short with only an end-hole designed for infusion, but from the femoral vein will only reach into the low IVC and lead to recirculation.
- Cannula insertion:
  - If a two-cannula system is used, it is generally recommended that both guidewires should be in the correct location before proceeding with cannula insertion, to prevent thrombosis of one cannula. It is also generally recommended to assure both wires are in place before systemic heparinization.
  - Incise the skin at the guidewire insertion site.
  - Sequentially dilate the tract from the skin to the vein with the dilators provided in the kit.
  - Insert the cannula over the guidewire (under fluoroscopic imaging if available)
    - "Arterial" cannula's tip should terminate at the cavoatrial junction.
    - "Venous" cannula's tip should terminate at the diaphragm.
  - It is ESSENTIAL that the cannulas move over the guidewire and that the guidewire is not moving forward with the cannula. Remove the inner obturator and guidewire together while placing your thumb over the end of the cannula opening, and then clamp the cannula at the designated site without the wire reinforcement. Heparin locks the cannula if the second cannula is not inserted simultaneously.

- Insertion of the dual-lumen VV ECMO cannula: These cannulas are generally placed through RIJ access, although both the LIJ and the left subclavian routes have been used successfully. These cannulas drain both proximally and from the tip, with the inflow "arterial" lumen exiting in between the two drainage sites on the "medial side" of the cannula. (This requires proper orientation of the cannula with the arterial side connection being placed medially at the exit site.) Proper positioning of these cannulas includes placement of the tip well into the intrahepatic IVC, assuring that the "arterial" or inflow port is stationed ABOVE the eustachian valve of the IVC to prevent problematic recirculation of the oxygenated blood directly back into the circuit (Fig. 13.5A,B).

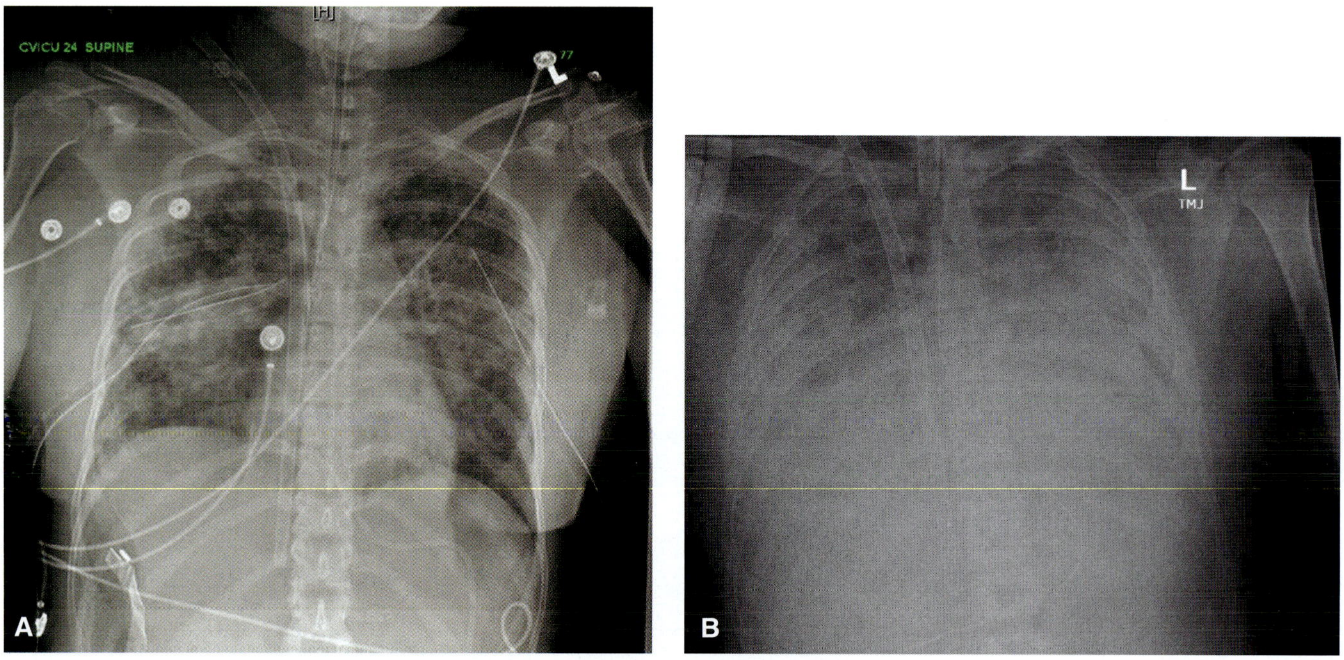

FIGURE 13.5 ▌ **A:** Ideal radiographic position of a dual lumen cannula (Avalon), pediatric. **B:** Ideal radiographic position of a dual lumen cannula (Crescent), adult.

  - Most experienced operators strongly recommend the use of fluoroscopy during this procedure which allows visualization of the entire wire within the field of vision during tract dilation and cannula insertion.
- Deair the cannulas and create a wet-to-wet connection:
  - Tubing of the circuit and the cannula remain clamped.
  - An assistant drips saline over the connections as you marry the ends
    - A common practice in cardiac surgery is to fill the end of the cannula connector and the free end of the circuit tubing with saline, then squeeze the tubing gently as the connector is inserted into the tubing. This prevents capture or entrainment of air into the line.
  - No significant air should be present in the circuit following the connection, particularly with VA ECMO. If air is present, keep clamps in place and repeat the connection.
- Secure the cannula(s) using a heavy suture of 0 or #1 Ethibond or Silk sutures at the insertion site and in additional sites along the cannula.
  - Optional: Utilize the provided device to secure the cannula to the leg/neck as appropriate. Femoral cannulas can be further supported with a loose ace or gauze wrap around the thigh.

VA ECMO

- In VA ECMO, blood is drained from the venous circulation, usually one of the femoral veins, and the oxygenated blood is returned into an arterial cannula, usually placed in a common femoral artery (CFA). Generally femoral arterial and venous cannulas are placed in adjacent positions on the ipsilateral side. However, there is no reason that they cannot be placed in the vessel on the contralateral side.

TIP

In the circumstances where the femoral veins are not accessible, such as extensive deep vein thrombosis or hematomas from pelvic fractures, the RIJ can be accessed for venous drainage for VA ECMO. However, a large "venous" multi-holed cannula must still be used, and care must be taken to secure proper placement in the RA, usually with the tip down into the intrahepatic IVC.

- Femoral artery access:
  - Prep and drape the patient with ability to identify all necessary landmarks
    - Anterior superior iliac spine
    - Pubic tubercle
    - Inguinal ligament
  - Identify the CFA, superficial femoral artery, and deep femoral artery
  - Access the CFA with a needle using ultrasound guidance. It is essential to access the CFA to accommodate the catheter and allow flow around the catheter to reduce the risk of distal ischemia.
  - Insert the guidewire into the aorta (under fluoroscopic guidance if available).
  - Light pressure may be applied over the insertion site to minimize bleeding while the venous access is obtained.
- Femoral vein access (as above for VV cannulation)
  - Insertion of cannula in the same fashion as VV ECMO (see above), except that there is no specific target for the tip of the arterial cannula.

TIP

While it is sometimes necessary to dilate the femoral tract as large as, or slightly larger than, the venous femoral cannula, you should avoid "overdilation" of the femoral artery tract (e.g., dilating with a 22-Fr dilator for a 21-Fr cannula, as this commonly leads to continued bleeding around the cannula during the ECMO run.

Initiation of ECLS Therapy

- Communication with the ECLS Specialist is key.
- The ECLS Specialist, typically a perfusionist or specialized nurse or respiratory therapist, will direct the initiation of therapy.
- Reconfirm there is no air trapped between the clamps of the cannula and sterile circuit tubing.
- Remove the clamps from the cannulas and circuits on the sterile field and communicate this to the ECLS Specialist.
- ECLS Specialist will remove their clamps from the circuit as they are increasing the RPMs.
  - Remember that the centrifugal pump is nonocclusive, and in VA configuration, when the clamps are all removed and the circuit is not yet running, the patient can pump blood into the arterial cannula and backward through the circuit into the venous side.
  - It is very common to see systemic vasodilation and hypotension from bradykinin release (kallikrein–kinin system) with the initial exposure of the blood to the circuit. This is almost always a transient event that responds to a fluid bolus, occasionally requiring calcium, and rarely epinephrine. Thus, it is a good idea to have those three items ready at initiation.

Confirmation of ECMO Therapy at the Time of Procedure

- VV ECMO
  - Adequacy of oxygenation:
    - Look for improvement in patient peripheral noninvasive oxygen saturation.
      - Frequently, the oxygen saturation will rise to 100% with a gradual decrease after the ventilator has been reduced to "rest" settings. Peripheral saturation goal is typically in the 80s, but with high native cardiac outputs, saturations in the mid to high 70s are not uncommon.
    - Obtain a blood gas post-oxygenator to confirm proper oxygenator function and calibrate any in-line gas monitoring devices as appropriate.

- Evaluation of recirculation (VV ECMO only), which is defined as oxygenated blood from the reinfusion cannula crossing directly into the drainage cannula rather than passing through the right heart and into the lungs.
  - Confirm position of the cannulas with fluoroscopy, chest radiograph, or flat plat of the abdomen.
  - Recirculation is highly positional, for both the cannulas and the patient, including intracardiac streaming, and is diagnosed physiologically, not radiologically.
    - It is not uncommon to see cannulas that look to be "too close" on CXR without any evidence of recirculation by saturations. In those circumstances, repositioning of the cannulas is NOT indicated (Fig. 13.6).

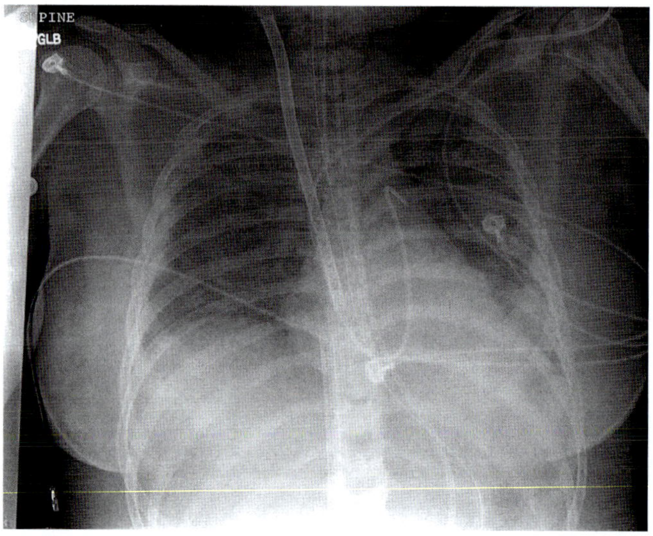

FIGURE 13.6 ▌ Radiograph showing close proximity of cannulas without the presence of recirculation.

  - Obtain a preoxygenator blood gas to calibrate in-line monitoring. With a peripheral saturation above 90%, A venous saturation <75% indicates minimal recirculation.
    - In patients with arterial saturations in the 70s, due to high native cardiac outputs, it is not usual to have venous saturations in the 50s.
    - In general, the venous return saturation should be significantly below the patient's arterial saturation. If they are equal or higher, there is significant recirculation.
  - Concern for recirculation with the dual-lumen cannulas can be easily assessed with transthoracic echo (TTE) or transesophageal echo (TEE), which is excellent at demonstrating the inflow patterns of blood flow and their relationship to the eustachian valve.

TIP

Recirculation is not only a product of the circuit and cannula configuration. Anything that lowers the patient's cardiac output, including primary cardiac failure, tamponade, tension pneumothorax, for example, will increase the amount of time that blood sits in the right atrium, which will increase the amount of oxygenated blood that is drawn back up into the ECMO circuit. It is not uncommon that the first sign of these hemodynamic problems is new recirculation issues noted by rising venous saturation.

- VA ECMO
  - Blood flow
    - Determine the maximum blood flow capable of the ECMO circuit given the current cannulation size and position.
    - In general, it is recommended for early VA ECMO management to maintain the highest flow possible with the lowest possible RPM, that is, no "wasted" RPM.
    - The physiologic goals (mean arterial pressure, arterial saturation) are set, and the blood flow is regulated to meet the goals. The flow is commonly set to maintain the SvO_2 >75%
    - If there is inadequate flow to meet goals (i.e., rising lactate), this should be corrected by increasing (1) VA ECMO flow or (2) hemoglobin or (3) circulating volume.

Troubleshooting

- Inability to pass the wire. The wires should slide freely in the vasculature. Resistance may mean you are not actually in the vessel.
  - Try to use a wire with more or less stiffness
  - Evaluate the vessel for calcifications (arterial wire resistance)
  - Convert to open cutdown procedure
- Inability to insert the cannula
  - Evaluate the skin incision for ability to accommodate the cannula size
  - Make sure you are not trying to cannulate through the inguinal ligament
  - Spin the cannula gently as it is inserted over the wire to minimize friction with the skin
  - Make sure the wire is NOT moving with the cannula but is guiding its movement.
    - If there is any kink in the wire that catches at the tip, and it moves with the cannula, it is no longer a guidewire, and there is significant risk of perforation of the vessel.
  - Consider that you might be placing a cannula that is too large for the patient and consider placing a smaller size cannula.
    - If you are confident that the cannula is the appropriate size for the patient, reassess the size of the vessel with US. If needed, consider opting for a different vessel.
  - Consider converting to open cannulation (Fig. 13.7) to directly assess the vessel size, or in the case of the arterial cannula, placement of a side graft to insert the cannula.

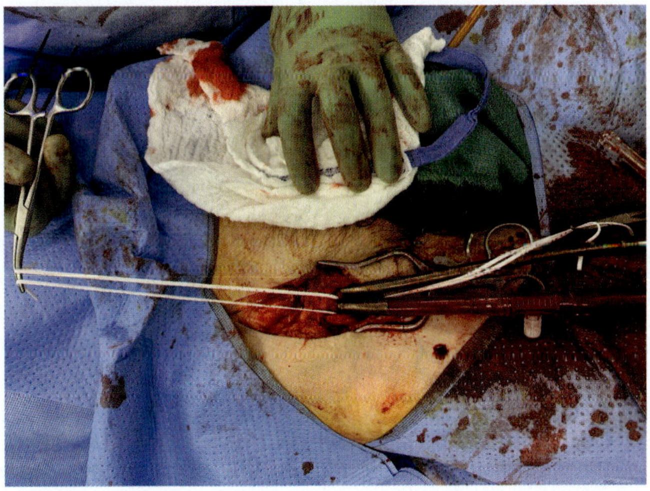

FIGURE 13.7 ❚ Right femoral artery and vein exposure for open cannulation of the common femoral artery and vein for VA ECMO.

- Deairing the connection
  - Do not release the clamps. Instead break the connection and repeat the wet-to-wet connection process
  - Have an assistant squirt the saline over the connection as it is made with a 60-mm toomey syringe.
    - It is not necessary to worry about a few small bubbles on VV ECMO in urgent circumstances.
  - Many arterial cannulas have built in connectors with Luer ports that can also be used to withdraw remaining air prior to initiating flow.
- Limb-threatening ischemia (VA ECMO) is a significant risk of femoral artery cannulation and should be recognized and corrected within about 4 hours or less of cannulation and initiation of ECMO support. There are several options to correct (or prevent) leg ischemia:
  - A retrograde dorsalis pedis (Fig. 13.8) or posterior tibial catheter connected to the arterial limb of the circuit via a Leur connector using a high-pressure arterial line without a stopcock.

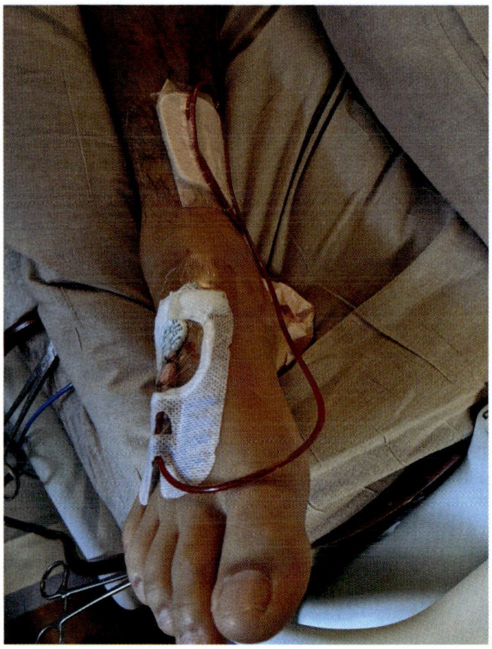

FIGURE 13.8 ▌ Retrograde dorsalis pedis arterial catheter for distal perfusion.

- In the absence of peripheral vascular disease, this will almost always provide sufficient flow to the lower leg to prevent ischemia.
- An antegrade superficial femoral artery (SFA) cannula can be placed either percutaneously or via cutdown to provide flow down the leg to prevent ischemia.
  - This method has several problems:
    - It can obstruct collateral flow coming in from the profunda branch, making the sheath the only source of blood flow to the leg.
    - Second, it only provides flow via the infusion side port which is connected to the arterial limb of the circuit, and by design has a stopcock that reduces the flow considerably.
- Cutdown of the contralateral CFA with placement of a tunneled side graft, and insertion of a cannula directly into the graft to allow bidirectional flow into the CFA, with subsequent removal of the ipsilateral original cannula and arterial repair, thrombectomy, etc., as necessary.
- Fem-Fem bypass grafting connected from the contralateral artery to the ipsilateral artery below the cannulation site has been used to treat limb ischemia.
- Graft access of the axillary artery can be very useful in patients with known or encountered extensive lower extremity PVD, either in response to leg ischemia after cannulation, or as a primary option to avoid femoral arterial cannulation.

- Inability to generate or maintain ECMO flow.
  - In the resistance-dependent centrifugal pump, obstruction of any kind, at any level will reduce, or eliminate flow through the circuit.
    - With a properly functioning pump, the causes of low flow are assessed along the path of the circuit as follows:
      - Decreased venous return can be due to:
        - hypovolemia, particularly in VA ECMO support, but is also commonly due to "obstruction" of the venous inflow which causes vibration of the venous line, often called "chatter" or "chugging."
          - It can also be caused by excessive RPMs and increased negative inlet pressure, but in its most problematic form is due to a low-lying IVC cannula sucking the vessel wall against the cannula.
          - It can be corrected by inserting a new venous cannula in the contralateral vein with the tip in the intrahepatic IVC.
    - Venous line obstruction, usually from kinking of the nonwire reinforced circuit tubing. This will show up as low inlet pressures, along with a drop in both pre- and postmembrane pressures.

- Membrane resistance, usually from thrombus, fibrin, or lipid build-up.
  - Hallmarked by a rise in the premembrane pressure, potentially a drop in the post membrane pressure, depending on severity of the resistance rise, and thus a rise in the TRANS-membrane pressure.
    - This can occur slowly (with fibrin or lipid) or very quickly (with acute thrombosis of the membrane).
    - The decrease in flow will at some point be accompanied by decrease in gas exchange as well.
- Arterial line obstruction, usually from kinking of the tubing.
  - Identified with a rise in both pre- and postmembrane pressures with a minor increase in the transmembrane pressures as the centrifugal pump attempts to force more flow through the arterial side of the circuit.
- Hypertension in patients on VA ECMO.
  - Any sudden rise in the patients systemic vascular resistance (SVR) due to pain, agitation, delirium, etc., will result in a decrease in the flow through the ECMO circuit.
  - If the flow has been reduced in an attempt to wean support, the patient can actually pump blood into the arterial line, backwards through the circuit, including the oxygenator, and into the venous system, usually the RA or IVC. This should be recognized by the clinical state of hypertension, particularly if sudden, but in more gradual causes of rising SVR such as hypovolemia, it may only be noted by clinical exam consistent with poor perfusion, prolonged capillary refill, decreased urine output, rising lactate, etc.
    - This is usually easily fixed with combination of volume, sedation, treatment for delirium, vasodilator therapy, etc. As the SVR falls, the centrifugal pump can produce more forward flow.

Suggested Readings

Combes A, Hajage D, Capellier G, et al. Extracorporeal membrane oxygenation for severe acute respiratory distress syndrome. *N Engl J Med.* 2018;378(21):1965–1975.

Guglin M, Zucker MJ, Bazan VM, et al. Venoarterial ECMO for adults: JACC Scientific Expert Panel. *J Am Coll Cardiol.* 2019; 73(6):698–716.

Peek GJ, Mugford M, Tiruvoipati R, et al. Efficacy and economic assessment of conventional ventilatory support versus extracorporeal membrane oxygenation for severe adult respiratory failure (CESAR): a multicentre randomised controlled trial. *Lancet.* 2009;374(9698):1351–1363.

Pranikoff T, Hines MH. Vascular access for extracorporeal support. In: Annich L, MacLaren W, Bartlett, eds. *ECMO Extracorporeal Cardiopulmonary Support in Critical Care.* 4th ed. 2005. Publisher: Extracorporeal Life Support (June 1, 2012).

Schmidt M, Bailey M, Sheldrake J, et al. Predicting survival after extracorporeal membrane oxygenation for severe acute respiratory failure. The Respiratory Extracorporeal Membrane Oxygenation Survival Prediction (RESP) score. *Am J Respir Crit Care Med.* 2014;189(11):1374–1382.

Chapter 14

Surgical Stabilization of Rib Fractures

FREDRIC M. PIERACCI

PERIOPERATIVE CONSIDERATIONS

Procedure Rationale

Selection of Ribs for Fixation

- Fractures of ribs 3 to 10 should be considered for fixation. Anterior fractures of the second rib may also be considered for repair in select circumstances.
- Fractures of the first and second ribs are more difficult and morbid to expose, and contribute minimally to chest wall stability.
- Fractures of the 11th and 12th ribs do not contribute substantially to chest wall stability. In rare circumstances such as impalement, the fractured segment may simply be excised.
- Posterior fractures within 3 cm of the transverse process should not be approached due to proximity to the spine and disruption of investing ligaments and muscles (Fig. 14.1).

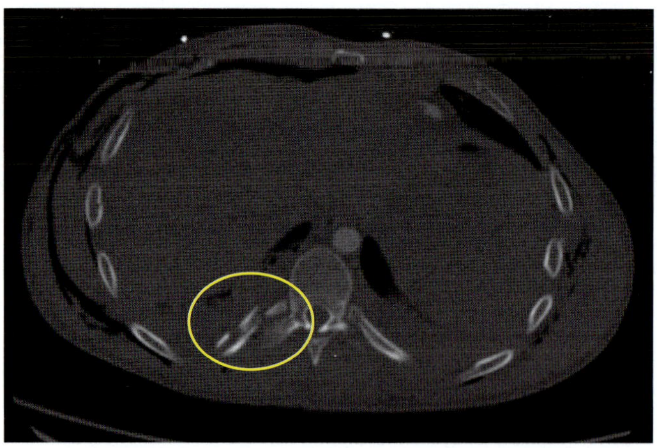

FIGURE 14.1 | Very posterior right ninth rib fracture.

- Anterior fractures within 3 cm of the cost-chondral junction may be considered for fixation to either the costal cartilage or sternum (Fig. 14.2).

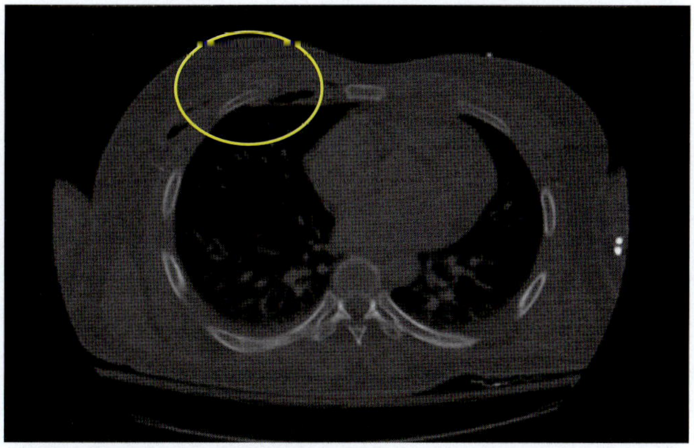

FIGURE 14.2 ❙ Very anterior right fourth rib fracture.

- We suggest using a preoperative planning sheet, on which fractures intended for repair are marked and then crossed off intraoperatively (Fig. 14.3).

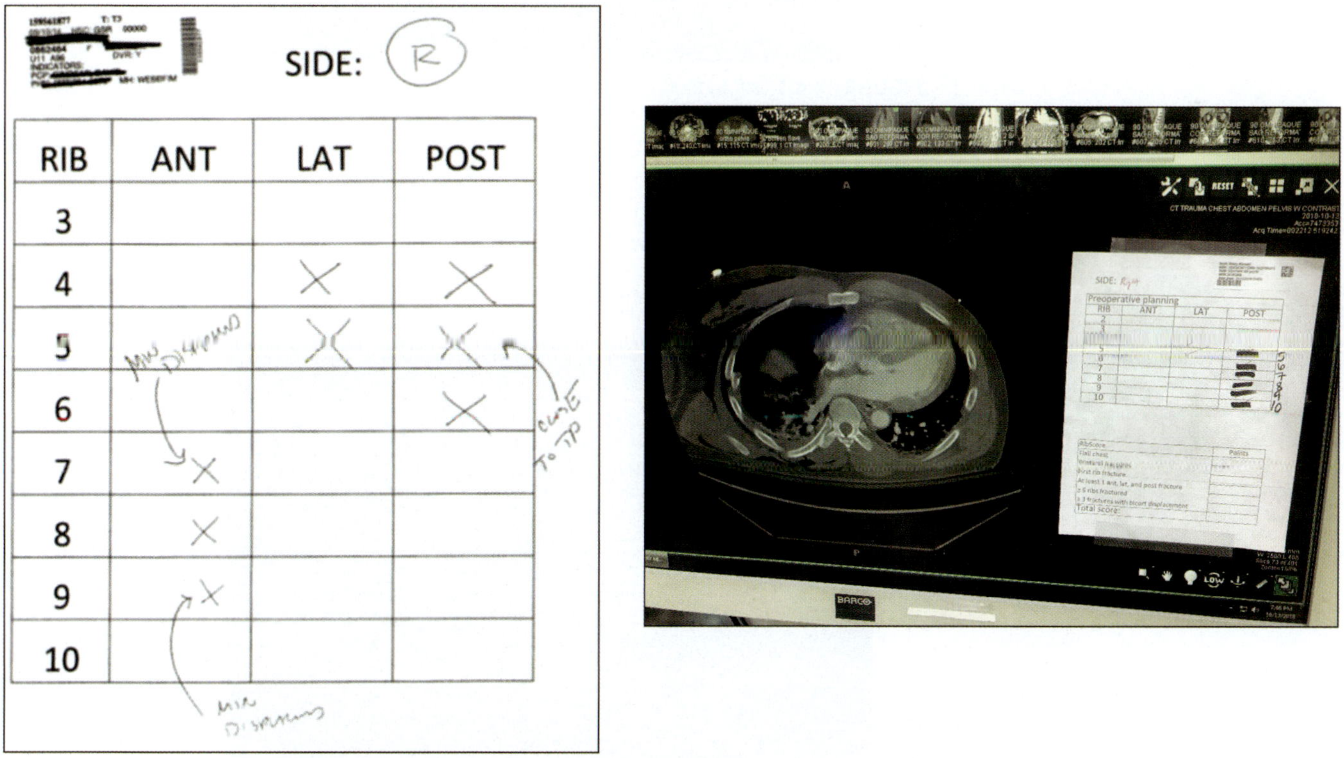

[redacted]

SIDE: R

RIB	ANT	LAT	POST
3			
4		X	X
5		X	X
6			X
7	X		
8	X		
9	X		
10			

FIGURE 14.3 ❙ Preoperative planning sheet for surgical stabilization of rib fractures.

Assessment of the Pleural Space

- Hemothorax and pneumothorax are common in patients with severe chest wall injuries. These injuries should be noted preoperatively.
  - Excessive subcutaneous air on CT imaging, persistent air leak, and evidence of lung parenchymal impalement with a rib fracture (Fig. 14.4) should be noted preoperatively.

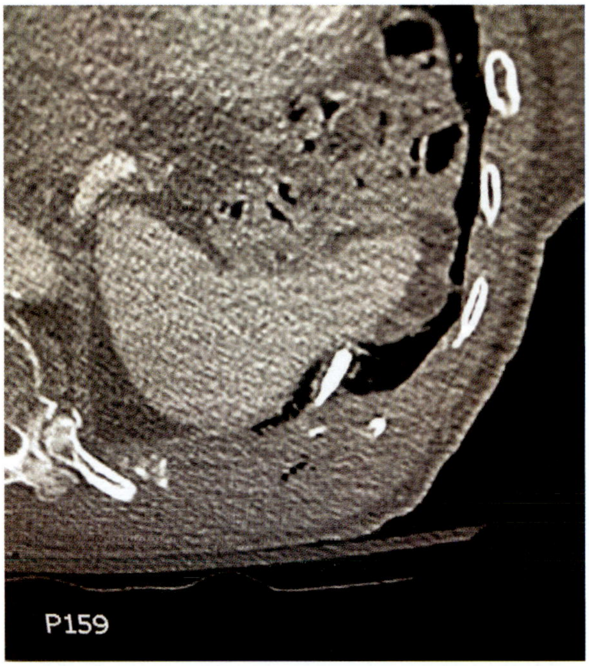

FIGURE 14.4 ▌ Left tenth rib fracture impaling lung parenchyma on CT imaging.

Assessment of the Diaphragm

- Diaphragm lacerations are difficult to diagnose on CT imaging.
- Fractures of ribs 7 to 10 are associated with diaphragm lacerations and should raise index of suspicion (Fig. 14.5).

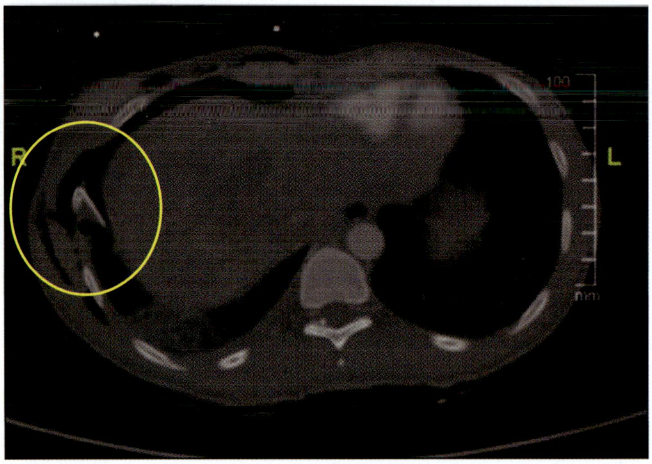

FIGURE 14.5 ▌ Right eighth rib fracture impaling diaphragm.

Essential Equipment

- Several commercially available, rib-specific fixation systems are available; no system has been shown to be superior to another.
- A peiatric Bookwalter self-retaining retraction system is useful for exposure (Fig. 14.6).
- Self-retaining wound protectors are useful for placement under the superficial muscles of the chest wall to gain exposure.

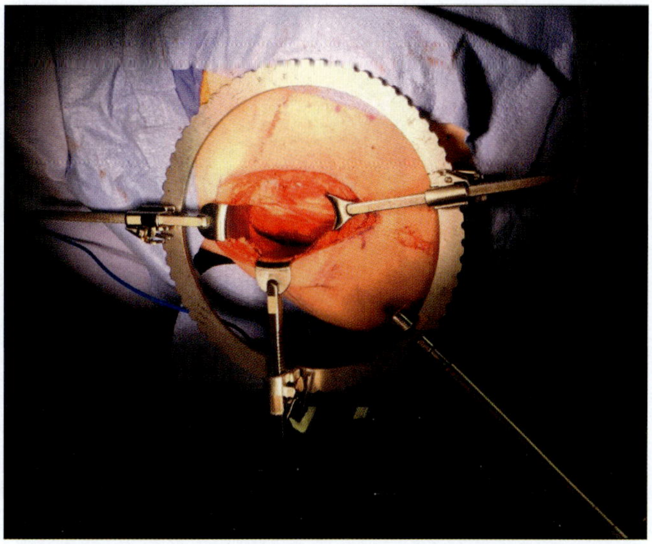

FIGURE 14.6 ▍ Use of a self-retaining retraction system to aid in exposure of posterior fractures.

- Peanut dissectors are useful for cleaning off rib surfaces without devascularizing them, as well as for holding plates in place.
- Right-angle retractors are useful for rib reduction and maintenance of countertraction during drilling and screw placement.
- Video-assisted thoracic surgery (VATS) equipment: A 5-mm thoracoscope, two 5-mm trocars, insufflation tubing, 5-mm suction irrigator, Maryland dissector, 7-inch, 22-gauge mediastinal needle.
- 19-Fr Blake drain for pleural drainage.
- Antimicrobial prophylaxis: Cefazolin 2 g IV, unless risk factors for methicillin-resistant staphylococcus aureus (MRSA), in which case vancomycin 1 g IV.
- Venous thromboembolism (VTE) prophylaxis: unfractionated heparin 5,000 U subcutaneous (SQ).
- Bronchoscopy.
- Severe chest wall injuries result in impaired secretion clearance.
- Flexible bronchoscope is performed to the level of the segmental bronchi in order to clear mucous, blood, foreign bodies (e.g., teeth), as well as access for traumatic airway injuries (Fig. 14.7).

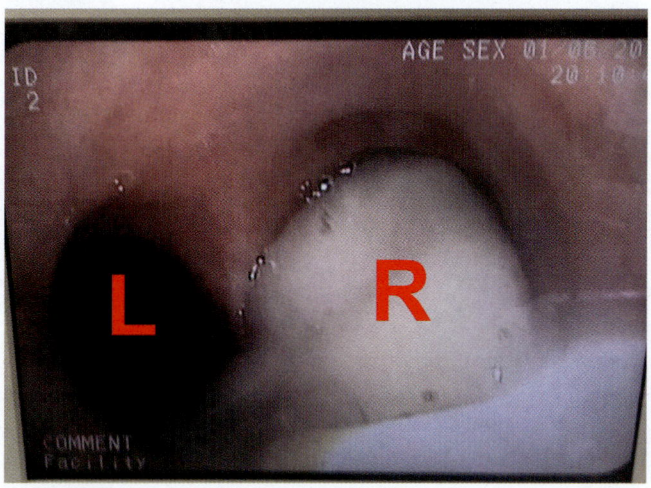

FIGURE 14.7 ▍ Right main stem bronchial plug identified on routine, intraoperative bronchoscopy.

TECHNIQUE

Lung Isolation

- Several methods are available. We utilize a bifurcated bronchial blocker, which straddles the carina and can be used to achieve rapid lung isolation (Fig. 14.8).
- The blocker is placed at the termination of the bronchoscopy.

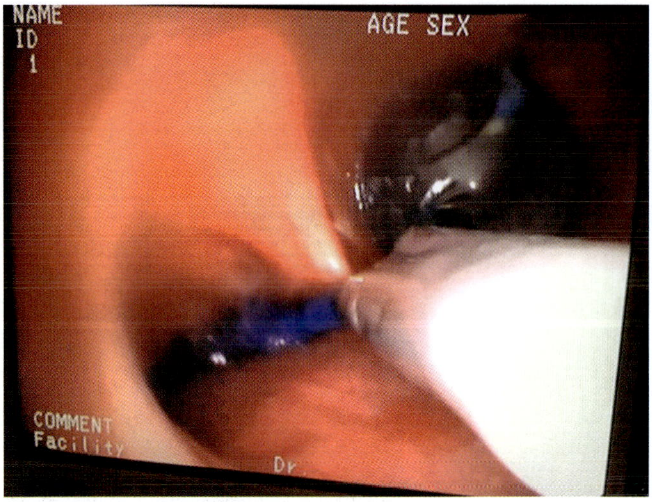

FIGURE 14.8 ▌ Bronchial blocker straddling the carina with right main stem balloon inflated.

Positioning and Incisions

Anterior Approach

Anterior fractures are approached in the supine position (Fig. 14.9).

- The ipsilateral arm may be hung in order to improve access
- For fractures of ribs 3 to 7, an inframammary incision is made beginning medially and curving up toward the axilla (Fig. 14.10).

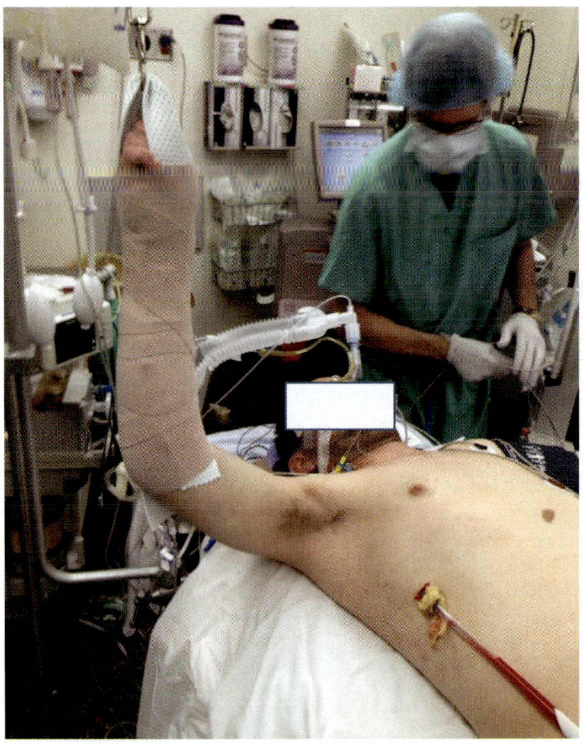

FIGURE 14.9 ▌ Positioning for repair of anterior fractures.

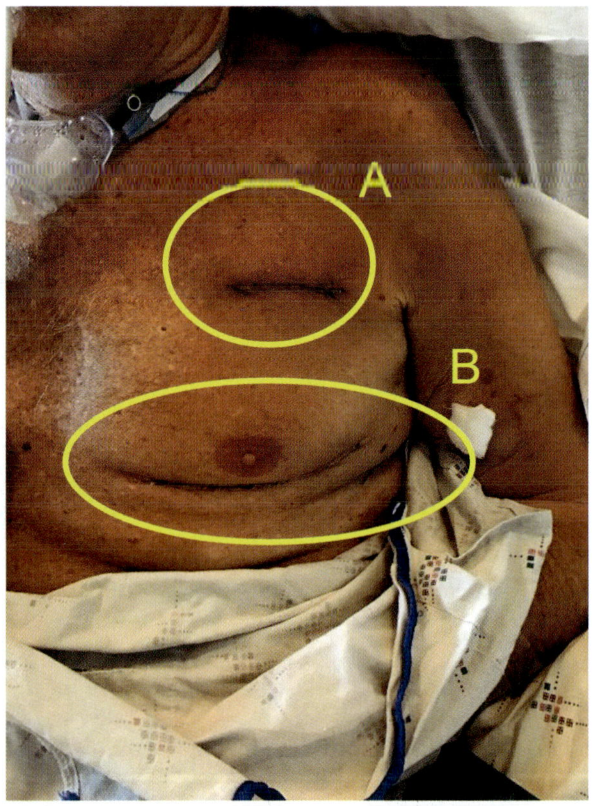

FIGURE 14.10 ▌ Infraclavicular (**A**) and inframammary (**B**) incisions for exposure of anterior rib fractures

- A subpectoral flap is raised, and the fibers of the pectoralis minor are either split or transected.
- Exposure of the anterior second rib may be difficult via the subpectoral flap. In this case, a transverse, 4-cm, infraclavicular incision is made, and the fibers of both the pectoralis major and minor are split.

Lateral Approach

- See Figure 14.11.
- Lateral fractures are approached in the lateral decubitus position.
- Regardless of fracture location, an oblique incision is made along the anterior border of the latissimus dorsi muscle.

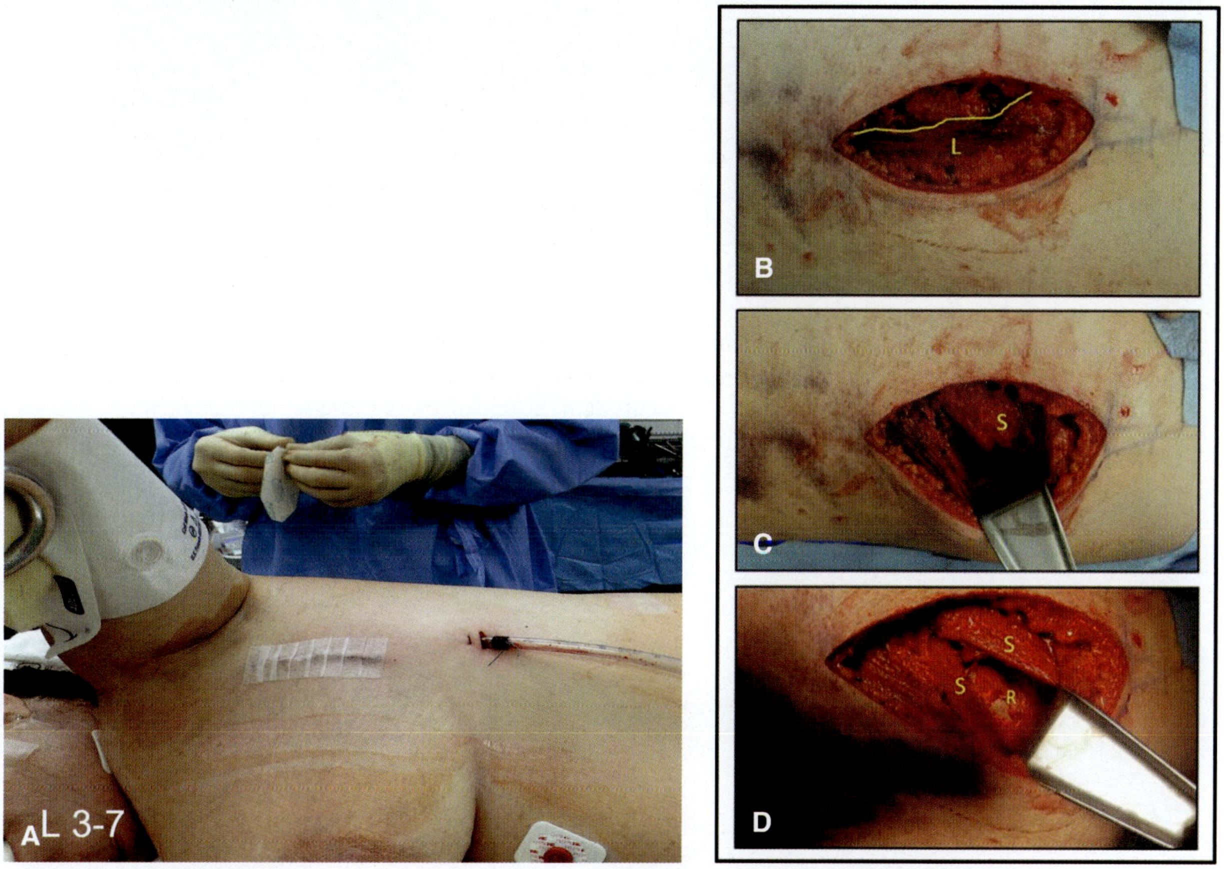

FIGURE 14.11 ▌ A–D: Incision and muscle-sparring exposure of lateral rib fractures 3-7. L, lattisimus dorsi; S, serratus anterior; R, rib fracture.

TIP

In order to avoid muscle division, make the incision along the anterior border of the latissimus dorsi muscle, not directly over the rib fractures.

- Develop a latissimus dorsi muscle flap by dissecting the muscle free of subcutaneous fat anteriorly and the serratus anterior muscle posteriorly.
- Identify the serratus anterior muscle and the long thoracic neurovascular bundle coursing directly over it.
- Split the fibers of the serratus anterior muscle over the fractures and away from the long thoracic neuro vascular bundle.
- Place the self-retaining wound protector under the serratus anterior muscle, and set up the self-retaining retraction system.
- Usually, fractures of three ribs may be repaired through a single split of the serratus muscle. To repair additional fractures, make a second (or third) split in the serratus anterior muscle over those fractures.

Posterior Approach

- Position the patient prone with the ipsilateral arm supported on an arm board approximately 4 to 6 inches below the body. This maneuver serves to lateralize the scapula (Fig. 14.12).

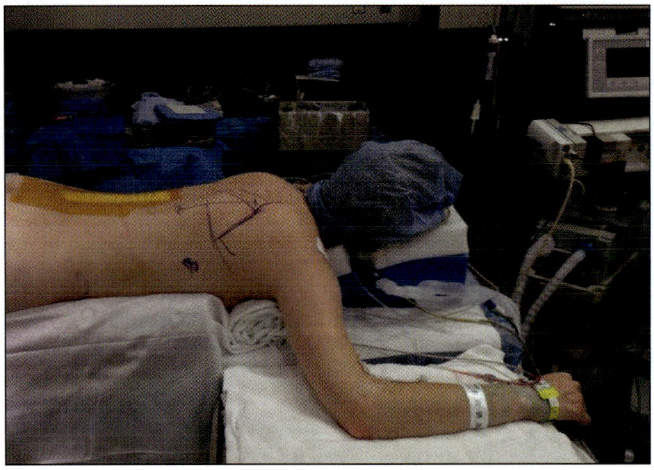

FIGURE 14.12 ❙ Prone positioning for exposure of posterior rib fractures.

- Make a longitudinal incision midway between the tip of the scapula and the spine, centered at the tip of the scapula, and adjusted either superiorly or inferiorly depending on the ribs fractured.
- Identify the triangle of auscultation, bounded by the inferior border of the trapezius muscle, the superior border of the latissimus dorsi, and the medial border of the scapula (Fig. 14.13).

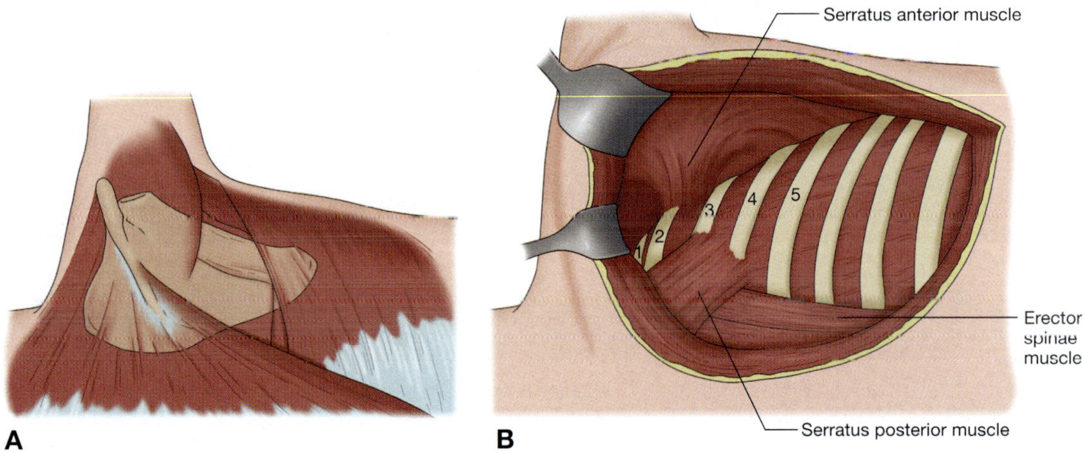

FIGURE 14.13 ❙ Development of the triangle of auscultation for exposure of posterior rib fractures.

- Develop flaps under both the trapezius and latissimus muscle.
- Either split or transect the rhomboid muscles.
- Develop a flap underneath the erector spinae muscle complex if additional medial exposure is needed.
- Caution: Be aware that the spinal accessory nerve (cranial nerve XI) courses on the posterior surface of the trapezius muscle.

Reduction and Fixation

- Usually, a right-angle clamp is the easiest tool to use to reduce rib fractures.
- Reduction typically results in entry into the pleural space, albeit via a small puncture.
- The rib diameter is measured using a bicortical fixation system.
- The rib plate is contoured to match the surface of the rib. This step is particularly important when repairing posterior fractures, as the sharp angle of the rib mandates additional bending. A plate template may be useful in gauging the necessary degree of bend for the plate.
- Typically, the screw furthest from the exposure (i.e., the posterior-most screw in a lateral exposure and the anterior-most screw during a posterior exposure) is placed first, as the rib "dives away" from the exposure at this point, and placement of the margin of the plate "flush" with the rib is most difficult at this location.

- The minimum number of screws per fracture side is achieved as dictated by the fixation platform.
- Nonlocking (lag) screws may be used to temporarily achieve fixation but should eventually be replaced with locking screws.

Evaluation of the Pleural Space

- VATS may be performed easily from either the supine or lateral decubitus position. VATS is technically more challenging from the prone position, and the surgeon may elect to reposition the patient in lateral decubitus at this stage of the procedure.
- Following SSRF, a 5-mm trocar is placed in the anterior axillary line at the site of the eventual chest tube.
- The trocar is brought through the skin stab incision and into the SSRF wound, such that it may be placed through the intercostal space under direct visualization.
- The SSRF wound is covered with a wet gauze, and pleural insufflation at 8 mm Hg is commenced.
- The scope is introduced, and a second, 5 mm port is placed along the posterior axillary line and under direct visualization.
- Retained hemothorax is evacuated, and the pleural surfaces, lung, and diaphragm are inspected for injury. Injuries are addressed as encountered.
- The pleural space is irrigated with 1 L of sterile saline.

Locoregional Anesthesia

- The 5-mm camera is moved to the posterior port
- A 7-inch, 22-gauge mediastinal needle is introduced directly through the skin and approximately the 7th interspace, posterior axillary line.
- Using a Maryland dissector through the anterior port, the needle is grasped and directed into the subpleural space of the 3rd to 10th intercostal spaces (Fig. 14.14).

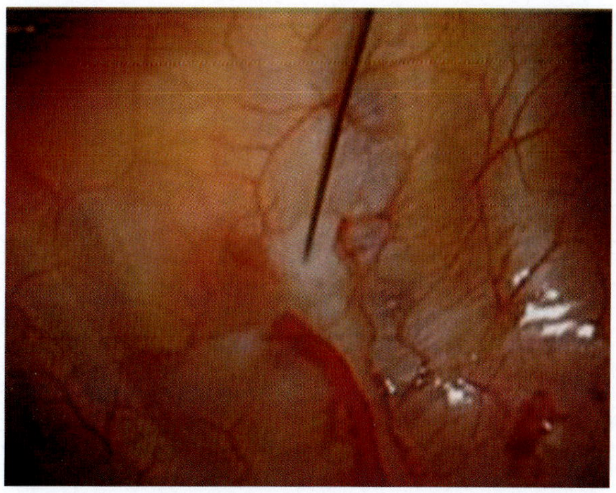

FIGURE 14.14 ▮ VATS intercostal nerve blocks with liposomal bupivacaine.

- A mixture of short-acting and long-acting (liposomal) anesthetic is instilled into each intercostal space.
- Care must be taken to avoid the intercostal artery and vein, and remain directly subpleural. The correct place is confirmed by visualization of a wheel of fluid under the pleura.

Pleural Drainage

- A 19-Fr Blake drain is placed through the anterior port and terminated posteriorly at the apex under direct, thoracoscopic visualization.
- The drain is connected to a water sealant system.

Closure

- Meticulous hemostatis is imperative, particularly since large potential spaces are created between muscle layers.

- The wound is closed in layers, beginning with the deep muscles (e.g., serratus anterior splits), followed by the superficial muscles (e.g., lattisimus dorsi), followed by the skin.

Suggested Readings

Bemelman M, Poeze M, Blokhuis TJ, Leenen LPH. Historic overview of treatment techniques for rib fractures and flail chest. *Eur J Trauma Emerg Surg*. 2010;36:407–415.

Pieracci FM, Johnson JL, Stovall RT, Jurkovich GJ. Completely thoracoscopic intra-pleural reduction and fixation of severe rib fractures. *Trauma Case Re*. 2015;4:39–43.

Pieracci FM, Rodil M, Stovall RT, et al. Surgical stabilization of severe rib fractures. *J Trauma Acute Care Surg*. 2015;78:883–887.

SECTION IV Abdominal Injuries

Chapter 15

Liver

HUNTER B. MOORE, ELIZABETH A. POMFRET, AND ERNEST E. MOORE

PERIOPERATIVE CONSIDERATIONS

Procedure Rationale

Due to its size, the liver is the most common organ injured after trauma. Treatment is best considered in the framework of the American Association for the Surgery of Trauma (AAST) anatomic grading severity from I to V. Most blunt injuries of the liver disrupt venous structures which become hemostatic when clot forms within the injury site. Consequently, grade I–III parenchymal injuries are managed nonoperatively. In contrast, half of grade V injuries require urgent operative intervention and the mortality for associated retrohepatic vena cava injuries exceeds 80%. Successful treatment of grade IV–V injuries requires a comprehensive knowledge of hepatic anatomy (Fig. 15.1) including ligamentous attachment, parenchymal segments, extrahepatic and intrahepatic vascularity, and the biliary system to employ an effective rapid step-up operative approach.

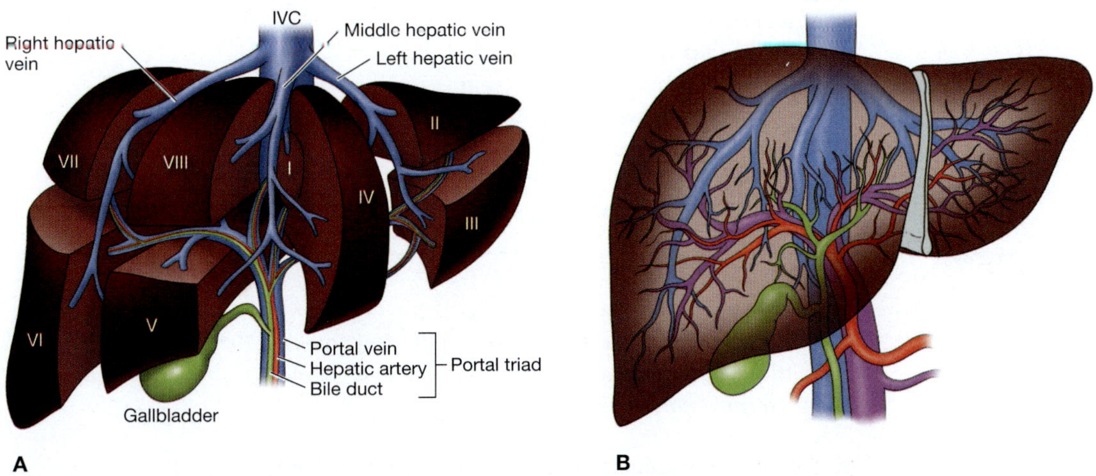

FIGURE 15.1 | Knowledge of hepatic anatomy is essential for effective management of major liver trauma. **A:** Segmental. **B:** Arteries and veins.

Essential Equipment

TIP

Availability of extensive equipment is important because the severity of liver injury is unknown at the time of exploratory laparotomy.

- Headlight
- Loupe magnification 2.5 glasses
- Argon beam coagulator
- Vascular stapler, triple level
- Ligasure device
- Gel foam and Surgicel
- Fibrin sealant and BioGlue
- Castroviejo needle driver
- Microvascular Gerald forceps
- Potts–Smith scissor
- Angled vascular clamps
- Bulldog vascular clamps
- Satinsky clamps
- Silastic vessel loops
- Rummel tourniquet (red rubber catheter and umbilical tape)
- 15-cm Pruitt-Inahara shunt with T port (8, 9, 10 Fr)
- Sutures
  - 6-0 Prolene on a C1 or BV1 needle
  - 4-0 Prolene on a C1 or BV1 needle
  - 3-0 silk plain and stick ties
  - Clips, small and medium
- Sterile 8- to 10-MHz Doppler probe
- Heparinized saline 50 to 100 units in 1,000 mL saline
- Papaverine 30 mg/mL, 10 mL vials
- Tissue plasminogen activator, 2 mg vial
- Fogarty embolectomy catheters #2, #3, #4
- Bulldog vascular clamps
- Three-way stopcock and A-line extension tubing
- 10-, 20-cc syringes of heparin saline on 18-gauge IV catheter with blunt needle (Olive) tip
- Contrast agent 50 mL (Omnipaque 240, GE Healthcare, Inc., Chicago, IL)
- Linear 8- to 10-MHz Doppler probe
- Viscoelastic hemostatic assay
- Cannulae for venovenous bypass
  - Femoral vein, 24 Fr
  - Jugular/subclavian vein, 24 Fr
  - Inferior mesenteric vein (IMV), 14 Fr

Patient Positioning

TIP

The complexity of liver injury is usually unknown at the time of emergent laparotomy. Consequently, the patient manifesting refractory shock should be prepped extensively, including the ability to perform venovenous bypass.

- Patient is positioned supine with both arms extended
- Prep includes the neck, chest, abdomen, and both legs to the knee
- Radial arterial line and large upper torso venous access
- Bair hugger on lower extremities
- Blood products available

TECHNIQUE

Abdominal Incision (Fig. 15.2)

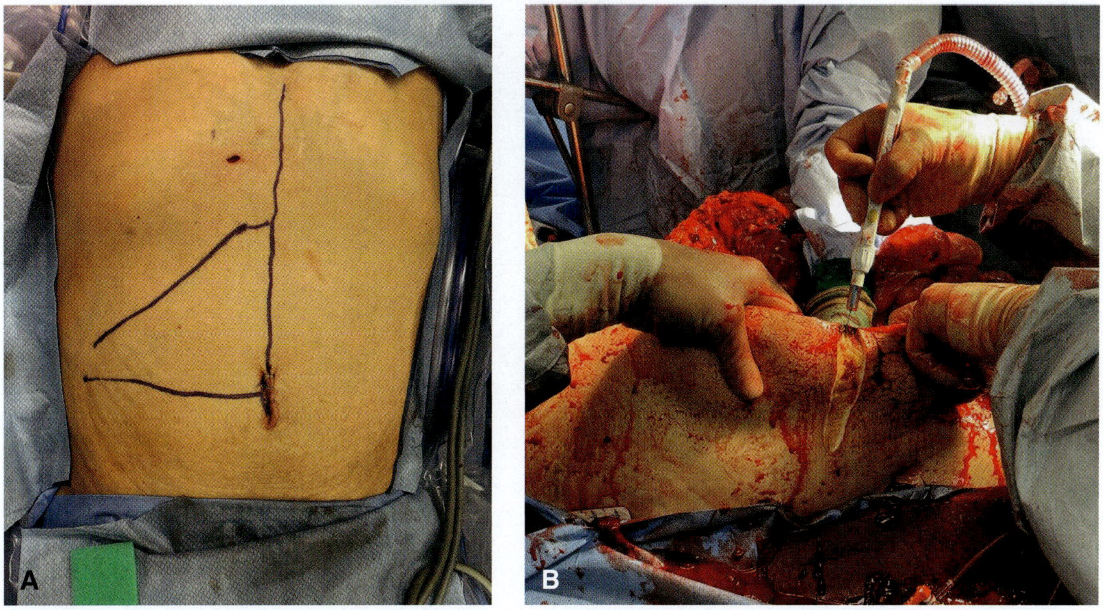

FIGURE 15.2 ▌ **A:** Following a standard midline incision a subcostal or lateral extension provide enhanced exposure to the liver. **B:** Note the right upper quadrant GSW. A lateral extension was made in this patient.

- Standard midline laparotomy incision
- Extension for major hepatic injury is either right subcostal or lateral T just above the umbilicus

Rapid Control of Liver Bleeding

- Perihepatic packing (Fig. 15.3) is the first critical technique to control active bleeding. Packing should be done to restore the anatomic position of the liver fragments as much as possible.

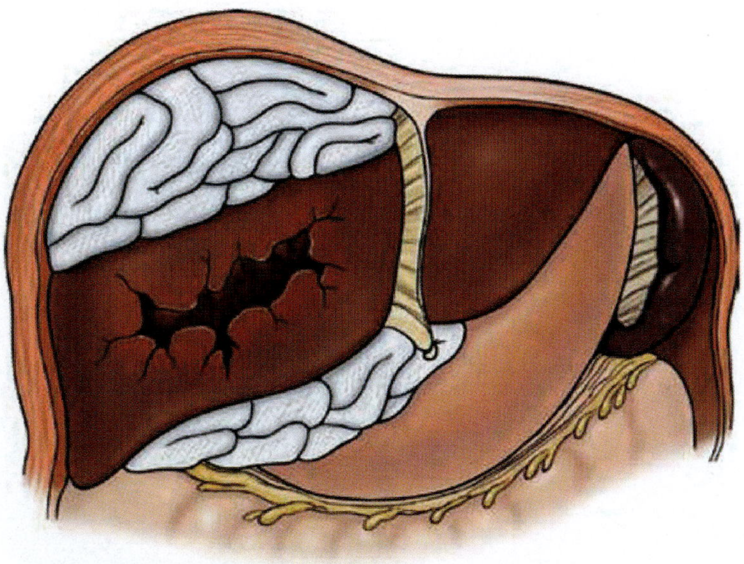

FIGURE 15.3 ▌ Perihepatic packing is done with the goal of reestablishing anatomic position of the liver fragments and bimanual anterior–posterior compression. From Abdomen and Pelvis. In: Feliciano DV, Mattox KL, Moore EE. eds. *Trauma, 9e*. McGraw Hill; 2021. Figure 44.

- For refractory bleeding, the porta hepatis is controlled with the Pringle maneuver. This is accomplished with a 1-inch Penrose drain around the liver hilum through the foramen of Winslow to encompass the hepatic artery, portal vein, and common bile duct (CBD). Tension to occlude blood flow is completed by applying a clamp to sinch the Penrose around the hilum (Fig. 15.4).

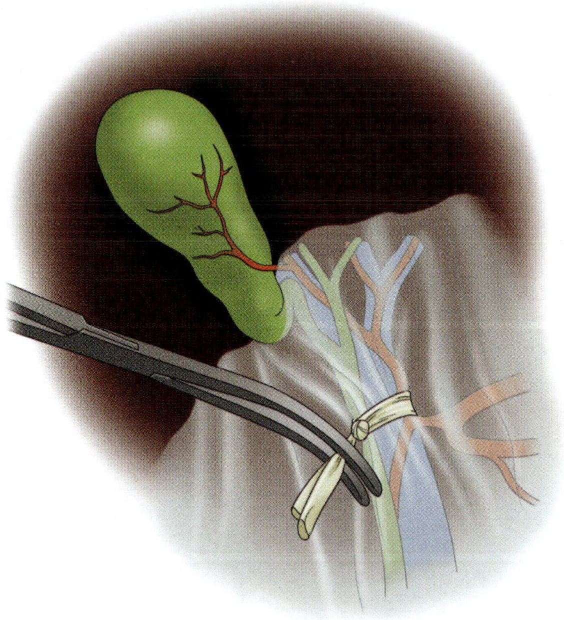

FIGURE 15.4 ❙ The Pringle maneuver is done to arrest vascular inflow to the liver, and includes encircling the hepatic artery, portal vein, and common bile duct.

- This is preferred over a vascular clamp or Rummel for Pringle, because both of those can fracture the intima of the hepatic artery when you are in a hurry and apply too much tension. The width of the Penrose will reduce this risk of injuring the artery. The tolerance to warm ischemia due to the Pringle maneuver is debated, most agree that the safe time is up to 30 minutes and can be reapplied with refractory bleeding after the liver is given time to recover after prolonged hilar occlusion.
- In patients who are hemodynamically unstable after attempted packing and Pringle has been applied, the best way to get control of bleeding from the liver when the source is unclear is total hepatic isolation (Fig. 15.5).

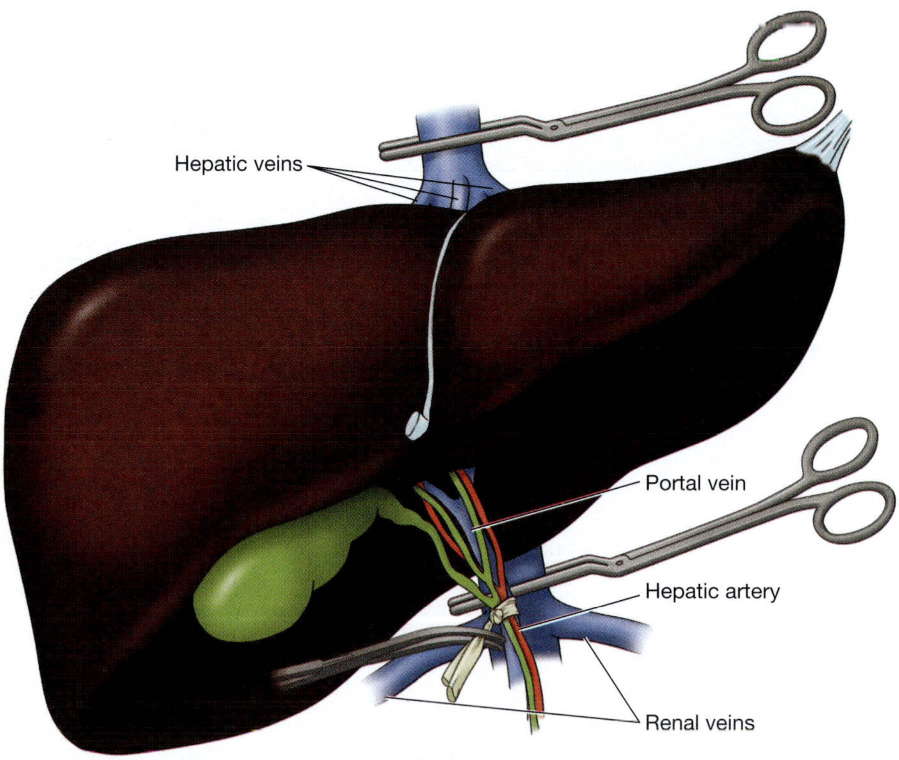

FIGURE 15.5 ❙ Total hepatic isolation to stop bleeding and identify the cause when packing and Pringle have failed.

This is accomplished by quickly cleaning off the inferior vena cava (IVC) above and below the liver to allow placement of vascular clamps (or Rummel tourniquets). The location of the lower clamp should be above the renal veins. The upper clamp is placed above the hepatic veins and will require taking down the falciform ligament and clearing the bare area of the liver to confirm the appropriate placement. These three occlusions (including Pringle) give total vascular control of the liver and allow time to figure out what and where the injury is located. If a large vena cava injury is identified, this should prompt urgent venovenous bypass if prolonged total liver isolation is anticipated (reviewed later).

Mobilization of the Liver

- Adequate mobilization of the liver is key to access for advanced surgical hemostasis. Systematic division of the right and left triangular and coronary ligaments as well as the falciform ligament (Fig. 15.6) are essential to enable manual delivery of the liver into the operative field.
- Extension into the chest is rarely required with appropriate ligamentous separation. A self-retaining retractor facilitates exposure (Fig. 15.7).

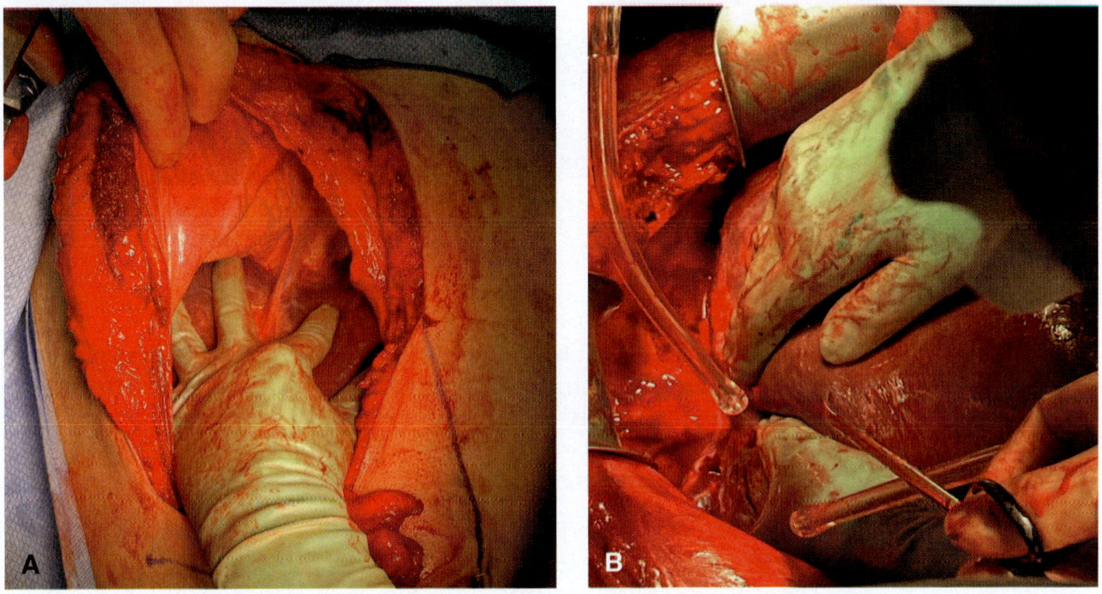

FIGURE 15.6 | Adequate mobilization of the liver for hemostasis requires division of the left (**A**) and right (**B**) triangular ligaments as well as the falciform ligament.

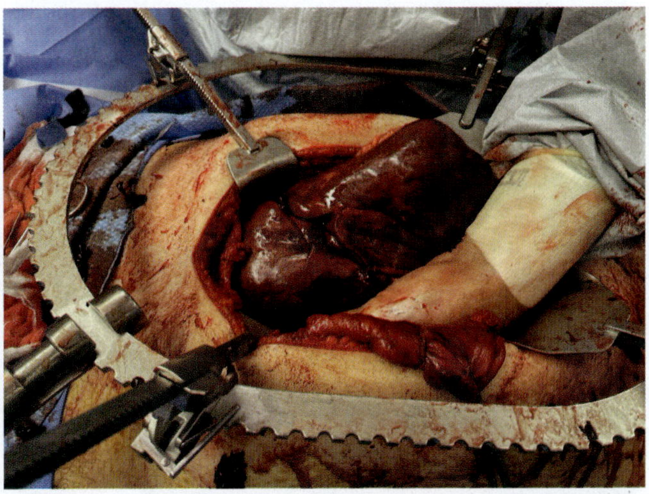

FIGURE 15.7 | A self-retaining retractor facilitates exposure of the seriously injured liver.

Nonanatomic Staple Resection of the Liver

- If parenchymal bleeding persists, direct access to the bleeding sites is the next step. While tractotomy was promoted a decade ago, the more effective approach is nonanatomic resection.
- The most expedient is staple resection of the fragmented liver (Fig. 15.8) with additional suturing of exposed vessels and bile ducts (Fig. 15.9).

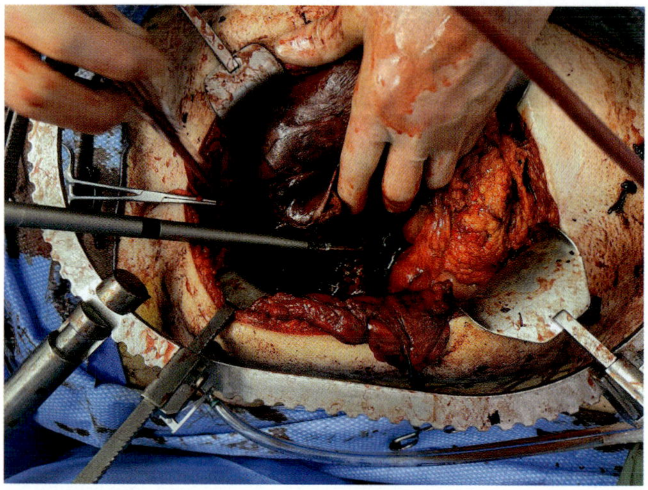

FIGURE 15.8 ▮ Nonanatomic hepatic resection is a rapid method to control complex parenchymal bleeding.

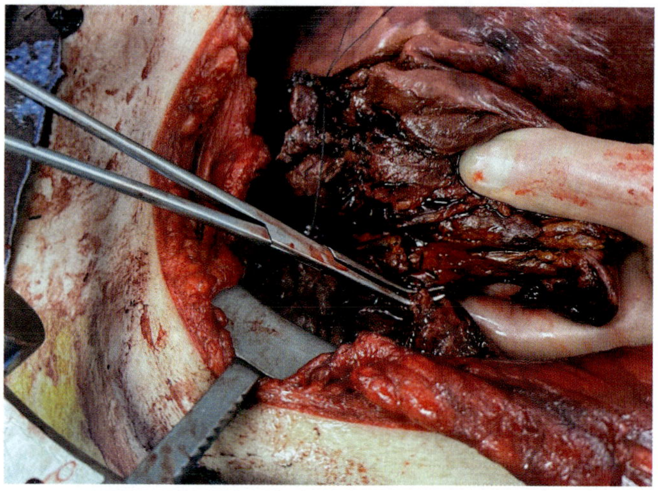

FIGURE 15.9 ▮ Individual blood vessels and bile ducts are suture ligated after exposure of the injury site.

- We prefer 2-0 silk tie sutures to clips for durability. An alternative approach for more peripheral injuries such as the left lateral lobe is to apply a Pringle and set the Bovie cautery to 100 and complete the parenchyma transection with suture ligation of vascular structures and argon beam for smaller bleeding vessels.

Porta Hepatis Isolation

- In the infrequent scenario of refractory lobar bleeding despite the previous efforts, selective hepatic arterial ligation should be considered.
- This is accomplished after hilar dissection and isolation of the lobar vessels (Fig. 15.10), and confirmation that selective occlusion controls the bleeding.
- Delayed lobar resection may be necessary if collateral blood flow and portal vein perfusion are disrupted due to the liver injury.

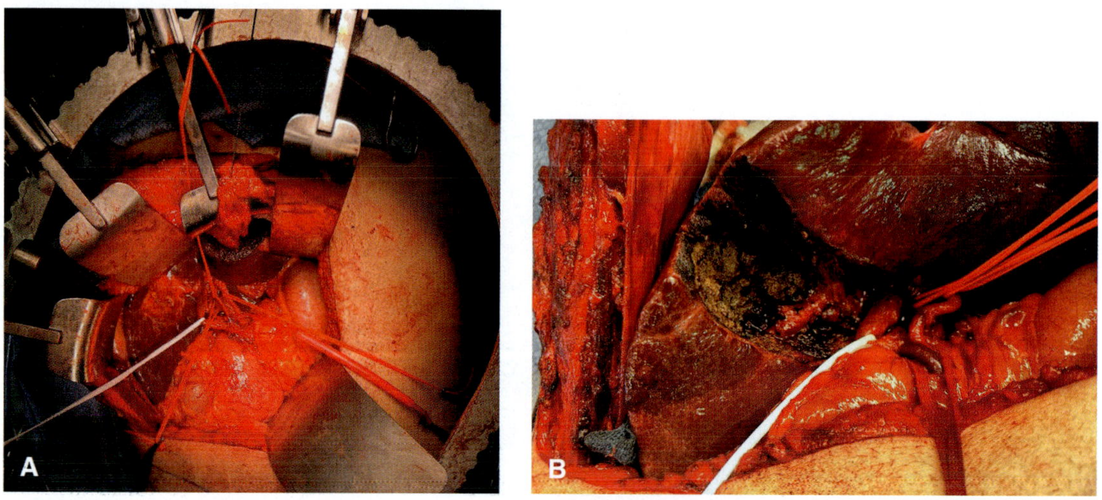

FIGURE 15.10 ▮ For refractory parenchymal bleeding, the portal structures should be separated and temporary hepatic arterial lobar occlusion done to determine if bleeding will respond to selective hepatic arterial ligation.

- The right and left branches of the hepatic artery provide arterial inflow to their respective halves of the liver.
- However, arterial supply to segment 4 can come originate from the right hepatic artery, which should be assessed if there is persistent bleeding from the left half after temporary occlusion of the left hepatic artery (Fig. 15.11).

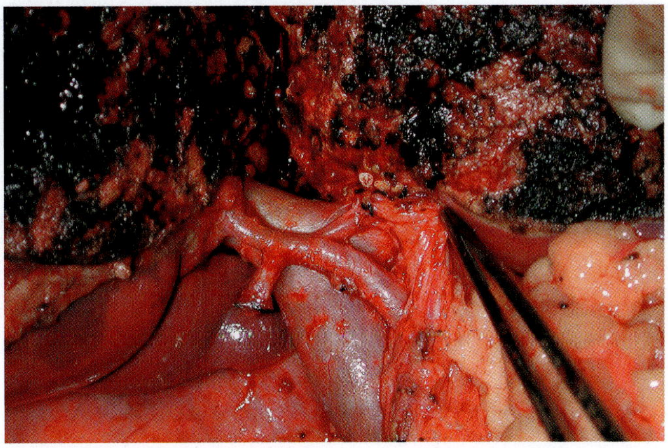

FIGURE 15.11 ▌ Example of a segment 4 artery branching from the right hepatic artery.

Transhepatic Balloon Occlusion

- A relatively common injury pattern following a hepatic gunshot wound (GSW) is a deep wound traversing the liver.
- The quickest and most effective method to control bleeding with an intact wound track is to place a balloon tamponade (Fig. 15.12).

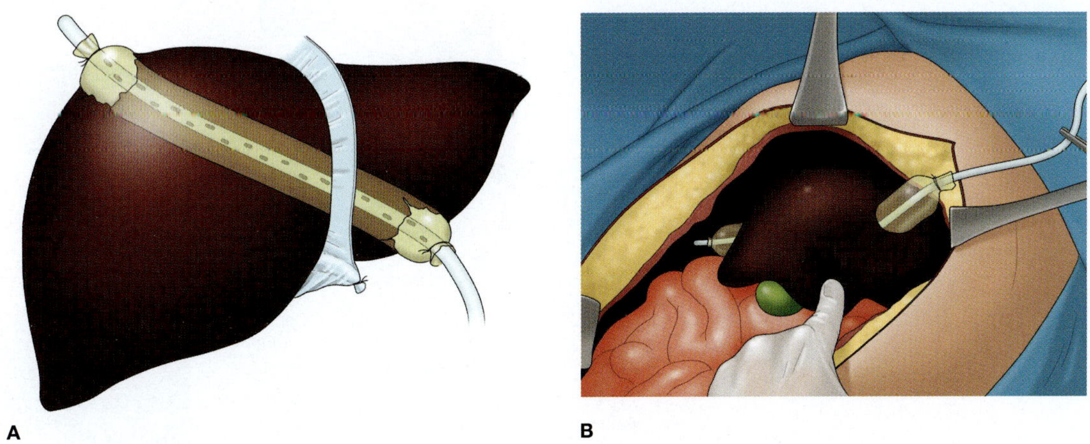

FIGURE 15.12 ▌ Transhepatic balloon occlusion (**A**) is effective for deep GSWs to the liver (**B**).

Evaluating the Biliary System

- Bile leaks after nonanatomic liver resection are common. There are multiple methods for identifying open biliary ducts.
- The least invasive technique is to squirt half-strength hydrogen peroxide on the cut edge of the liver.
- Open bile ducts will stain foaming peroxide with bile, making identification easier.
- If there is concern for additional leaks, infusion of methylene blue via the gallbladder while compressing the distal CBD is another effective technique (Fig. 15.13).
- If this method fails and there is still concern for ongoing leak, performing a cholecystectomy, and injecting air in the cystic duct with a 10-cc syringe with distal CBD compression can be performed to assess for air bubbles on the cut edge. This can be augmented via intraoperative cholangiogram if there are concerns for proximal large duct injury.

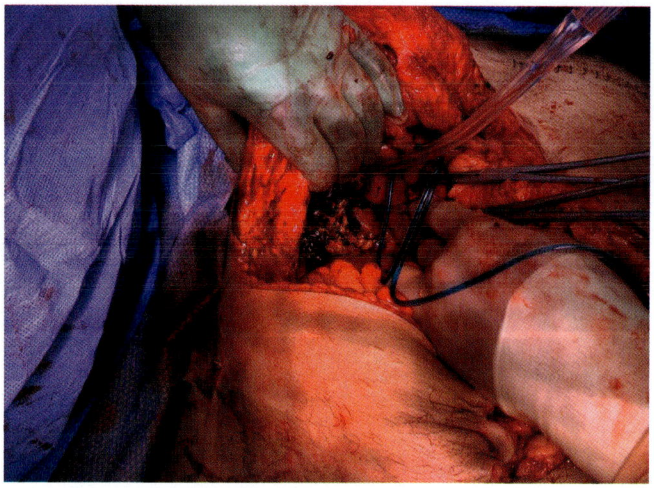

FIGURE 15.13 ▍ Evaluation for residual bile duct leaks can be accomplished by injecting methylene blue into the gall bladder while compressing the distal CBD.

Repair of Retrohepatic Vena Cava

- The reported mortality for retrohepatic IVC injury continues to exceed 85%, but much of that is due to late recognition.
- Lack of bleeding control with the Pringle maneuver is the hallmark of this infrequent injury. Injury of the retrohepatic IVC is challenging, and we believe is best approached with early venovenous bypass (Fig. 15.14) once hepatic bleeding is controlled with total hepatic vascular isolation, perihepatic packing and the patient is hemodynamically stable.

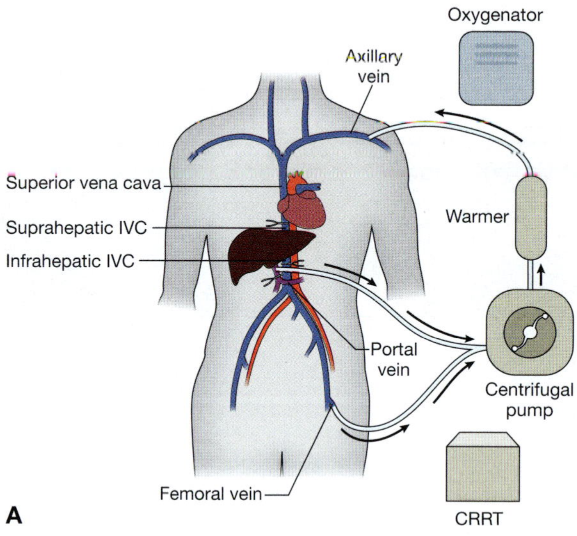

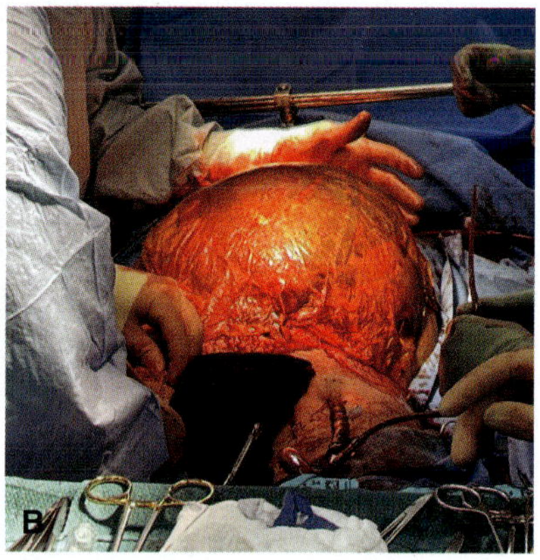

FIGURE 15.14 ▍ Management of the retrohepatic IVC can be very challenging, and we believe best approached with early venovenous bypass. (**A**) Schematic, (**B**) operative photograph.

- The approach to hemorrhage control in patients that are not amenable to surgical packing was previously described in the rapid control of liver bleeding.
- Most IVC injuries in patients who arrive alive to the hospital should be amenable to temporary packing control due to the low pressure of the venous system.
- With the demands for simultaneous effective compression of the liver to control bleeding and rapid initiation of venovenous bypass, a multidisciplinary team of trauma and transplant surgeons (Fig. 15.15) is optimal.
- Decompression of the portal system is accomplished with placement of a cannula in the IMV.
- The left femoral vein is accessed percutaneously and connected together with the IMV cannula. This provides outflow of the lower body for bypass and portal system. The left subclavian vein is then accessed for returning blood to the systemic circulation.

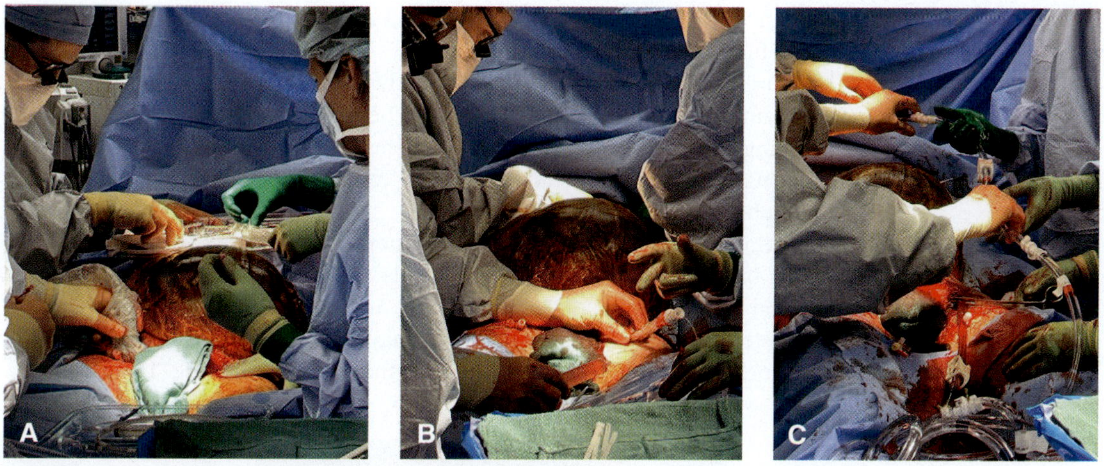

FIGURE 15.15 ▮ Due to the multiple challenges of controlling hepatic bleeding and initiating venovenous bypass, a multidisciplinary approach with trauma and transplant surgeons is optimal (as depicted in **A–C**).

- Bypass is initiated at a rate of 2.5 L/min and adjusted based on the patient's hemodynamics.
- Next, the suprahepatic IVC can be isolated and controlled between the liver and diaphragm (Fig. 15.16).
- A REBOA can be employed for control of the IVC above or below the liver (Fig. 15.17) when venous access is obtained in the right groin or neck.

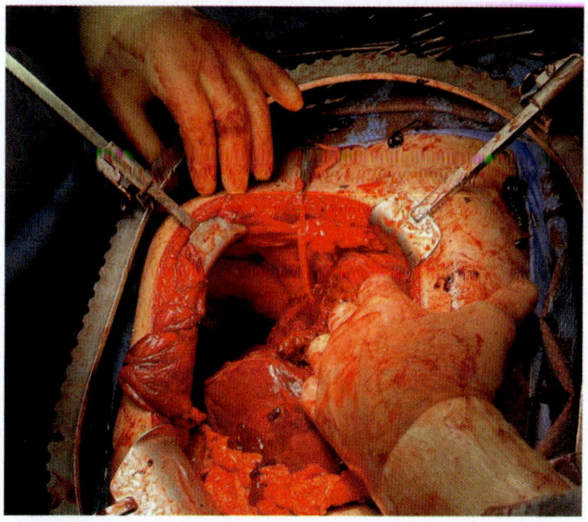

FIGURE 15.16 ▮ Occlusion of the suprahepatic IVC can be done between the liver and the diaphragm.

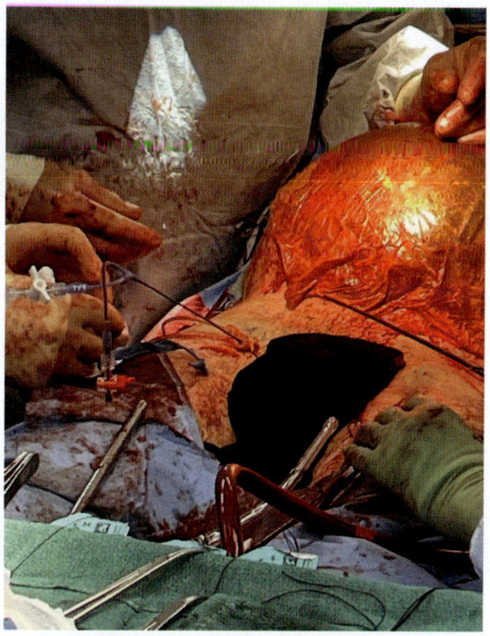

FIGURE 15.17 ▮ A REBOA can be used to occlude the IVC above or below the liver.

- When this is not available, Rummel tourniquets (or vascular clamps) above the left renal vein on the infrahepatic vena cava and above the hepatic veins on the suprahepatic vena cava can be accomplished in an expedited fashion.
- The approach to the retrohepatic IVC depends on the location of the injury.
- Almost all injuries will require mobilization of the right lobe of the liver for optimal visualization. Extrahepatic injuries can be repaired without a major resection of the liver, and once identified, IVC occlusion should be isolated to the area of injury to allow drainage of the hepatic veins.
- Intrahepatic injuries require extensive mobilization of the right lobe with ligation of the short hepatic veins.
- Adequate visualization may also require mobilization of the caudate lobe from the left side of the patient. When feasible, placing an additional Rummel tourniquet below the hepatic veins, and

release of the suprahepatic occlusion will allow for intermittent Pringle release to allow the liver to reperfuse while addressing the repair.

- IVC injuries in this region can be directly repaired with 4-0 Prolene suture if the injury is minimal in diameter, often associated with short hepatic vein injuries.
- Closing in a transverse orientation reduces the risk of stenosis.
- Alternatively, large injuries of the vena cava can be repaired with a bovine pericardium patch or interposition PTFE graft.
- Bleeding from the liver side can be temporarily addressed with manual compression.
- Most of the bleeding from the liver side is venous and can be suture ligated with the adjunct of topical hemostatic agents if needed.
- Persistent bleeding from the liver side may warrant a hepatectomy and may be indicative of hepatic vein or accessory hepatic vein injury in the parenchyma (Fig. 15.18).

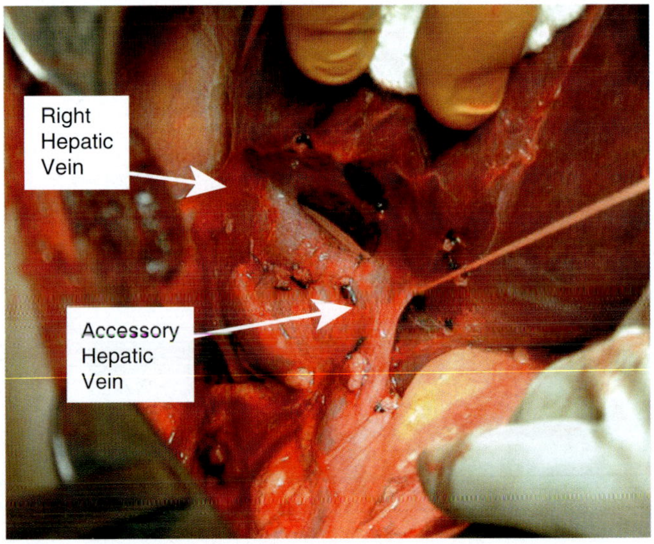

FIGURE 15.18 ▌ Example of an accessory segment 5 hepatic vein that if injured can be a source of refractory liver side bleeding after repair of the IVC.

HEPATIC TRANSPLANTATION

- Hepatic transplantation for prolonged ischemia or destructive injuries to the porta hepatis is well documented.
- Patients that lack traumatic brain injury or other major central nervous system injuries should be referred early to a transplant center for evaluation.
- Historically, these patients are referred late, as the determination of nonrecoverable hepatic injury is difficult to predict, due to the liver's regenerative properties.
- Delaying referral can result in the patient developing an infection or multiorgan failure making them ineligible for transplantation.
- Guidelines on transplant referral after traumatic liver injury are lacking and warrant evaluation, as the current outcomes in liver transplant posttraumatic injury are dismal.

Suggested Readings

Biffl WL, Moore EE, Franciose RJ. Venovenous bypass and hepatic vascular isolation as adjuncts in the repair of destructive wounds to the retrohepatic inferior vena cava. *J Trauma*. 1998;45(2):400–403.

Buckman RF Jr, Miraliakbari R, Badellino MM. Juxtahepatic venous injuries: a critical review of reported management strategies. *J Trauma*. 2000;48(2):978–984.

Kaltenborn A, Reichert B, Bourg CM, et al. Long-term outcome analysis of liver transplantation for severe hepatic trauma. *J Trauma Acute Care Surg*. 2013;75(5):864–869.

Kozar RA, Moore FA, Moore EE, et al. Western Trauma Association critical decisions in trauma: nonoperative management of adult blunt hepatic trauma. *J Trauma*. 2009;67(6):1144–1148.

Poggetti RS, Moore EE, Moore FA, Mitchell MB, Read RA. Balloon tamponade for bilobar transfixing hepatic gunshot wounds. *J Trauma*. 1992;33(5):694–697.

Chapter 16
Spleen

ERIC CAMPION AND ERNEST E. MOORE

PERIOPERATIVE CONSIDERATIONS

Procedure Rationale

- The spleen is one of the most commonly injured organs in the body. The first consideration during treatment of splenic injury is the hemodynamical stability of the patient. A hemodynamically stable patient with a splenic injury affords the treating surgeon the ability to thoughtfully choose among several therapeutic options. The most common treatment modality for the injured spleen is careful observation as the majority of splenic injuries are managed without surgery, and angioembolization should be considered for patients with severe splenic injuries or active contrast extravasation.
- Patients who have persistent hemodynamic compromise or bleeding requiring ongoing transfusion, warrant emergent operative evaluation. The younger the patient the more effort should be made to preserve as much spleen as possible, and autotransplantation if splenectomy is required.

Essential Equipment

- Headlight
- Ligasure device
- Argon beam coagulator
- Gel foam and Surgicel
- Large Zatinsky and assorted angled vascular clamps
- PDS, vicryl and silk suture

Positioning and Prepping

- Patient is positioned supine with both arms extended.
- Prep of the patient with unknown injuries includes the neck, chest, abdomen, and both legs to the knee.
- Radial arterial line and large upper torso venous access
- Bair hugger on lower extremities
- Blood products available

TECHNIQUE

Abdominal Incision

- Standard midline laparotomy incision is used for exploration of hemodynamically unstable patients.
- Left upper quadrant oblique incision is an option when injury is known prior to operation and limited to the spleen and distal pancreas.

Rapid Control of Splenic Bleeding

- Perisplenic packing is typically not effective in arresting hemodynamically significant bleeding from the spleen. Rapid mobilization and control of splenic vessels is preferred. With extensive bleeding a large Zatinsky clamp can be placed across the hilum for rapid control of bleeding, although this is a risk for pancreatic tail injury.

Mobilization of the Spleen

- Adequate mobilization of the spleen is key to evaluate a splenic injury (Fig. 16.1).

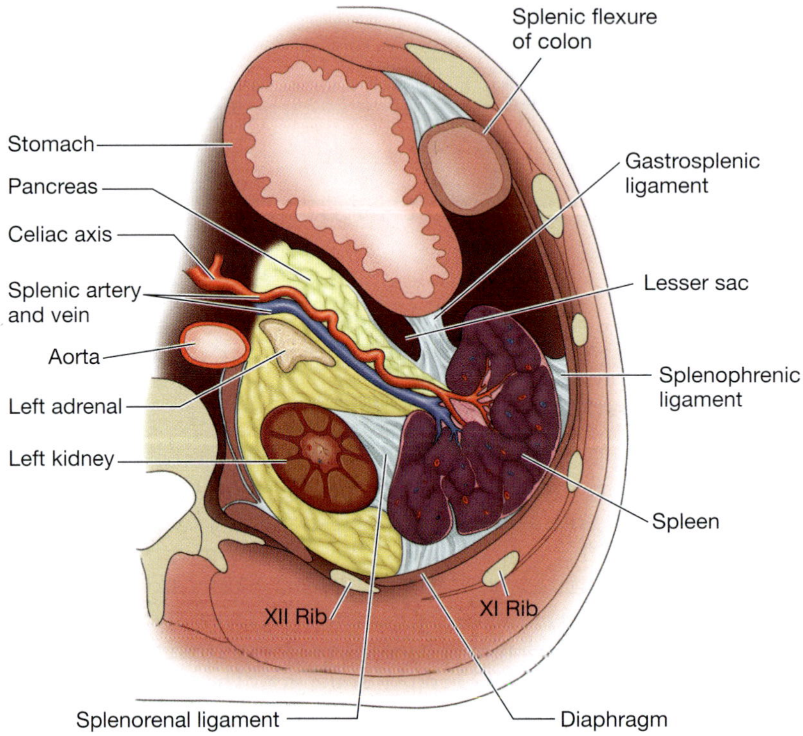

FIGURE 16.1 ❙ Anatomic relationship of the spleen to other structures.

- Mobilization of the spleen can be accomplished in a rapid fashion with the surgeon putting each of the splenic attachments on tension and exposing them for division sharply or with electrocautery by the assistant (Fig. 16.2).

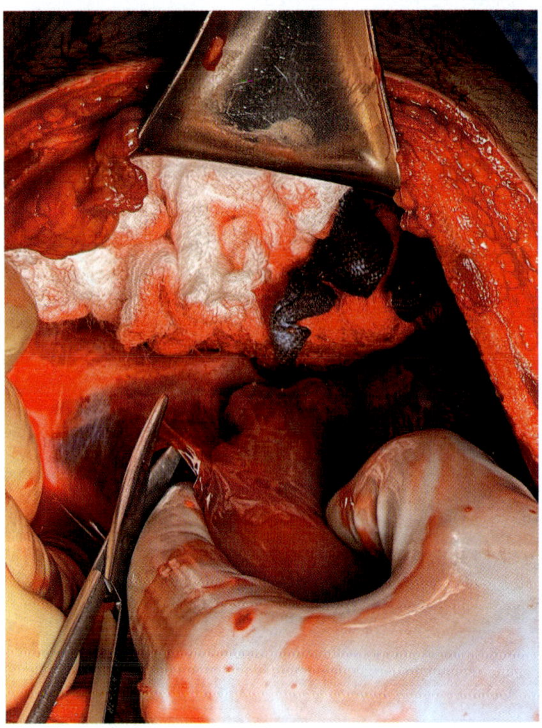

FIGURE 16.2 ❙ Retroperitoneal attachments to the splenic capsule are divided under visualization.

- The peritoneum should be divided 2 cm from the border of the spleen to avoid further injury to the spleen. The length and strength of these attachments can be highly variable. Careful exploration and division under visualization are advisable, particularly if splenic preservation is being entertained. This can be accomplished for the splenocolic, splenorenal, and splenophrenic ligaments.
- The short gastric vessels from the stomach need formal division which can be accomplished with clamps and ties or with an energy device such as the ligasure (Fig. 16.3).

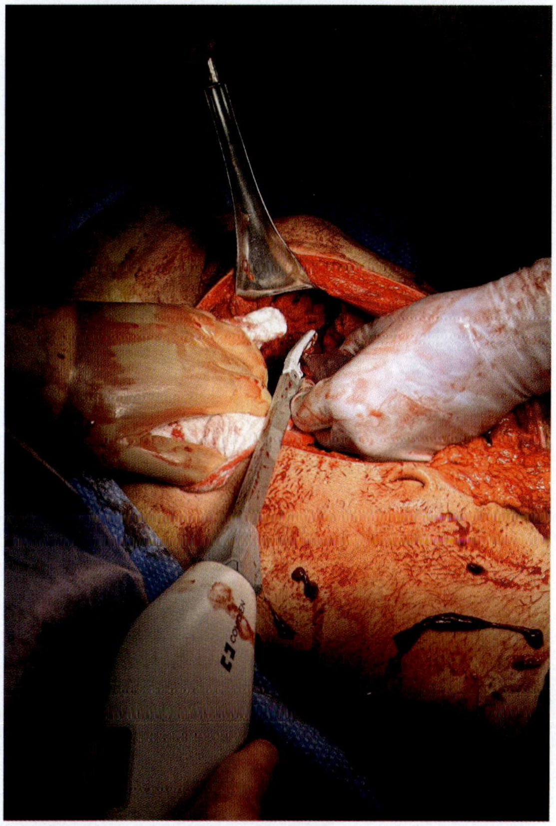

FIGURE 16.3 ▎Division of short gastric vessels with energy device.

- However, division of the short gastrics should be delayed until full inspection of the spleen has been performed if splenic preservation is being considered. When dividing the short gastrics care must be taken not to include the stomach wall in the ligature or energy device to avoid gastric injury.

Splenectomy versus Splenic Preservation

Once the spleen is mobilized it should be fully visualized, including the posterior hilum. The extent of splenic injury as well as the hemodynamic status of the patient should be taken into account to determine whether splenectomy or splenorrhaphy should be undertaken. While splenic preservation is preferred, rapid splenectomy is preferred in patients with multiple serious injuries or severe hemodynamic instability refractory to resuscitation.

Splenectomy

TIP

The anatomic relation of the splenic artery and vein with respect to the pancreas is variable (Fig. 16.4). While the splenic artery is often separated superiorly, the splenic vein is typically within the pancreatic capsule inferiorly.

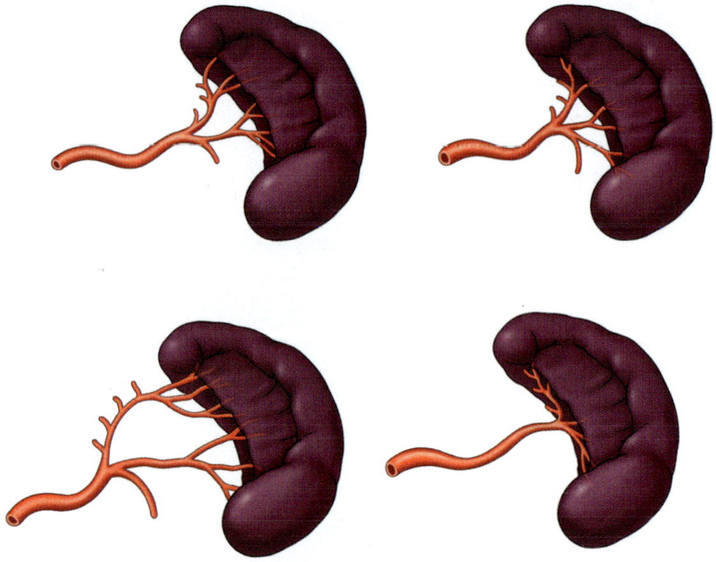

FIGURE 16.4 ■ Splenic artery anatomy variability.

- If not previously done, rapid suture ligation or division of the short gastrics with an energy device should be performed. The splenic artery and vein should be individually ligated to prevent arteriovenous fistula. In order to accomplish rapid control, a large Zatinsky vascular clamp (or surgeon's hand) is placed at the hilum to control major bleeding from the spleen. The vessels can then be individually clamped and suture ligated. If visualization is difficult with the spleen in situ, the spleen can be resected with a large vascular clamp across the hilum or a gastrointestinal anastomosis (GIA) stapler can be used in emergent situations in which rapid control is needed (Fig. 16.5).

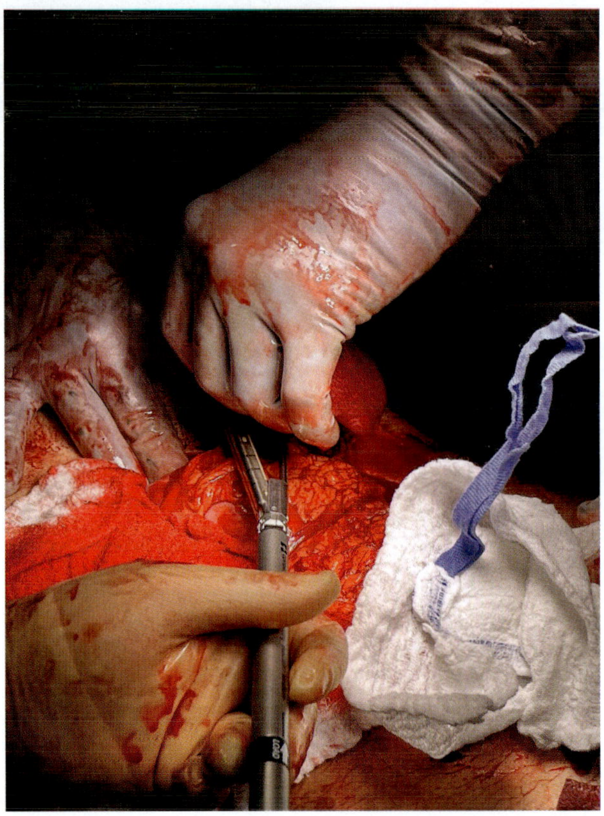

FIGURE 16.5 ■ Stapler ligation of splenic artery proximal to clamp.

- This can aid in visualizing the distal splenic vessel which can be ligated just proximal to the clamp. If a stapler is used, consideration for individually ligating the vein and artery once the clinical situation allows can prevent arteriovenous fistula. Care is taken to avoid any damage to the tail of the pancreas. Drains are not advisable unless significant injury to the pancreatic tail is suspected.

Splenorrhapy

- If in the surgeon's judgment the patient is sufficiently stable and the situation allows for splenorrhaphy, that is the preferred approach. Splenorrhaphy should be approached in a stepwise fashion.

Regional Hemostasis

- If the spleen has capsular tear this may be able to be controlled with simple measures such as argon beam coagulator with or without hemostatic adjuncts. A variety of topical hemostatic adjuncts including Surgicell, evarrest, Gel foam, and thrombin spray can be employed for surface bleeding.

Partial Splenic Resection

- Deeper injuries to the spleen can be managed with a combination of techniques. Fractures of the spleen can be repaired with pledgeted sutures or a partial splenectomy can be performed. Partial splenectomy takes advantage of the spleens typically segmental vascular supply in which damaged part of the spleen can be resected while remaining splenic parenchyma survives on a separate blood supply.
- Pledgeted mattress sutures are used to repair the cut edge the partial splenectomy (Fig. 16.6).

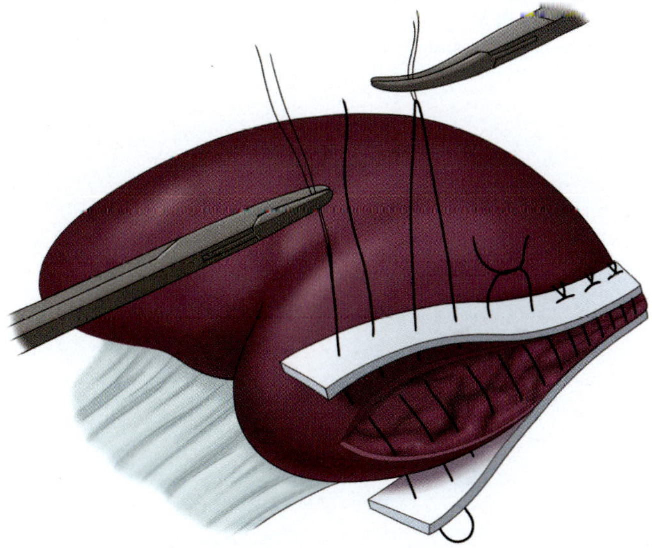

FIGURE 16.6 ▌ Pledgeted suture placement across cut edge of spleen.

Splenic Autotransplantation

- An option after splenectomy is autotransplantation of splenic tissue in small pieces into multiple pouches of the omentum. The parenchyma of the spleen is divided into five segments 20 mm × 20 mm × 5 mm in size.
- These segments are secured in greater omental pouches and secured with silk suture (Fig. 16.7).
- Clips should be attached to the borders of the omental pouch for later identification.

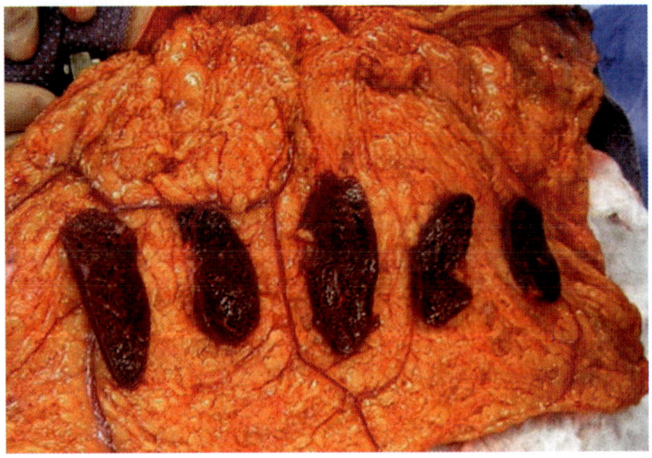

FIGURE 16.7 ▌ Autotransplantation of the spleen into small pouches.

Suggested Readings

Coccolini F, Montori G, Catena F, et al. Splenic trauma: WSES classification and guidelines for adult and pediatric patients. *World J Emerg Surg*. 2017;12:40.

Senekjian L, Cuschieri J, Robinson BRH. Splenic artery angioembolization for high-grade splenic injury: Are we wasting money? *Am J Surg*. 2021;221(1):204–210.

Skattum J, Naess PA, Gaarder C. Non-operative management and immune function after splenic injury. *Br J Surg*. 2012;99(Suppl 1):59.

Surendran A, Smith M, Houli N, et al. Splenic autotransplantation: a systematic review. *ANZ J Surg*. 2020;90(4):460–466.

Zarzaur BL, Kozar R, Myers JG, et al. The splenic injury outcomes trial: an American Association for the Surgery of Trauma multi-institutional study. *J Trauma Acute Care Surg*. 2015;79(3):335–334.

Chapter 17
Duodenum and Pancreas

NICOLE L. WERNER AND ERNEST E. MOORE

PERIOPERATIVE CONSIDERATIONS

Procedure Rationale

- The duodenum and pancreas are retroperitoneal structures conveying bioactive digestive contents and are surrounded by major vascular conduits.
- Injuries to these structures are relatively infrequent due to the protection by the spine, retroperitoneal musculature, and overlying abdominal viscera.
- On the other hand, penetrating wounds to the duodenum and pancreas are often associated with life-threatening bleeding, and delayed recognition of blunt injuries of the duodenum and pancreas may result in major complications.
- A thorough knowledge of the regional anatomy (Fig. 17.1) is essential for rapid exposure of associated bleeding and systematic evaluation of the duodenum and pancreas to exclude an occult injury.

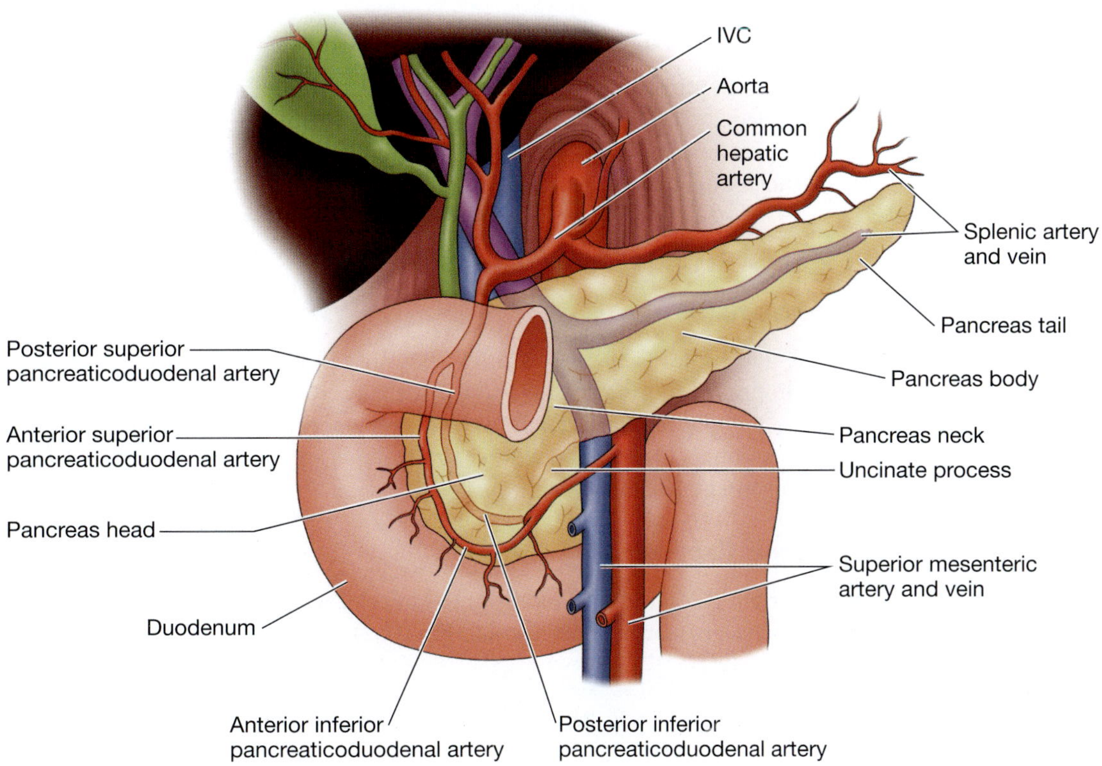

FIGURE 17.1 ▎The duodenum and pancreas are retroperitoneal structures surrounded by major blood vessels.

Essential Equipment

TIP

All of the items should be readily accessible, but not all must be opened immediately upon patient entry into the operating room.

- Standard laparotomy set
- Laparotomy pads
- GIA and TA staplers (Coviden, Mansfield, MA)
- Vascular shunts, in a variety of sizes: Pruitt-Inahara, 8 to 10 Fr (LeMaitre Vascular, Inc., Burlington, MA)
- Impact LigaSure (Coviden, Mansfield, MA)
- Harmonic scalpel (Ethicon, Raritan, NJ)
- Coagulation agents including QuikClot hemostatic dressing (Z-Medical, Wallingford, CT) and Evarrest fibrin sealant patch (Ethicon, Inc., Somerville, NJ)
- 2-0 and 3-0 silk sutures and ties
- 2-0, 3-0, and 4-0 Prolene sutures
- 0, 3-0, 4-0, 5-0, 6-0 PDS sutures
- Fogarty embolectomy catheters Size 2 & 3 Fr.
- Metzenbaum scissors (blunt tipped for dissection)
- Potts scissors (for incising and excising vascular wall)
- No. 11 scalpel blade
- Castroviejo needle driver
- Microvascular forceps
- Bulldog soft vascular clamps (small vessels)
- Profunda vascular clamps (right angled and straight)
- Satinsky-shaped clamps (side biting)
- DeBakey clamps (serrated rows of interdigitating teeth)
- Moistened umbilical tape, thin rubber catheters, and silastic vessel loops
- BioGlue surgical adhesive (CryoLife, Kennesaw, GA)

Patient Positioning

- Patients should be positioned and prepped for a standard laparotomy for trauma, with both arms extended.
- An upper midline incision is employed. A self-retaining retractor is helpful due to the deep location of the duodenum and pancreas.

TECHNIQUE

Duodenum

- The duodenum is 30 cm (12 fingerbreadths) in length and consists of four segments. D1 is intraperitoneal beginning at the pylorus to a point where it crosses the common bile duct (CBD) and the gastroduodenal artery (GDA). D2 is retroperitoneal and includes the ampulla of Vater. D3 is the retroperitoneal transverse section to the superior mesenteric vein (SMV). D4 is from the SMV to the ligament of Treitz.

Duodenal Exposure

- The right colon is mobilized from the inferior aspect of the duodenum.
- A Kocher maneuver is performed (Fig. 17.2).

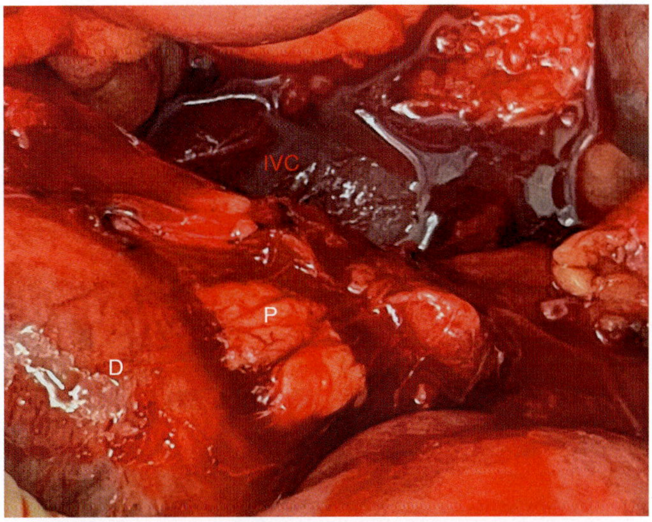

FIGURE 17.2 | The Kocher maneuver allows for posterior inspection of the C-loop of duodenum (D) and pancreatic head (P). Shown is the pancreaticoduodenal complex that has been mobilized and rotated medially, exposing the IVC.

- The lateral peritoneal attachments of the C-loop of the duodenum are divided with scissors.
- The retroperitoneal attachments between the C-loop of the duodenum, pancreatic head, and CBD are divided with blunt dissection. Dissection continues until the inferior vena cava is visualized.
- The Cattell–Braasch maneuver may be required to allow additional mobilization of the duodenum beyond the Kocher maneuver.
  - The right colon from the cecum through hepatic flexure is mobilized starting laterally at the white line of Toldt.
  - The retroperitoneal membrane is detached from the posterior aspect of the small bowel mesentery, starting at the ileocecal region and extending toward the ligament of Treitz.
- The ligament of Treitz should be sharply divided for full exposure of D4 when needed.

TIP

The superior mesenteric artery and vein prevent complete mobilization of the duodenum and should be carefully avoided during exposure of the duodenum. The duodenum is well vascularized allowing for repair in most circumstances.

Duodenal Repair

- Primary repair is preferred for most partial circumference injuries (Fig. 17.3).

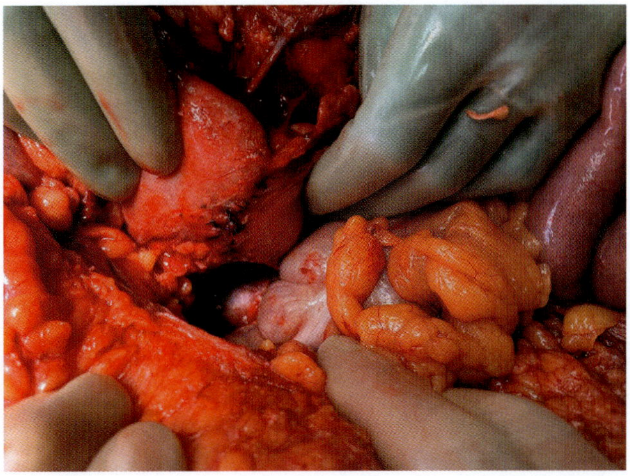

FIGURE 17.3 | Primary repair is preferred for most partial circumference injuries of the duodenum. Shown is antimesenteric suture repair of a D2 injury.

- Devitalized tissue is debrided sharply.
- Primary anastomosis is done with single-layer running 3-0 PDS. The wound should be closed in a direction that results in the largest residual lumen.
- Omental pedicle can be used to buttress repair if the tissue is tenuous.

- For near-complete transections without involvement of the ampulla, end-to-end duodenoduodenostomy may be performed if the ends can be mobilized without tension:
  - Complete the transection of the duodenum, after confirming where the ampulla is located.
  - Debride any devitalized tissue.
  - End-to-end, single-layer anastomosis is created with a running 3-0 PDS (Fig. 17.4).

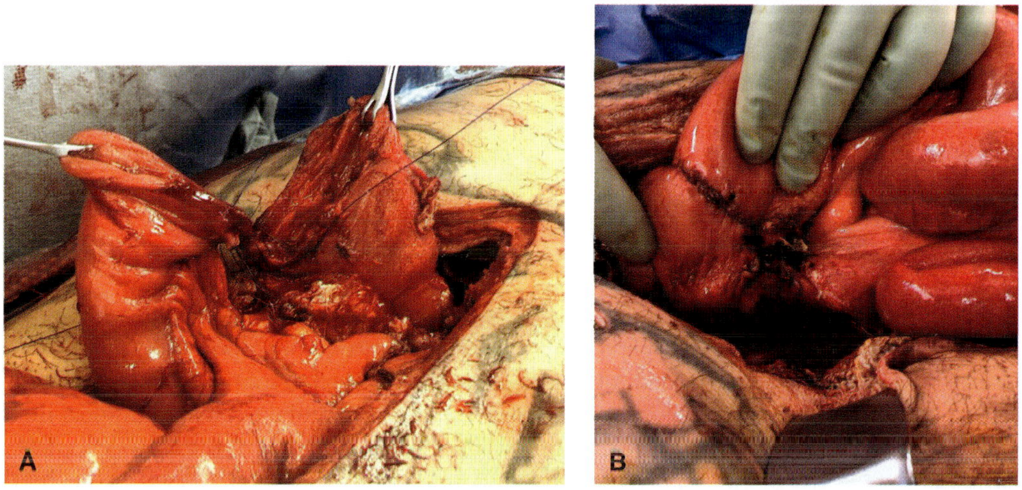

FIGURE 17.4 ▌ **A:** The two ends of duodenum grasped with babcock forceps. **B:** Primary anastomosis with running 3-0 PDS. The transected duodenum should be reanastomosed if the ampulla is intact; that is, pancreatic duct and CBD are intact.

- Consideration is given to placing a feeding tube past the site for extensive injuries.
- There should be no tension on the repair after completion; if there will be tension, the duodenum should be reconstructed with a Roux limb (see below).

Duodenal Reconstruction with Roux Limb

- The Roux limb reconstruction of the duodenum is ideal for large antimesenteric injuries in D1 to D3 (Fig. 17.5).

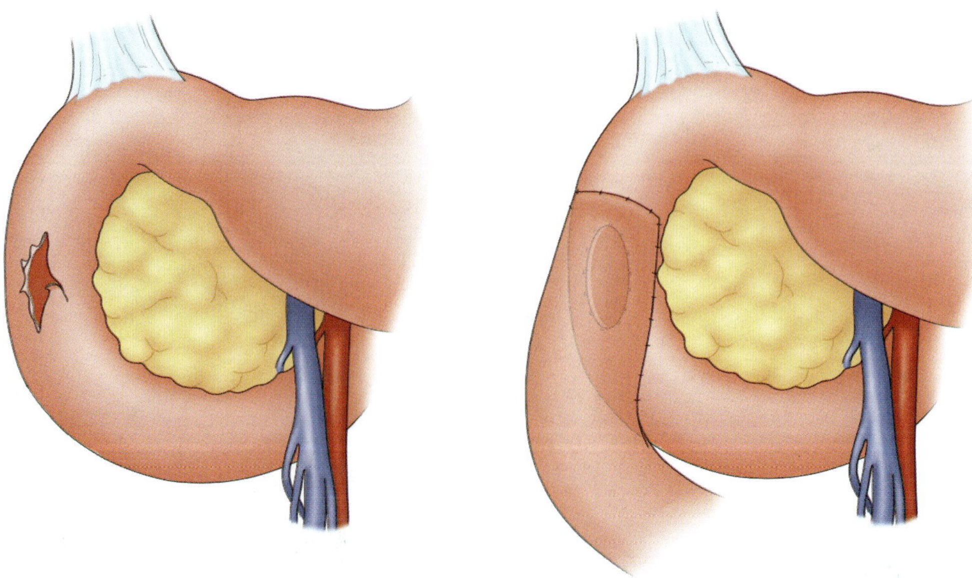

FIGURE 17.5 ▌ Roux-en-Y duodenojejunostomy is useful for closure of large duodenal injuries involving the antimesenteric D1 to D3 when primary repair is not feasible.

- Debride the edges of the wound back to viable tissue.
- Divide the jejunum 30 cm distal to the ligament of Treitz to form a Roux limb.
- The colonic mesentery is opened to the right of the middle colic artery and the Roux limb is brought through this defect.
- The Roux limb is sewn to the duodenal defect in an end-to-side fashion to maximize the duodenal lumen.
  - The Roux limb should be positioned over the duodenal defect in a configuration without tension.
  - The Roux limb enterotomy is created with electrocautery to match the size of the duodenal defect.
  - A single-layer anastomosis is sewn with a running 3-0 PDS suture.
- The jejunojejunostomy is created in an end-to-side fashion.
  - 3-0 Silk sutures are used as stay sutures to align the two pieces of bowel.
  - A single-layer anastomosis is sewn with a running 3-0 PDS suture.
- The colonic mesentery defect is closed with running 3-0 Vicryl suture to prevent internal hernia formation.
- A feeding tube is guided past the duodenal reconstruction into the proximal jejunum.

Pancreas

- The pancreas is 15 to 20 cm in length, 3 to 4 cm in width, and 1 to 1.5 cm in depth. The head of the pancreas is within the C-loop of the duodenum and surrounds the distal CBD. The uncinate process partially encloses the SMV and SMA.
- The neck of the pancreas is the thinnest portion and overlies the superior mesenteric vessels. The tail is posterior to the stomach and extends into the splenic hilum. The main pancreatic duct transverses the entire length of the pancreas and is roughly in the center of the gland.
- The main duct enters the left side of the CBD to form the ampulla of Vater. The accessory duct of Santorini enters the duodenum separately at the minor papilla.

Pancreatic Exposure

- Anterior pancreas (Fig. 17.6):

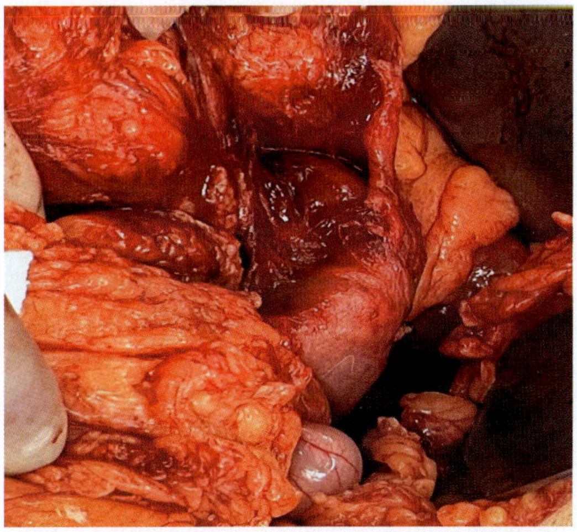

FIGURE 17.6 | Anterior exposure of the pancreas is accomplished via the lesser sac. Anterior exposure of the head of the pancreas with blunt injury.

  - The right colon and transverse mesocolon are mobilized from the head of the pancreas.
  - The lesser sac is entered by dividing the gastrocolic ligament with LigaSure and retracting the transverse colon and omentum inferiorly. This exposes the body and tail.
- Posterior pancreas:
  - The posterior pancreatic head is evaluated with a Kocher maneuver (see Duodenal exposure).
  - For the body of the pancreas, divide the retroperitoneal attachments to the pancreas starting at its inferior border and working superiorly, being careful to avoid the splenic vein, which is positioned posterior and inferior to the gland. The splenic artery is typically separated from the pancreas superiorly, but may be within the pancreatic capsule.
  - The spleen can be mobilized medially to evaluate the posterior pancreatic tail.

Distal Pancreatectomy

- In emergent conditions, distal pancreatectomy is completed with the attached spleen (Fig. 17.7).

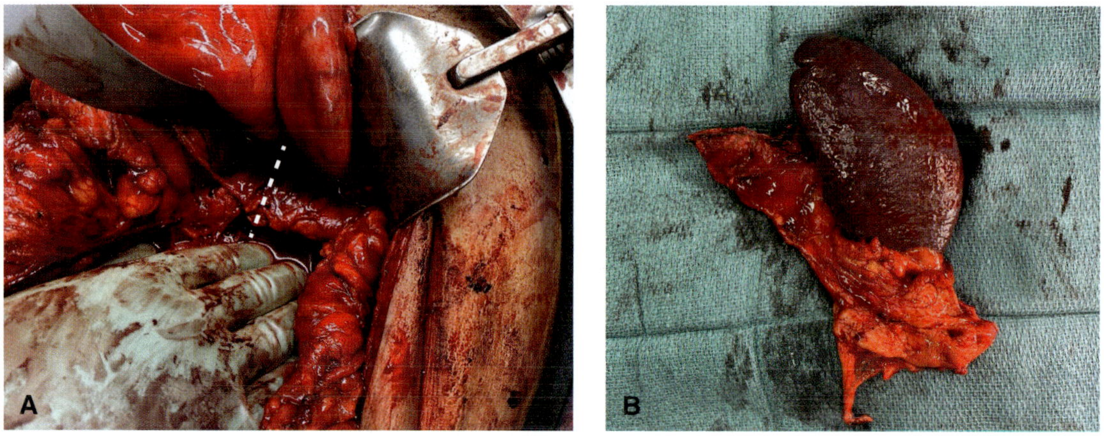

FIGURE 17.7 ❙ Distal pancreatectomy is performed for pancreatic duct injuries distal to the neck of the pancreas. The pancreatic resection line is shown in (**A**) and specimen containing the distal pancreas and spleen in (**B**). Distal pancreatectomy with splenectomy is appropriate in hemodynamically unstable patients, but splenic preservation is preferred for all others.

- Exposure to the body and tail of the pancreas is obtained.
- The splenic artery is dissected and encircled with a vessel loop to avoid injury and for rapid occlusion in the event of bleeding.
- Identification of the laceration is critical and facilitated by imaging prior to laparotomy.

TIP

If integrity of the pancreatic duct is uncertain, a needle cholangiogram can be performed by placing an 18-gauge angiocatheter in the fundus of the gallbladder and secured with a purse-string suture. Pressure is applied to the CBD proximal to the juncture of the cystic duct, while 30 mL of full strength contrast is injected. A pancreaticogram is obtained more than 75% of the time.

- The short gastric vessels are divided using the LigaSure.
- Dissect the pancreas from its retroperitoneal attachments, starting from the inferior border. The splenic vein is identified during this dissection as it lays on the posterior surface of the pancreas. The splenic vein is elevated with the pancreas.
- The lienorenal and lienophrenic attachments are divided and the spleen is freed from the posterior abdominal wall. (See Chapter 16.) This should allow the spleen and distal pancreas to be reflected medially.
- Suture ligation of the splenic artery and vein are done 1 cm proximal to the level of planned transection. The artery is doubly secured with a stick tie and free tie. A medium clip placed at the splenic artery stump can be helpful postoperatively for identification.
- Pancreatic transection is performed with a TA stapler using a 4.8-mm staple load fired just proximal to the site of injury.
- If the duct is visible, it should be ligated with a 4-0 PDS horizontal mattress suture.
- BioGlue can be placed over transected end of the pancreas if there is tenuous tissue.
- The role of drains following pancreatic resection is controversial, but most evidence supports placing a drain with early removal. A 10-Fr flat Jackson-Pratt drain is placed in the resection bed.

Spleen Preserving Distal Pancreatectomy

TIP

Splenic preservation is desirable when performing a distal pancreatectomy due to reduced infectious complications.

- Identifying the injury and mobilizing the body and tail of the pancreas are done as described above.
- The spleen is left in situ with its various ligaments to facilitate dissection and prevent subsequent torsion.
- The splenic vein is carefully preserved by elevating the pancreas and leaving the vein in place.
- Branch vessels from the splenic artery and vein are controlled as they are encountered with 3-0 silk suture ligation or harmonic scalpel.
- Dissection of the pancreas from the retroperitoneal attachments is continued cephalad until the superior border is reached. Often there is a space between the splenic artery and the superior aspect of the gland. The remainder of the splenic artery along the body and tail of the pancreas is dissected out.
- Pancreatic transection is performed as described above.
- In the event the splenic artery and vein cannot be preserved, the spleen can be salvaged by maintaining the short gastric blood supply.

Midpancreatic Resection with Roux Limb

- Exposure to the head, body, and tail of the pancreas is done as described above.
- The proximal splenic artery is encircled with a vessel loop.
- The pancreas is dissected from its retroperitoneal attachments, starting from the inferior border, with careful attention to leave the splenic vein in place.
- The proximal pancreas is transected with a TA stapler using a 4.8 mm staple load.
- The distal pancreas is transected with a scalpel.
- The jejunum is divided 30 cm distal to the ligament of Treitz using a GIA Blue (3.5-mm) load stapler.
- The colonic mesentery is opened, and the Roux limb is brought through this defect.
- The Roux limb is sewn to the distal pancreas using an ink-well technique in an end-to-end two-layer anastomosis, after placing a 5-Fr pediatric feeding tube into the pancreatic duct and securing it in place with a 4-0 PDS suture.
  - The inner row consists of anterior and posterior 2-0 PDS traction sutures approximately 1 cm from the cut edge of the pancreas. The sutures are then placed 2 cm from the edge of the jejunal limb to facilitate ink-well of the pancreas, and tied once the outer posterior sutures are placed (Fig. 17.8).

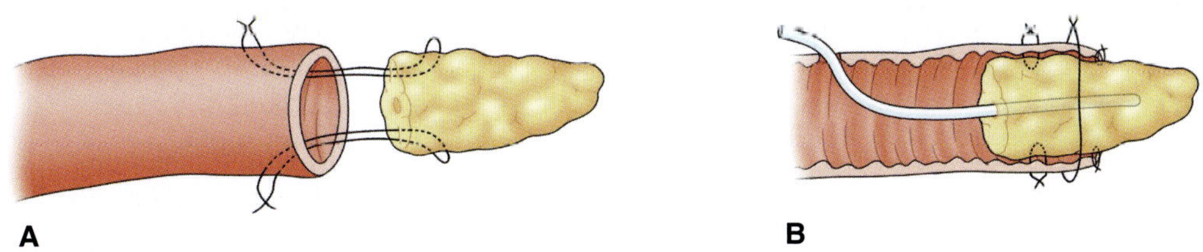

FIGURE 17.8 ▌ The inkwell technique for a pancreaticojejunostomy is shown in (**A**). Due to high risk of pancreatic leak following trauma, we add pancreatic banding to an exteriorized pancreatic duct stent (**B**).

  - The outer posterior row is 3-0 silk 2 cm from the pancreatic edge to the end of the jejunal limb.
  - The outer anterior row is 3-0 silk suture placed between pancreatic parenchyma and Roux limb approximately 2 cm from the cut edge. This completes the ink well.
  - For pancreas that have a high risk for leak; that is, soft gland and <3 mm duct, which is typical following injury, we place a 5-Fr feeding tube into the duct and exteriorize it via the jejunal limb and place a banding suture of 2-0 PDS over the ink-well portion of the pancreas (Fig. 17.8).
- The jejunojejunostomy is created in an end-to-side fashion.
  - 2-0 Silk sutures are used as stay sutures to align the two pieces of bowel.
  - A single-layer anastomosis is sewn with a running 3-0 PDS suture.
- The colonic mesentery defect is closed with running 3-0 Vicryl suture to prevent internal hernia formation.
- An alternative is pancreaticogastrostomy, which has equivalent results.

Duodenal Preserving Pancreatic Head Resection

TIP

Duodenal preservation can be accomplished when there is a destructive injury to the head of the pancreas but preserved CBD.

- The CBD enters the ampulla superior and posterior, integrity is critical to confirm for duodenal preservation. A cholangiogram can be performed via the gall bladder as described above.
- Exposure of the pancreas to head and body is performed.
- Identify the SMV at the inferior border of the pancreas and develop the plane posterior to the pancreatic neck.
- Transection line is determined by the extent of the injury.
- 2-0 PDS stay sutures placed on superior and inferior borders of the pancreas are followed by sharp dissection of the pancreatic neck with a scalpel. The sutures on the distal side can be used for the ink-well pancreaticojejunal anastomosis as described above.
- The pancreatic head is removed with a Harmonic scalpel with careful dissection to avoid injury to the CBD.
- A Roux limb is created as described above and placed over the distal pancreas.
- The distal pancreaticojejunal anastomosis is completed as discussed above.
- The necessity for a proximal pancreaticojejunal anastomosis is controversial, but we prefer a second opening in the Roux limb to the pancreatic head remnant: One layer, running 3-0 PDS suture. Alternatively, if the pancreatic duct is clearly visible and the remnant pancreas is small, the pancreatic duct can be ligated with a 4-0 PDS and the second anastomosis avoided.
- A 10-Fr flat Jackson-Pratt is placed adjacent to the pancreaticojejunostomy.

Combined Injuries of the Duodenum and Pancreas

- The C-loop of the duodenum and head of the pancreas have a shared blood supply through the superior and inferior pancreaticoduodenal arteries (Fig. 17.1).
- Consequently, a destructive injury to the C-loop or pancreatic head often necessitates a combined resection. However, nonresectional alternatives can be employed for less severe injuries.

Pyloric Exclusion with Gastrojejunostomy

- A 6-cm gastrostomy incision is made on the greater curvature of the stomach adjacent to the pylorus.
- The pylorus is identified through the interior of the stomach and grasped with a Babcock forceps (Fig. 17.9).

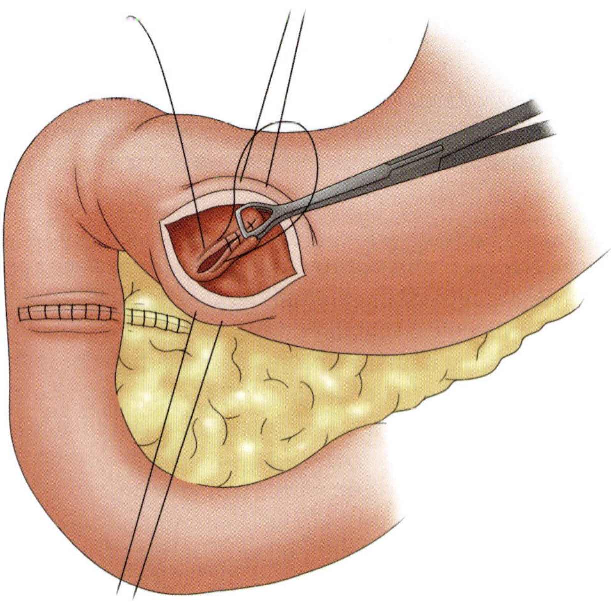

FIGURE 17.9 ▌ Pyloric exclusion consists of closing the pylorus to divert gastric contents, and creating a loop gastrojejunostomy for gastric emptying.

- A 0 PDS purse string is placed around the pylorus and tied to close off the gastric outlet. Sutures should be placed full thickness.
- A side-to-side gastrojejunostomy is formed by bringing up a loop jejunum (approximately 30 cm from the ligament of Treitz) to anastomose to the gastrostomy. The anastomosis is formed using a single-layer, continuous 3-0 PDS suture.
- Consideration is given to placing a feeding tube distal to the gastrojejunostomy.

Pancreaticoduodenectomy (First Stage)

- Pancreaticoduodenectomy (Whipple procedure) may be necessary for destructive wounds of the head of the pancreas and adjacent duodenum, particularly with ampullary involvement. Due to the typical associated bleeding and physiologic consequences, the trauma Whipple is usually considered damage control where resection is completed at the initial operation followed by a second operation for delayed reconstruction.

TIP

The priority of the initial operation for a trauma Whipple is to terminate bleeding and, thus, the approach differs from an elective resection where the extent of malignancy is critical to define. While there has been enthusiasm for a pylorus-preserving resection, the advantages have not been confirmed.

- Wide exposure of the pancreaticodudenal complex is essential to determine the extent of injuries and access-associated bleeding. The hepatic flexure is mobilized and a complete Kocher maneuver is completed.
- The easiest transection is the gastric antrectomy, accomplished with a long linear stapler (Endo GIA Purple [3.0, 3.5, 4.0 mm] load).
- The jejunum is then divided 10 cm distal to the ligament of Treitz with a GIA Blue (3.5-mm) load.
- The CBD should be transected close to the duodenum, well below the cystic duct juncture, to preserve an optimal CBD remnant for later reconstruction. The CBD is ligated with a 2-0 silk to control the bile drainage and theoretically encourage CBD dilation.
- The pancreas is divided after creating a tunnel anterior to the portal vein, initiated at the inferior edge of the pancreas at the level of the SMV. 3-0 PDS sutures are placed at the superior and inferior edges of the pancreas to minimize bleeding from the small superior and inferior pancreaticoduodenal arteries.
- Resection of the pancreatic head is begun superiorly by 3-0 silk suture ligation of the GDA. If there is any question of the arterial anatomy (Fig. 17.1), a bulldog can be placed on the presumed GDA until hepatic artery integrity is ensured.
- The duodenum and adjacent pancreas are freed from the underlying SMV and SMA by suture ligation of the intervening small vessels.
- The mesentery of the proximal jejunum is taken as close to the bowel wall as possible with a LigaSure. Division of the mesentery is continued proximally to D3.
- The devascularized duodenum and jejunum are reflected beneath the mesenteric vessels.
- The uncinate process attachments to the retroperitoneum are freed using a LigaSure and 3-0 silk ties for visible vessels.
- Two 10-mm Jackson-Pratt drains are placed to exteriorize pancreatic secretions.

Pancreaticoduodenectomy (Second Stage)

TIP

Reconstruction following a trauma Whipple is often more challenging than an elective resection because the CBD and pancreatic ducts are typically small. Loupe magnification is advisable.

- The jejunal end is brought behind mesenteric vessels and laid in C-shape.
- The pancreaticojejunal is accomplished as described in the Midpancreatic resection with Roux Limb section. Due to the high risk of pancreatic fistula, we generally employ two preventive measures:

(1) we exteriorize a 5-Fr pancreatic stent via the jejunal limb (Fig. 17.10), and (2) place a 2-0 PDS "binding suture" around the end of the jejunal limb that contains the pancreas (Fig. 17.8).

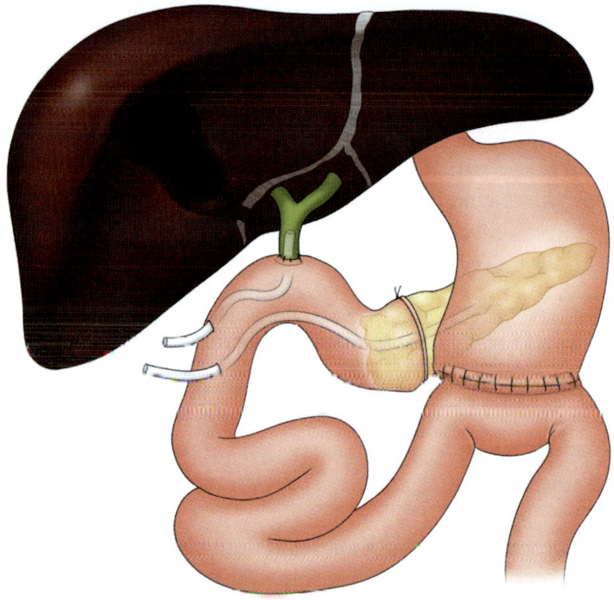

FIGURE 17.10 ▌The completed pancreaticoduodenectomy for trauma consists of an end-to-end pancreaticojejunostomy, end-to-side choledochojejunostomy, and exteriorized stents from the pancreatic and common bile ducts.

- For the biliary–jejunal anastomosis, the CBD is transected just above the cystic duct juncture and the duct sewn end to side into the jejunum with interrupted 4-0 PDS sutures. If the CBD is less than 3 mm, a second stent is placed in the duct and exteriorized via the jejunal limb.
- The gastrojejunostomy anastomosis is antecolic, one layer, and created end to side using 3-0 PDS. The staple line on stomach is cut away with heavy scissors to create the gastrostomy. Approximately 30 to 40 cm of jejunum is maintained between the biliary and gastric anastomoses.
- A feeding tube is guided through the gastrojejunostomy anastomosis for feeding distal to the three anastomoses.

POSTOPERATIVE CARE

- Distal feeding can be started once physiologic restoration (normothermia, correction of metabolic acidosis, and restoration of the coagulation status) is accomplished in the intensive care unit.
- A high level of vigilance is required to assess for biliary, pancreatic, and gastric leaks from the reconstruction. The options for their management are beyond the scope of this chapter.

Suggested Readings

Ball CG, Biffl WL, Moore EE. Time to update the American Association for the Surgery of Trauma (AAST) pancreas injury grading lexicon? *J Trauma Acute Care Surg.* 2021;92(3):e38–e40.

Biffl WL, Ball CG, Moore EE, et al; WTA Multicenter Trials Group on Pancreatic Injuries. Don't mess with the pancreas! A multicenter analysis of the management of low-grade pancreatic injuries. *J Trauma Acute Care Surg.* 2021;91(5):820–828.

Biffl WL, Zhao FZ, Morse B, et al; WTA Multicenter Trials Group on Pancreatic Injuries. A multicenter trial of current trends in the diagnosis and management of high-grade pancreatic injuries. *J Trauma Acute Care Surg.* 2021;90(5):776–786.

Bredbeck BC, Moore EE, Barnett CC Jr. Duodenum preserving pancreatic head resection (Beger procedure) for pancreatic trauma. *J Trauma Acute Care Surg.* 2015;78(3):649–651.

Malhotra A, Biffl WL, Moore EE, et al. Western Trauma Association Critical Decisions in Trauma: Diagnosis and management of duodenal injuries. *J Trauma Acute Care Surg.* 2015;79(6):1096–1101.

Moore EE, Cogbill TH, Malangoni MA, et al. Organ injury scaling, II: Pancreas, duodenum, small bowel, colon, and rectum. *J Trauma.* 1990;30(11):1427–1429.

Peng SY, Wang JW, Lau WY, et al. Conventional versus binding pancreaticojejunostomy after pancreaticoduodenectomy: a prospective randomized trial. *Ann Surg*. 2007;245(5):692–698.
Poon RTP, Fan ST, Lo CM, et al. External drainage of pancreatic duct with a stent to reduce leakage rate of pancreaticojejunostomy after pancreaticoduodenectomy: a prospective randomized trial. *Ann Surg*. 2007;246(3):425–433.
Schellenberg M, Inaba K, Cheng V, et al. Spleen-preserving distal pancreatectomy in trauma. *J Trauma Acute Care Surg*. 2018; 84(1):118–122.
Seykora TF, Liu JB, Maggino L, et al. Drain Management Following Distal Pancreatectomy: Characterization of Contemporary Practice and Impact of Early Removal. *Ann Surg*. 2020;272(6):1110–1117.
Thompson CM, Shalhub S, DeBoard ZM, et al. Revisiting the pancreaticoduodenectomy for trauma: a single institution's experience. *J Trauma Acute Care Surg*. 2013;75(2):225–228.

Chapter 18
Abdominal Vascular Injury

CHARLES J. FOX

PERIOPERATIVE CONSIDERATIONS

Procedure Rationale

- Abdominal vascular injury is defined as a disruption of major intraperitoneal, retroperitoneal, and pelvic blood vessels. Rapid control of bleeding vessels located in the midst of viscera or deep in the retroperitoneum is necessary to prevent an exsanguinating cardiac arrest. While surrounding structures may impede operative access, they may also facilitate life-saving tamponade as not all injuries are immediately unstable. Unlike transections, pseudoaneurysms and large intimal tears may allow additional time for a diagnostic assessment and semiurgent endovascular repair. The incidence of penetrating abdominal hemorrhage remains high in urban trauma centers where low-velocity handguns are prevalent and prehospital transport is rapid. Common sites of bleeding are the viscera, mesentery, and blood vessels of the retroperitoneum. The trauma surgeon must have the knowledge and skill to quickly control and repair the aorta, inferior vena cava, and other important branch vessels.

TIP

It is important to recognize patterns of injury, particularly for a patient who appears clinically stable but may have profound metabolic derangements or a concerning mechanism of injury.

- Know the prehospital vital signs and trends.
- Recognize patterns of shock, shock index, thromboelastography (TEG) abnormalities, and admission lactate levels.
- Note seat belt contusions and fractures associated with vessel injury.
- Activate the massive transfusion protocol early.
- Communicate swiftly to the operating room staff so the room is ready when the patient arrives.

Essential Equipment

TIP

The entire team needs to know the proper positioning, how to prepare a wide surgical field, apply a warming blanket, open all major vascular instruments, correct graft materials, and verify large-bore intravenous access. Blood products need to be in the room and hemodynamic monitoring is mandatory. Do not open the abdominal cavity until the whole team is ready for massive bleeding and capable of a rapid transfusion of warmed blood.

- Headlight
- Loupe magnification 2.5 glasses
- Omni tract retractors
- Gel foam and surgical
- Fibrin sealant and BioGlue surgical adhesive
- Long Ryder and Castro needle drivers

- Microvascular forceps
- Potts-Smith scissors
- Silastic vessel loops
- Umbilical tapes
- Rummel tourniquets (red rubber catheter and umbilical tape)
- 3-0 Prolene on a C1 needle, 36 inches for parachuting anastomosis
- 4-0 Prolene on an RB1 needle, 36 inches for deep pelvic vessels
- 3-0 silk plain and stick ties
- Manually loaded Hemoclips, small, medium, and large
- Sterile 8- to 10-MHz Doppler probe
- Heparinized saline 50 to 100 units in 1,000 mL saline
- Fogarty embolectomy catheters no. 2, no. 3, no. 4
- DeBakey aortic clamp
- Large vascular (Henley) clamp
- Wiley hypogastric vascular clamps
- Satinsky side-biting vascular clamps
- Sponge sticks
- Vascular shunt
  - 15- or 31-cm Pruitt-Inahara shunt (with T port) 8 to 14 mm balloon diameter
- Grafts
  - 12 to 20 mm diameter Dacron, bifurcated
  - Cryopreserved artery if contamination
- Portable ultrasound machine
- Continuous wave Doppler with sterile probe

Positioning

TIP

Ensure that there is plenty of room for the surgical team to work and that blankets are not draped over the table rails that will prevent securely tightening the self-retaining retractor.

- Place upper body Bair warmer, urinary bladder catheter, and a radial arterial line.
- Supine position with arms extended.
- Prep abdomen nipples to knees.
- A full midline laparotomy incision is recommended.

TECHNIQUE

Surgical Approach

TIP

Get in the room early to go over the steps of hemorrhage control with the scrub technician in the room during the preparation phase. Omini tract retractor components, Prolene suture (36", SH), vascular clamps, silk ties, hemoclips, and sponge sticks are on the mayo stand and ready to pass. Have the team ask for more materials before the last of anything is passed to the surgeon. Consider the option of placing a 7-French sheath in the femoral artery and a REBOA in zone 1 before opening the abdomen.

Zone 1 Surgical Techniques: Aorta

- A midline retroperitoneal hematoma is approached differently depending on the likelihood of an injury to the suprarenal abdominal aorta (supramesocolic), or to the infrarenal abdominal aorta, left renal vein, or inferior vena cava (inframesocolic).
- Zone 1 hematomas, regardless of mechanism (blunt or penetrating), are opened (Fig. 18.1).

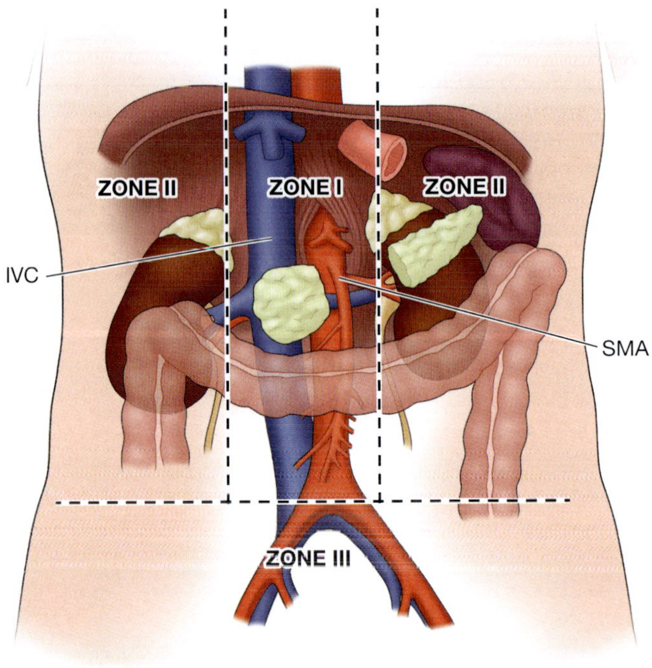

FIGURE 18.1 ▌Zones of the retroperitoneum.

- A left-sided medial mobilization is the preferred operative approach for injury to the suprarenal abdominal aorta (Fig. 18.2).

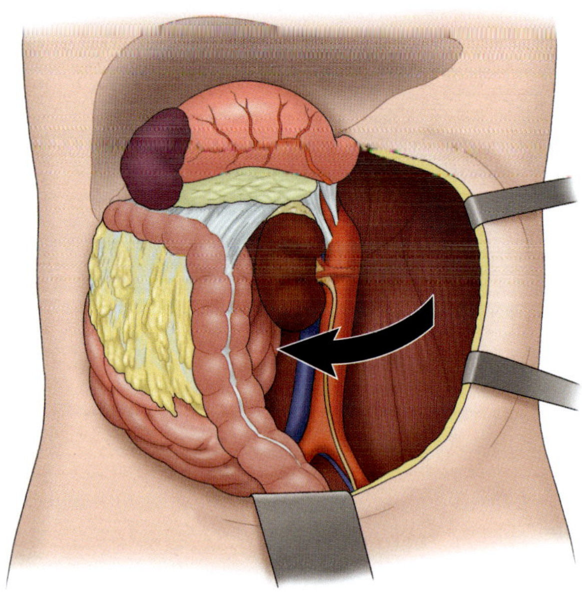

FIGURE 18.2 ▌Medial rotation of all left-sided intraabdominal viscera allows visualization of the entire abdominal aorta, including the hiatal or diaphragmatic, suprarenal or visceral, and infrarenal portions.

- Divide the lateral retroperitoneal attachments at the line of Toldt to reflect the left colon, kidney (or leave in situ), spleen, tail of the pancreas, and fundus of the stomach to the midline.
- The entire aorta from the diaphragm to the bifurcation of the iliac vessels is visualized.
- Ensure that the spleen is not injured.
- Time-consuming dissection of the celiac plexus is spared by transecting the left crus of the aortic hiatus of the diaphragm to expose and clamp the distal thoracic aorta.
- Active hemorrhage may require hasty manual compression for temporary proximal control.

- Alternatively dividing the lesser omentum, retracting the stomach and esophagus to the left, and manually separating the crura muscle fibers can control the supraceliac aorta.
- Small aortic tears are repaired using a long (36 in) 3-0 or 4-0 polypropylene suture.
- Patch aortoplasty using Dacron or Polytetrafluoroethylene (ePTFE) is used for larger perforations to avoid an iatrogenic stenosis.
- An end-to-end anastomosis is used for short segmental defects when a tensionless repair is possible.
- When a prosthetic conduit is necessary, a 14- to 16-mm Dacron or ePTFE graft (slight undersizing encouraged) is sufficient in the nondiseased adult aorta.
- If concomitant bowel injury exists, then the enteric contents are first controlled with clamps, followed by aortic repair, closure of the retroperitoneum, copious irrigation, and subsequent reconstruction of the gastrointestinal tract.

Zone 1 Surgical Techniques: Celiac Axis and Superior Mesenteric Artery

- Major injuries to the celiac trunk can be managed by ligation.
- The common hepatic artery may be amendable to a lateral repair.
- The left gastric and splenic arteries should be ligated when injured.
- Retrograde flow from the inferior pancreaticoduodenal artery will maintain hepatic viability when the common hepatic artery is ligated proximal to the gastroduodenal artery.
- Collateral flow should maintain midgut viability when the superior mesenteric artery is injured and subsequently ligated.
- Temporary arterial shunting and delayed repair may eliminate intestinal ischemia that results from distal vasoconstriction and impaired retrograde flow.
- Proximal exposure of the superior mesenteric can be performed using the left medial rotation described earlier and leaving the left kidney down in the retroperitoneum.
- When the injury is retropancreatic, then division of the pancreas will facilitate the exposure.
- For injuries distal to the pancreas between the middle colic and pancreaticoduodenal branches of the artery, ligation may be simpler than a repair challenged by pancreatic leaks.
- Injuries to the more distal superior mesenteric artery beyond the transverse mesocolon should be repaired to avoid ischemia to the distal midgut.
- Segmental branches are usually ligated with intestinal resection.
- Saphenous or prosthetic grafts to the superior mesenteric artery can be placed on the distal infrarenal aorta to avoid contamination by pancreatic injury.
- The grafts are configured in an end-to-side or end-to-end fashion and passed without tension through the posterior aspect of the mesentery to the mid or distal superior mesenteric artery.
- Cover the all-suture lines with retroperitoneal fat or an omental pedicle to avoid an aortoenteric fistula in the future.
- Proximal injury, transfusion, acidosis, and multiple organ failure portend a poor prognosis for these abdominal injuries.

Zone 1 Surgical Techniques: Renal

- Renal artery injuries when closer to the hilum of the kidney can be effectively controlled in the midline retroperitoneum.
- The transverse mesocolon is retracted superiorly and the small bowel is eviscerated to the right. The ligament of Treitz is then divided as the inferior mesenteric vein is retracted to the left.
- With extensive mobilization of the duodenojejunal junction, the anterior left renal vein is exposed crossing the abdominal aorta.
- The left renal vein can be mobilized by division of the adrenal, gonadal, and lumbar veins or ligated primarily when these venous tributaries are preserved. The left renal artery is found just superiorly and posteriorly to the left renal vein.
- The renal arteries can be controlled with vessel loops after dissection of the surrounding retroperitoneal tissue (Fig. 18.3).
- The inferior vena cava may require gentle retraction with a vein retractor to best expose the right renal artery. To expose the infrarenal inferior vena cava and right renal vein, the avascular line of Toldt is transected to mobilize the right colon and hepatic flexure while performing a Kocher maneuver by sweeping the pancreas and duodenum to the left and incising the retroperitoneal tissues that cover these vessels.

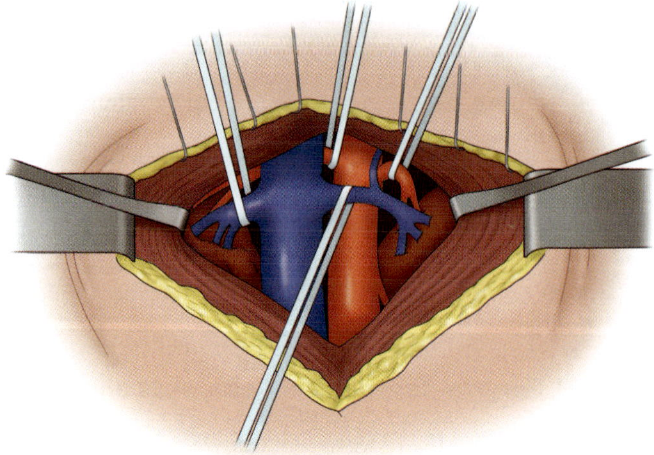

FIGURE 18.3 ▌Vessel loops are placed around the proximal renal vessels before perirenal hematomas are entered.

Zone 1 Surgical Techniques: Inferior Mesenteric Artery

- The inferior mesenteric artery can be ligated in young patients.

Zone 2 Surgical Techniques: Renal

- Hematomas in zone 2 are all explored in penetrating wounds but in blunt abdominal injury are only explored when hematomas are ruptured, rapidly expanding, or pulsatile.
- In the lateral retroperitoneum (zone 2), hemorrhage is often secondary to injury to the distal renal artery, renal vein, or parenchyma of the kidney.
- Those with penetrating wounds should have the hematoma carefully opened to examine the underlying kidney. Many surgeons prefer to first control the renal artery in the midline at the base of the mesocolon with a silastic vessel loop; however, one option is to simply open the retroperitoneum laterally, divide Gerota fascia and elevate the injured kidney into the wound. The vessels just proximal to the renal hilum can be easily controlled manually or with a large vascular (Henley) clamp.
- Repair of renovascular injury should be based on the patient condition and nephrectomy should be performed for those patients with multiple injuries, or prolonged ischemia time after an intraoperative palpation confirms a normal contralateral kidney.
- Renal arteries are small but maybe amendable to lateral arteriorrhaphy for small perforations. A time-consuming repair on these small vessels located in the deep retroperitoneum can be very challenging and should be carefully decided.
- When a repair is preferred, a saphenous vein interposition graft, prosthetic graft, or translocated splenic and hepatic arteries can be used for renovascular reconstruction. This repair is particularly important in those patients with a solitary kidney.
- Blunt renal artery thrombosis is easily diagnosed by a computed tomography angiography (CTA) showing a lack of contrast enhancement. Conflicting outcomes associated with both revascularization and observation has generated controversial opinion on the best management practice. Ischemia time, associated injuries, and the status of the contralateral kidney appear to influence the current surgical decision making. Patients not undergoing revascularization of one thrombosed renal artery need to be monitored for 6 to 12 months after injury to allow for the early detection of delayed hypertension. Intimal tears of the renal artery without thrombosis can be incidentally discovered and may be observed if there is no contrast extravasation.
- Early follow-up imaging is important, and anticoagulation should be considered on an individual basis depending on other associated injuries. In the endovascular era of catheter-based interventions, there is presently a very important role for the use of covered stents to treat intimal tears, pseudoaneurysms, arteriovenous fistulae, and thrombotic occlusions of the renal artery.

Zone 3 Surgical Techniques: Pelvic

- Hematomas in zone 3, the pelvic retroperitoneum are all explored in penetrating wounds but in blunt abdominal injury are only explored when hematomas are ruptured, rapidly expanding, or pulsatile.

- Pelvic hematomas associated with an absent ipsilateral femoral pulse are explored because of the potential for an iliac artery injury.
- Exposure of the vessels in zone 3 can be achieved by dividing the avascular line of Toldt of the left or right colon with medial displacement.
- The iliac vessels are exposed while carefully locating the ureter as it crosses the common iliac artery to avoid devascularization. Finally, the dissection is extended in a caudad direction, opening the retroperitoneum as necessary.
- Injuries to zone 3 also can be challenging to manage, as there are often associated colonic and genitourinary injuries, resulting in significant contamination.
- Injuries to the common iliac arteries can usually be suture repaired. Occasionally, resection and primary anastomosis can be performed.
- A balloon thrombectomy should be passed to remove any thrombotic debris, and heparinized saline irrigation should be used liberally.
- Autogenous and prosthetic grafts also can be utilized to repair common iliac arteries.
- Internal iliac artery injuries are generally managed by ligation.
- Injuries to the external iliac artery can be managed by suture repair or with an end-to-end anastomosis.
- Iliofemoral bypasses can be performed with autogenous or prosthetic grafts, although prosthetic grafts may be preferred if the iliac artery is large.
- Ligation is poorly tolerated by most patients and is associated with a high rate of limb loss. Extensive tissue destruction may require ligation, and, in some cases, extra-anatomic bypass (axillofemoral, femorofemoral) should be performed.
- A temporary luminal shunt will allow for delayed reconstruction when the patient's condition has stabilized.
- A lateral venorraphy should be attempted provided that the repair will not produce a significant stenosis and subsequent thromboembolism.
- Injury to any region of the iliac vein may require ligation and this is generally well tolerated, although massive edema and a compartment syndrome that requires a fasciotomy should be anticipated.
- Exposure of an injured iliac vein to control hemorrhage may occasionally question the need for transecting the overlying iliac artery, but this is rarely performed.

Surgical Techniques: Inferior Vena Cava

- Refer to the liver chapter for retrohepatic inferior vena cava injury.
- Hematomas from penetrating injury, unless retrohepatic, should be explored. The infrahepatic cava is best exposed by mobilization and medial rotation of the right colon, hepatic flexure, and the duodenum (Fig. 18.4).

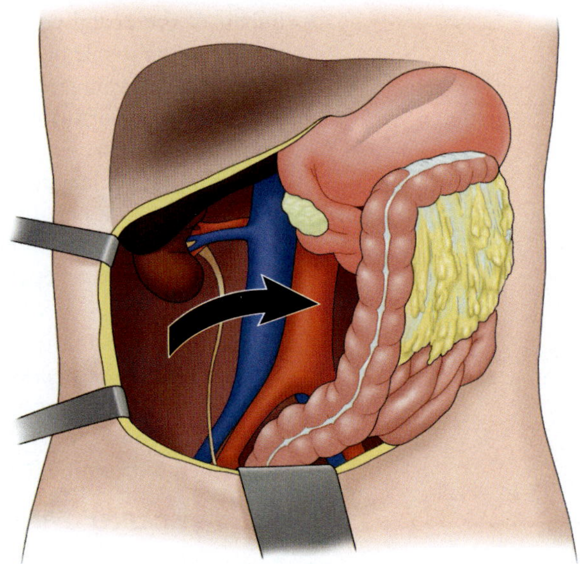

FIGURE 18.4 ▮ Medial mobilization of right-sided intra-abdominal viscera allows for visualization of the entire infrahepatic inferior vena cava.

- When exposure of a retrohepatic hematoma is necessary, division of the hepatic ligaments and mobilization of the liver is usually required. Extending the incision to include a subcostal incision, thoracotomy or sternotomy may be necessary for technically difficult cases when perihepatic packing is ineffective in controlling hemorrhage. More radical maneuvers include hepatic vascular isolation or placement of an atriocaval shunt.
- The management of injuries to the infrahepatic suprarenal inferior vena cava and the infrarenal inferior vena cava consist of lateral venorraphy with 3.0 or 4.0 vascular suture on large needles whenever feasible. If through-and-through injuries are found in these vessels, both anterior and posterior aspects of the vessel must be repaired. Although the infrahepatic suprarenal inferior vena cava has no venous tributaries, it is difficult to mobilize the posterior wall repaired by extending the anterior injury and performing a repair from within the lumen of the vein. When there has been massive destruction, ligation can be considered but reconstruction with a patch or ringed prosthetic graft is preferred to avoid renal failure.
- The management of injuries to the infrarenal inferior vena cava generally consists of lateral venorraphy while using sponge sticks or a partially occluding Satinsky vascular clamp.
- After verifying that there is no posterior defect, place stay sutures on either side of a long laceration to stop additional tearing of a traumatic venotomy.
- Care must be taken to avoid the avulsion of lumbar veins during hasty attempts at clamp control. Alternatively, intraluminal balloon occlusion can be effective in gaining proximal and distal control of hemorrhage. Tamponade with a tightly rolled pack and serial application of Babcock clamps as the pack is slowly moved distally is another effective method of preparing the wound for lateral venorraphy. In the presence of through-and-through injuries, primary repair can be accomplished, either by extending the laceration or by rotating the vessel. This may involve ligating many lumbar veins in the region. The infrarenal inferior vena cava can be ligated in cases of massive destruction and is generally well tolerated. Massive edema and the potential need for a fasciotomy mandate careful postoperative observation and wearing of compression garments. Venous thromboembolism should be anticipated in patients with a severe caval stenosis following repair and systemic anticoagulation should be considered.

Surgical Techniques: Portal Vein System

- The portal vein is formed by the confluence of the superior mesenteric vein and the splenic vein located behind the neck of the pancreas and to the left of the inferior vena cava. It passes behind the first part of the duodenum and enters the hepatoduodenal ligament. In the hilum of the liver, the portal vein divides into the right and left branches.
- Most patients present in hemorrhagic shock and require an emergent laparotomy to control hemorrhage. A Pringle maneuver is applied, and a careful dissection is performed to precisely define which structures in the porta hepatis have been injured.
- Back-bleeding may be controlled by having an assistant compress all three structures with forceps right next to the liver.
- Repair of the portal vein is made difficult by the challenges of an adequate exposure but remains similar to the repair of other venous injuries described above.
- When a lateral venorraphy can be achieved without prolonged bleeding, primary repair of the portal vein should be performed.
- Complex reconstruction (saphenous interposition) of the portal vein is discouraged unless there is concomitant injury to the hepatic artery. When a penetrating wound in the hepatoduodenal ligament injures the hepatic artery, options for treatment include various primary repair techniques, however, ligation is well tolerated when the portal vein remains intact.
- Ligation of both the hepatic artery and portal vein is not advised and one of these vessels should be repaired.
- Similarly, injuries to the superior mesenteric vein should be repaired primarily. Although ligation of these veins may be necessary, ligation of either the portal or superior mesenteric vein can threaten the viability of the large and small intestine.
- Abdominal compartment syndrome should be anticipated and a second look laparotomy should be performed to examine bowel viability.

Endovascular Management

- Endovascular techniques have advanced the contemporary management of abdominal vascular injuries. Many case reports now confirm emerging roles in selected cases of aortoiliac and renovascular injury.

- Endovascular stent placement following blunt injury with arterial dissection, false aneurysm, or arteriovenous fistula has established an alternative successful treatment option with a low complication rate.
- In selected cases, a catheter-based intervention may now be considered as a primary surgical therapy.
- Embolization of an internal iliac artery for pelvic bleeding can be approached from the ipsilateral or contralateral femoral artery to place proximal nonselective (Fig. 18.5) coils or hemostatic agents or advanced further into the anterior or posterior division to minimize the potential for ischemic complications.

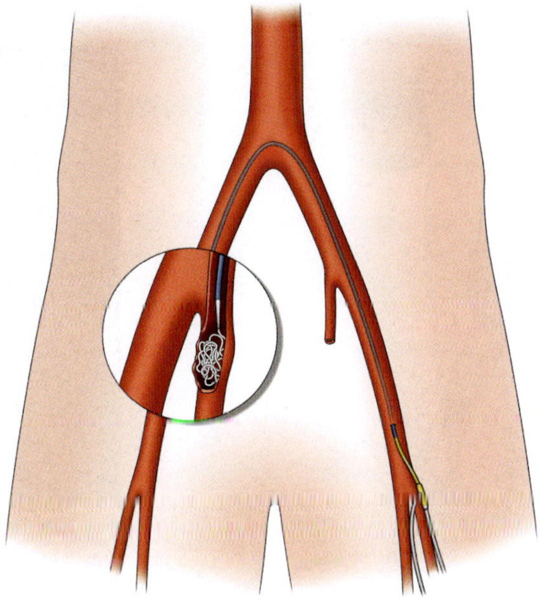

FIGURE 18.5 ▌ Contralateral transfemoral coil embolization of the right hypogastric artery is considered a nonselective embolization.

- Infrarenal covered stents used for endovascular aneurysm repair (EVAR) may be used to seal an abdominal aortic (Fig. 18.6) or iliac artery injury (Fig. 18.7).

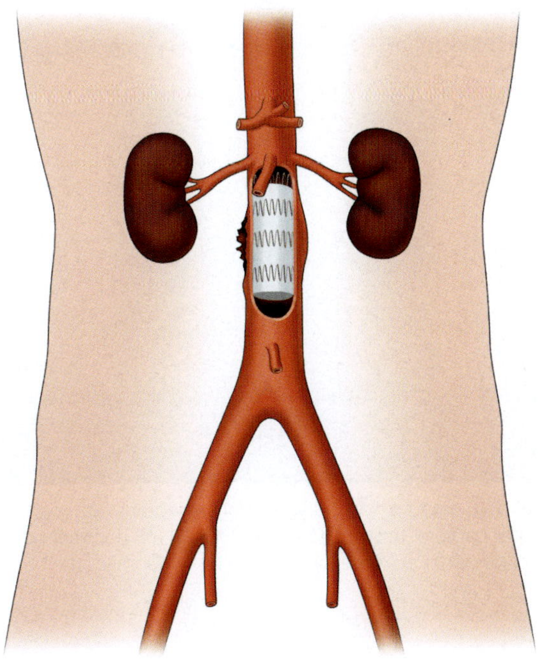

FIGURE 18.6 ▌ A main body or aortic cuff can be inserted in the infrarenal position to reline a dissection, cover a pseudoaneurysm, or prevent thromboembolism after blunt aortic injury.

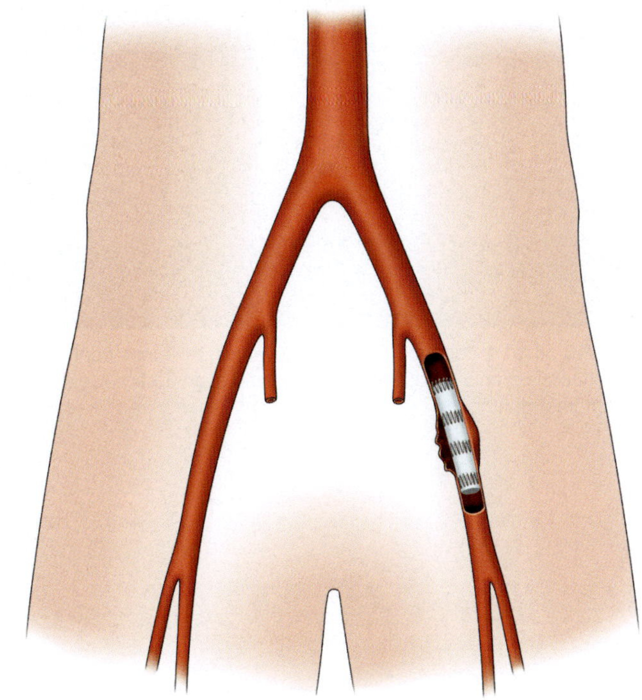

FIGURE 18.7 ▌ An iliac limb can be placed from the ipsilateral or contralateral femoral artery depending on the location of the injury.

- Modular (main body with limbs) components can treat the entire infrarenal aortoiliac segment or they can be modified with fenestrations (physician-modified endografts [PMEGs]) to preserve important arterial branches (renal, superior mesenteric, or subclavian) (Fig. 18.8).
- High-speed mechanisms of injury, often associated with seat belt sign or unstable spinal injury can also result in an aortic injury and should undergo CT angiography with 2.0-mm cuts on a high speed (64 to 128) multidetector row scanner (Figs. 18.9, 18.10) in preparation for endovascular management (Figs. 18.11, 18.12, 18.13).

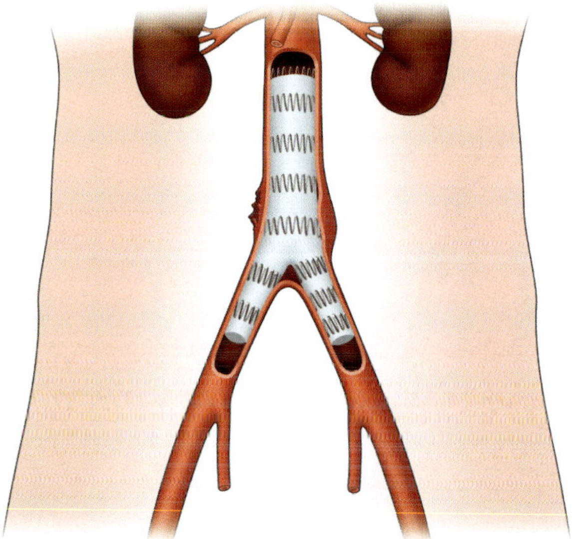

FIGURE 18.8 ❙ Illustration of a standard EVAR with suprarenal fixation and preservation of the internal iliac arteries.

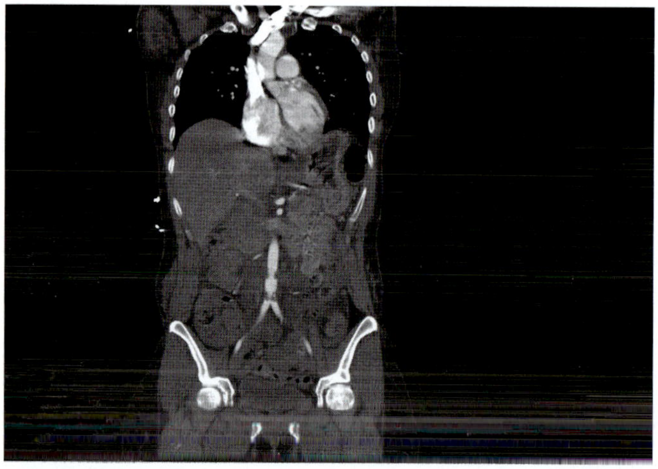

FIGURE 18.9 ❙ Coronal CT image following intravenous contrast depicts a pseudoaneurysm with intimal injury in the region of the aortic bifurcation.

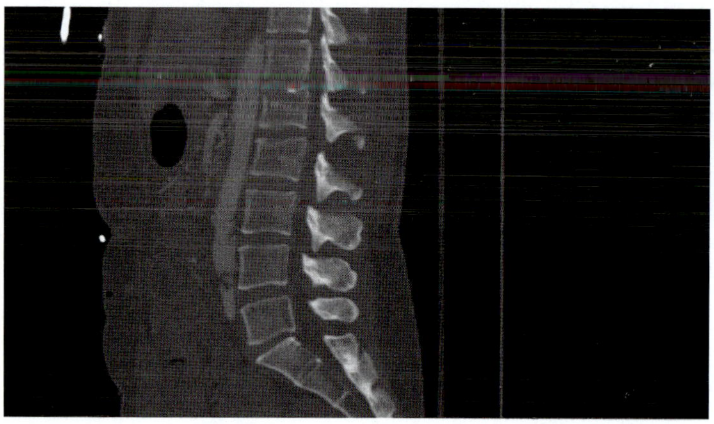

FIGURE 18.10 ❙ Sagittal CT image following intravenous contrast shows the external contour irregularity characteristic of an aortic injury that requires urgent treatment.

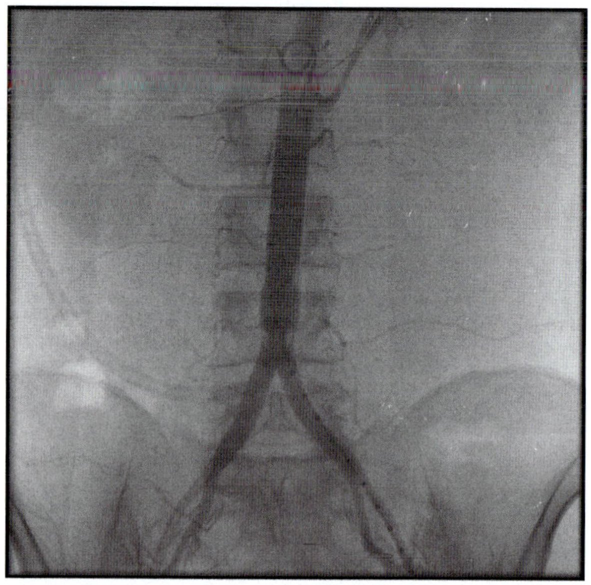

FIGURE 18.11 ❙ Left transfemoral angiogram with marking pigtail catheter delivers 15 mL/sec for 30 mL contrast bolus and demonstrated the injury at the L4 vertebral body.

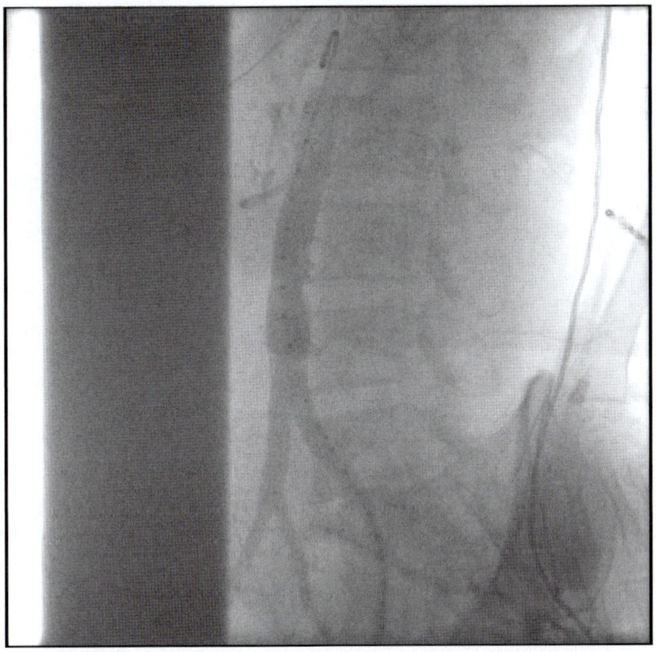

FIGURE 18.12 ▌ A lateral projection was performed to evaluate for thrombus extension not seen on the anterior–posterior projection before selecting a stent size.

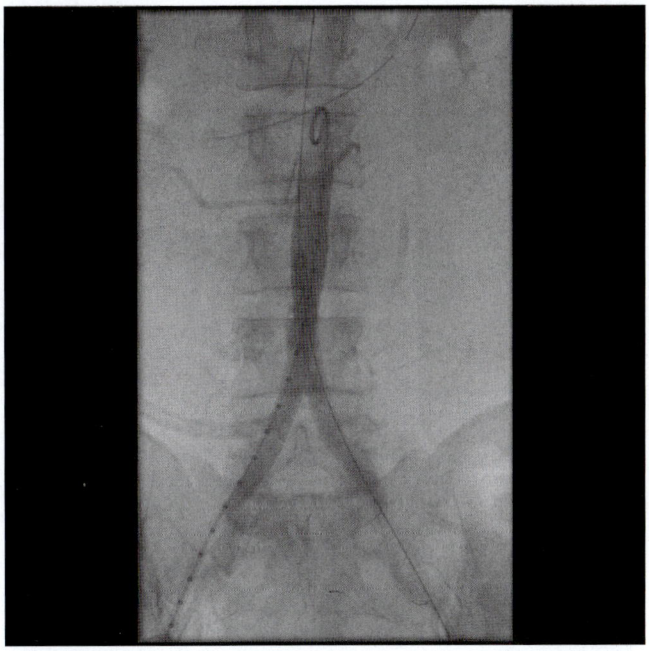

FIGURE 18.13 ▌ Completion angiogram following placement of two "kissing" 8 × 79 mm covered stents.

POSTOPERATIVE CARE AND COMPLICATIONS

- Abdominal vascular injuries are associated with high rates of morbidity.
- A second look operation within 12 to 24 hours following the restoration of blood pressure, temperature, and other physiologic derangements may be helpful to establish bowel viability and to verify patency of small vessel repairs with continuous-wave Doppler or intraoperative duplex sonography.
- Abdominal compartment syndrome is common in the presence of abdominal vascular injuries and should be monitored carefully and treated with negative pressure dressings and delayed abdominal closure.
- Dehiscence of a vascular suture line may occur in the postoperative period and should be carefully anticipated especially in those with pancreatic or gastrointestinal contamination.
- A CTA may be a useful adjunct for obtaining contrast-enhanced completion imaging following abdominal vascular reconstruction or endovascular interventions (Fig. 18.14).

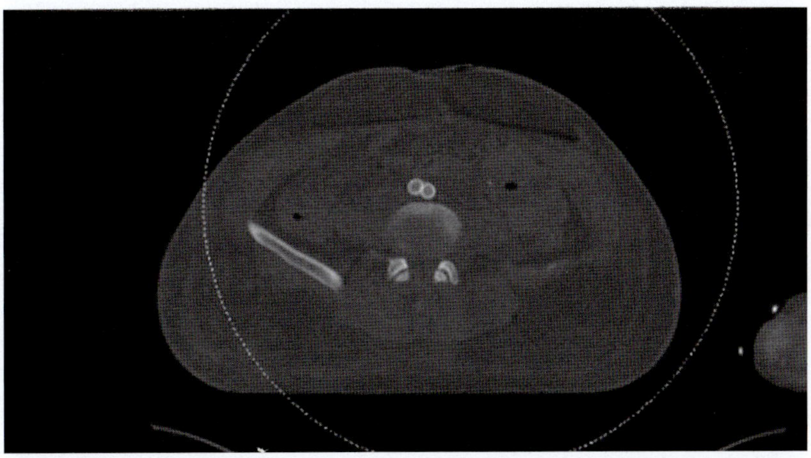

FIGURE 18.14 ▌ Predischarge axial CT with IV contrast showing opacification of the stents at the aortic bifurcation.

- Duplex ultrasonography should also be performed in the early postoperative period to establish graft patency and assess the velocity of blood flow useful in predicting the potential for a future graft failure.
- The role of anticoagulation for small vessels such as the mesenteric or renal arteries should be considered on a case-by-case basis.
- Complications following abdominal vascular reconstruction such as distal embolization and thrombosis suggest the possibility of an unrecognized intimal injury.

Suggested Readings

Asensio JA, Britt LD, Borzotta A, et al. Multiinstitutional experience with the management of superior mesenteric artery injuries. *J Am Coll Surg*. 2001;193(4):354–365.

Asensio JA, Chahwan S, Hanpeter D, et al. Operative management and outcome of 302 abdominal vascular injuries. *Am J Surg*. 2000;180(6):528–533.

Asensio JA, Forno W, Roldan G, et al. Abdominal vascular injuries: injuries to the aorta. *Surg Clin North Am*. 2001;81(6): 1395–416, xiii–xiv.

Fox CJ. Injury to abdomen. In: Fisher JE, Bland KI, eds. *Mastery of Surgery*. 6th ed. Lippincott Williams & Wilkins; 2010.

Fox CJ, Horer T, Moore EE. Abdominal vascular injury. In: Jose de Brito C, Murilo R, Loureiro E, eds. *Cirurgia Vascular*. 5th ed. Thieme Revinter; 2020.

Melmer PD, Clatterbuck B, Parker V, et al. Superior mesenteric artery and vein injuries: operative strategies and outcomes. *Vasc Endovascular Surg*. 2022;56(1):40–48.

Chapter 19

Damage Control Surgery/ The Open Abdomen

DANIEL DANTE YEH

PERIOPERATIVE CONSIDERATIONS

Procedure Rationale

- Damage control surgery (DCS) is a philosophical approach to emergency surgery that prioritizes temporary control of hemorrhage and enteric contamination over definitive repair in physiologically unstable patients suffering from hypothermia, coagulopathy, and acidosis (i.e., "the lethal triad" or "the bloody viscous cycle").
- Damage control resuscitation (DCR) or "hemostatic resuscitation" is a related concept which is equally as important in achieving successful outcomes.
- The decision to abbreviate the index operation should be made shortly after identification of all injuries and should be clearly communicated to the Anesthesia and nursing team.
- Return to the operating room for definitive repair of all injuries should be delayed until physiologic resuscitation is complete.
- The duration of open abdomen (or sternum or thorax) should be minimized and these cavities should be closed at the first available opportunity once injuries have been definitively repaired.

ESSENTIAL EQUIPMENT

- Standard trauma laparotomy set
- Laparotomy pads
- Surgical staplers
- Vascular shunts in a variety of sizes (Chapter 29)
- Energy coagulation devices such as Impact LigaSure (Coviden, Mansfield, MA), Harmonic Scalpel (Ethicon Endo-Surgery, Cincinnati, OH), and Argon Beam Coagulator (ABC)
- Hemostatic adjuncts such as QuikClot Combat Gauze® (Z-Medical, Wallingford, CT), Gelfoam® (Pfizer, New York, NY), Surgicel®, and Evarrest® Fibrin Sealant Patch (Ethicon, Inc., Somerville, NJ)
- Temporary abdominal closure options
  - Towel clips
  - "Barker" vacuum pack technique
    - 1010 Steri-Drape™ (3M Health Care, St. Paul, MN)
    - 10-French Jackson-Pratt (JP) drains × 2 (C.R. Bard, Inc., Covington, GA)
    - Ioban™, 23 × 17 inches (3M Health Care, St. Paul, MN)
  - Negative pressure wound therapy device such as V.A.C ULTA™ Therapy Unit (3M, St. Paul, MN)
    - V.A.C. GRANUFOAM™ (3M, St. Paul, MN)
    - AbThera™ Open Abdomen Dressing (3M, St. Paul, MN)

Subsequent Operations

- Sequential abdominal closure
  - No. 1 PDS sutures (Ethicon, Inc., Somerville, NJ)
  - V.A.C. WHITEFOAM™ (3M, St. Paul, MN)

  - V.A.C. GRANUFOAM™ (3M, St. Paul, MN)
  - V.A.C ULTA Therapy Unit (3M, St. Paul, MN)
- Mesh-mediated medial fascial tension
  - Vicryl 30- × 30-cm mesh (Ethicon, Raritan, NJ)
  - 2-0 Prolene (45 cm length) (Ethicon, Raritan, NJ)

POSITIONING

- Supine
- Arms extended at 90 degrees from the body

SURGICAL TECHNIQUE

TIP

The sterile prep should extend from the neck to the mid-thighs, as emergency procedures in the thorax or groin may be required.

Initial Operation

- Standard midline laparotomy incision.
- Control of major hemorrhage is the first priority upon abdominal entry
  - Vascular injuries (see Chapter 29)
    - Major arteries and veins (aorta, superior mesenteric artery, iliac arteries, femoral arteries, popliteal arteries, portal vein, hepatic vein, and suprarenal inferior vena cava [IVC]) should not be ligated. If unable to immediately and quickly repair the injury to these vessels, intravascular shunting should be performed (see Chapter 29).
    - All other arterial and venous injuries may be ligated for hemorrhage control during DCS.
  - Solid organs
    - Spleen—splenectomy should be performed without hesitation in an unstable patient. Transection of the hilum with a surgical stapler is faster than individual ligation of the vessels (see Chapter 16), but may increase the risk of injury to the tail of the pancreas.
    - Liver—packing above and below the liver with laparotomy pads is the first maneuver for liver injuries and will control bleeding in the majority of cases. Take care not to compress the IVC with overly aggressive liver packing. Techniques to manage major hepatic injuries are presented in Chapter 15.
    - Kidney—nephrectomy should be performed in unstable patients with a palpable contralateral kidney. Nonexpanding Zone 2 hematomas should not be explored at the index operation if they are not believed to be a source of life-threatening bleeding.
- Control of intestinal injuries
  - Stomach, small, and large bowel injuries (including duodenum) not requiring resection may be temporarily controlled with a rapid whip stitch using any suture material. This temporary suture will ultimately be cut and removed at a later time during definitive repair or reconstruction.
  - Destructive injuries to the gastrointestinal (GI) tract may be addressed by resection using a surgical stapler. In the absence of a stapler, the lumen may be occluded using umbilical tape ligature. Using clamps and surgical ties to divide the mesentery may be too time consuming in an unstable patient and this step may be more quickly completed using an energy coagulation device such as Ligasure™ or harmonic scalpel. The bowel is left in discontinuity at the index DCS operation.
  - Pancreas—major pancreatic head injuries should be packed for hemostasis and drained to control contamination, and destructive injuries to the body and tail of the gland may be resected with a surgical stapler. Ductal assessment should not be attempted in the setting of DCS.
- Temporary abdominal closure
  - Towel clip closure—in the absence of any other equipment, penetrating towel clips may be applied to the skin temporarily in the operating room (OR) while correcting shock and coagulopathy; that is, the "30-minute timeout" (Fig. 19.1). However, this method is not optimal for formal DCS because of the risk of abdominal compartment syndrome (ACS) and egress of fluid between the clamps.

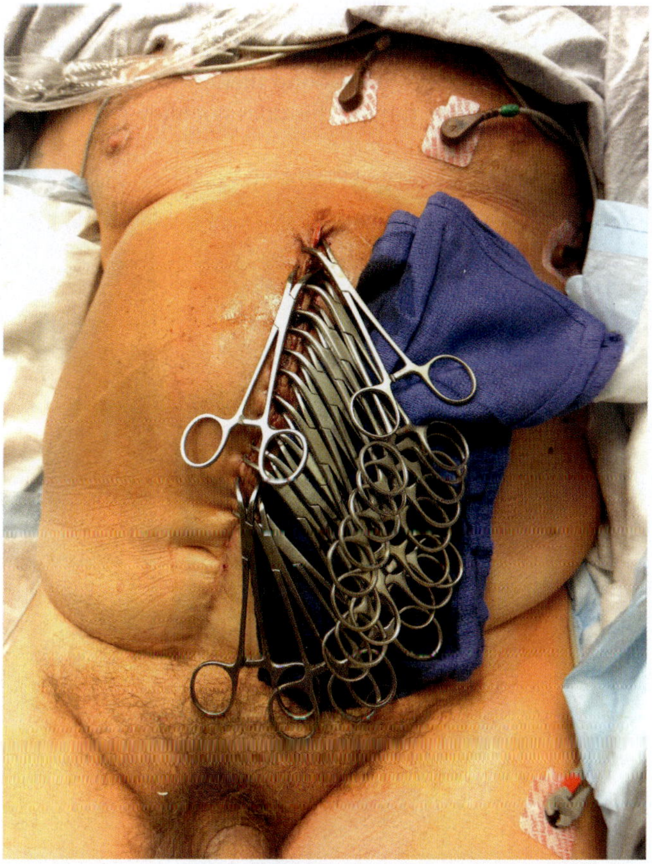

FIGURE 19.1 ▌ Towel clips can be applied to the skin for temporary abdominal closure.

- "Barker" method
  - The intestines are protected from injury using a fenestrated 1010 Steri Drape™. It is important to extend the drape laterally to the paracolic gutters to mitigate the risk of adhesions.
  - Two closed-suction drains are placed atop the Steri-Drape™ adjacent to the fascial edges and brought out at the cephalad-most aspect of the wound. The drains should be connected to continuous wall suction.

TIP

Exiting the drains at the caudal aspect of the wound increases the risk of leakage of the temporary dressing.

- An Ioban™ dressing is next placed atop the entire abdominal wall.

TIP

- *Placing pleats in the Ioban™ at this stage will accommodate for future bowel edema and expansion.*
- *To aid in tamponade of liver injury treated with packing, the skin of the upper portion of the incision may be reapproximated.*

- Alternative methods of temporary abdominal closure:
  - A fenestrated sterile x-ray cassette drape may be used instead of a 1010 Steri-Drape™ (Fig. 19.2).
  - A negative pressure wound therapy device (e.g., V.A.C. GRANUFOAM™ or V.A.C. AbThera™) may be used, though this does not allow visualization of the underlying bowel (Fig. 19.3).

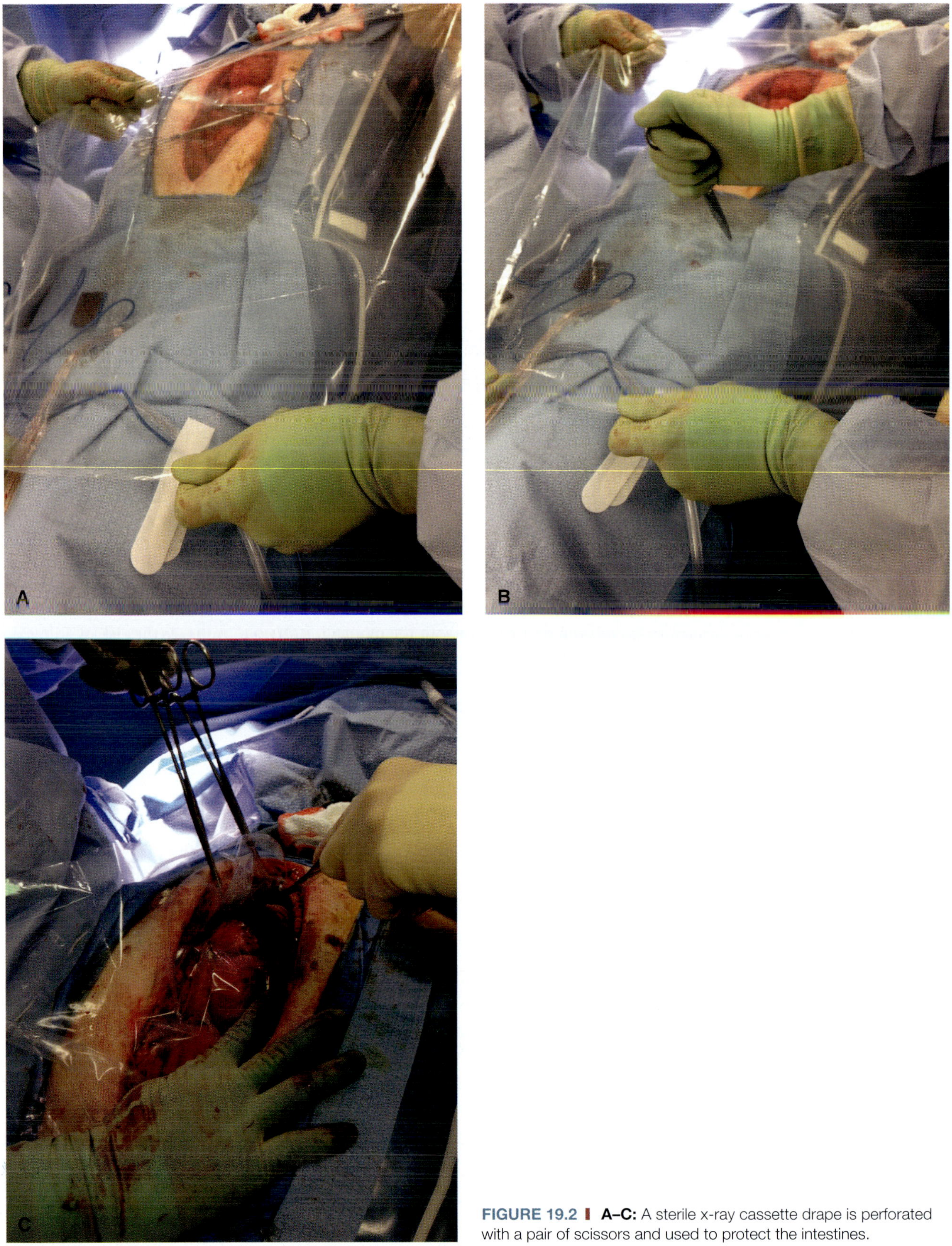

FIGURE 19.2 ▌ A–C: A sterile x-ray cassette drape is perforated with a pair of scissors and used to protect the intestines.

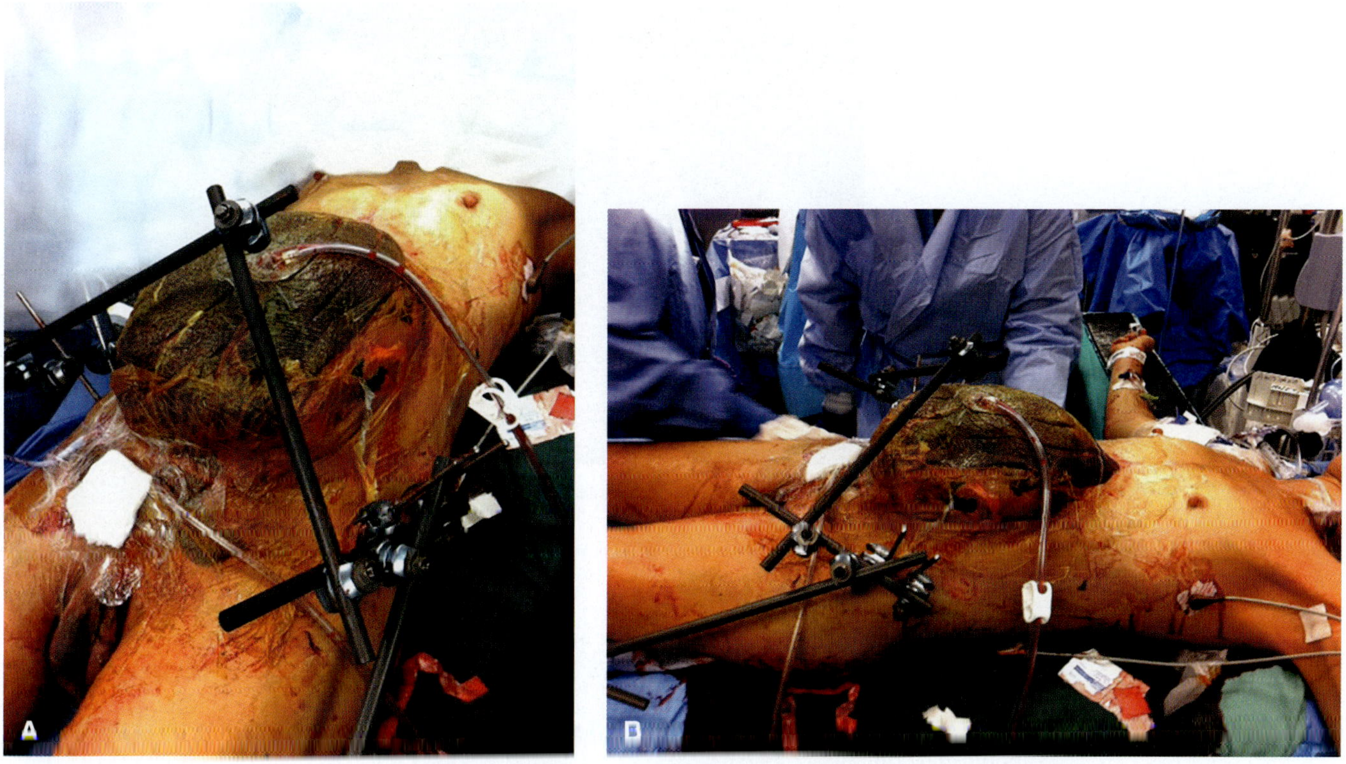

FIGURE 19.3 ▌ A, B: A V.A.C. may be used as a temporary abdominal closure.

Return After Physiologic Restoration

> **TIP**
>
> *Physiologic resuscitation is complete when the patient is normothermic, and all coagulation and metabolic derangements have been corrected.*

- Additional hemostasis procedures such as angioembolization and mechanical fracture stabilization may be required to control major bleeding.
- In the absence of ongoing bleeding, physiologic resuscitation should be complete within 12 hours.
- Upon return to the operating room:
  - Laparotomy pads are carefully removed.

> **TIP**
>
> *Irrigating with warm saline can help separate laparotomy pads from adherent bowel.*

  - Temporary vascular shunts are removed and vascular injuries are repaired using autologous vein, bovine pericardium, or prosthetic grafts (see Chapter 29).
  - GI continuity is restored with anastomosis or ostomy creation (if deemed high risk for anastomotic leak).
- Primary fascial closure is preferred, if possible, after definitive repair of injuries. This is guided by monitoring the peak airway pressure (PAP) by anesthesia. PAP <25 mm Hg is generally considered safe to avoid pulmonary barotrauma.
- If fascial closure cannot be accomplished due to inability to easily approximate the edges without undue tension, sequential closure can be performed. Interrupted fascial sutures starting from both the superior and inferior directions are placed until the tension is too great to continue (Fig. 19.4).

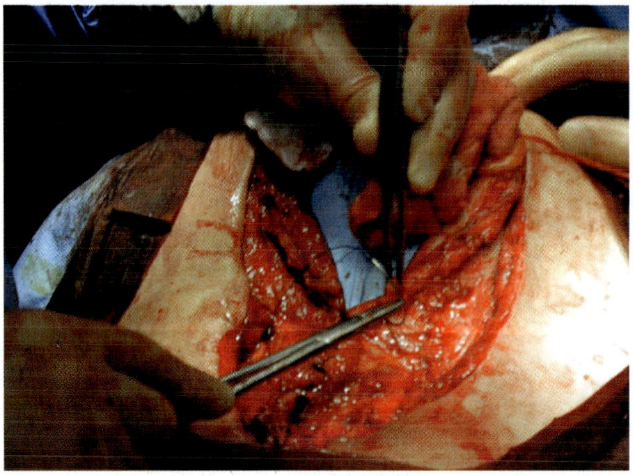

FIGURE 19.4 Interrupted fascial sutures are used to progressively close the midline.

TIP

Using figure-of-eight sutures (instead of simple interrupted) can distribute the tension and decrease the risk of the sutures pulling through the fascia.

- V.A.C. WHITEFOAM™ sponges are then placed (overlapping and stapled together) to cover the abdominal contents.
- Full-thickness fascial sutures are then placed and tied down atop the V.A.C. WHITEFOAM™ sponges to apply continuous medial fascial tension. This step is critical to avoid loss of domain.

TIP

These fascial tension sutures should be placed 2 cm from the fascial edge and spaced 5 cm apart.

- The skin can be stapled over the fascial closure sections. The remaining skin is protected using an occlusive dressing such as Ioban™ or V.A.C. Drape (3M, St. Paul, MN) and the center is trimmed to allow placement of V.A.C. GRANUFOAM™ (3M, St. Paul, MN) sponge atop the V.A.C. WHITEFOAM™ (Fig. 19.5). The whole apparatus is finally covered with another occlusive dressing before connecting to wall suction (Fig. 19.6).

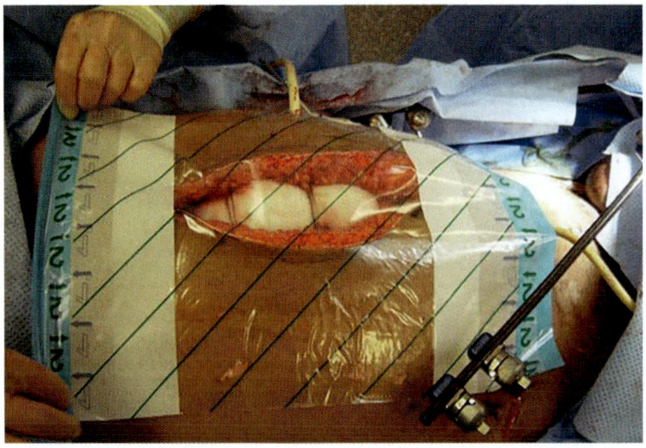

FIGURE 19.5 ❙ An occlusive dressing (with the center cut out) is used to protect the skin.

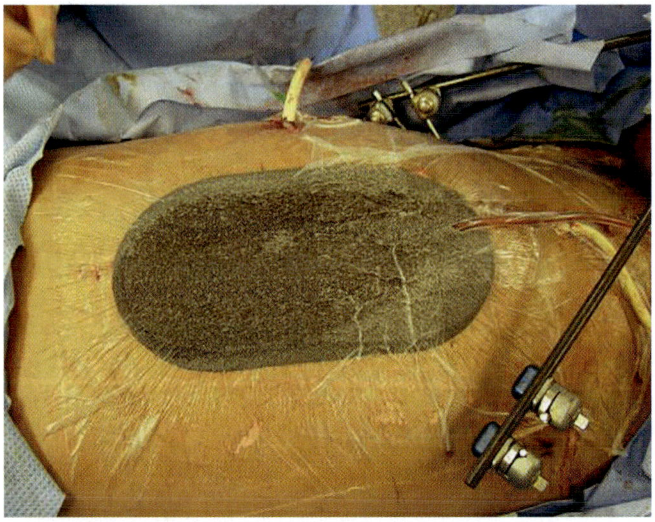

FIGURE 19.6 ❙ Black GRANUFOAM™ is placed atop the WHITEFOAM™ and covered with a second occlusive dressing before connecting to wall suction.

- The procedure is repeated every 24 to 48 hours with progressive closure attempted at the superior and inferior margins of the open wound using the above technique.
- Alternate methods of restoring abdominal domain:
  - Mesh-mediated medial fascial traction
    - A fenestrated drape (1010 Steri-Drape™ or sterile x-ray cassette drape) is used to protect the intestines from the mesh and mitigate adhesions to the abdominal wall.
    - A 30- × 30-cm Vicryl mesh is sutured using a 2-0 Prolene to bridge the fascial gap (Figs. 19.7 and 19.8).

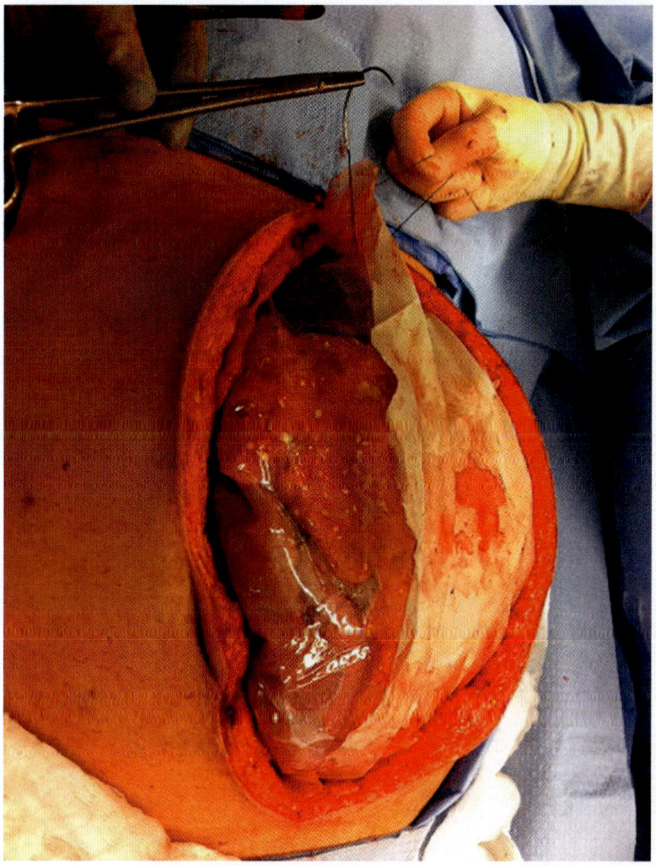

FIGURE 19.7 ▌ Vicryl mesh is sutured circumferentially to the fascia.

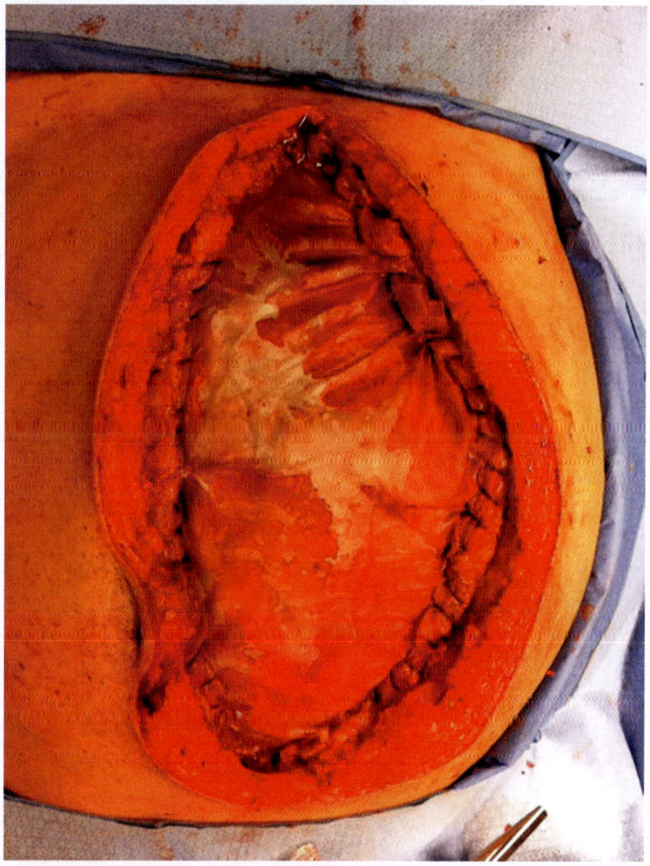

FIGURE 19.8 ▌ Traction is applied while suturing the mesh to the fascia to prevent loss of abdominal domain.

TIP

If excessive tension is applied, the mesh will rip or the Prolene will break, giving the surgeon immediate feedback.

- V.A.C. GRANUFOAM™ (3M, St. Paul, MN) sponge is placed atop the Vicryl mesh and covered with the occlusive dressing.

- Every 24 to 48 hours, the center of the Vicryl mesh is sliced open and the adjacent edges of the Vicryl mesh are drawn together, sutured, and trimmed (Figs. 19.9 to 19.11).

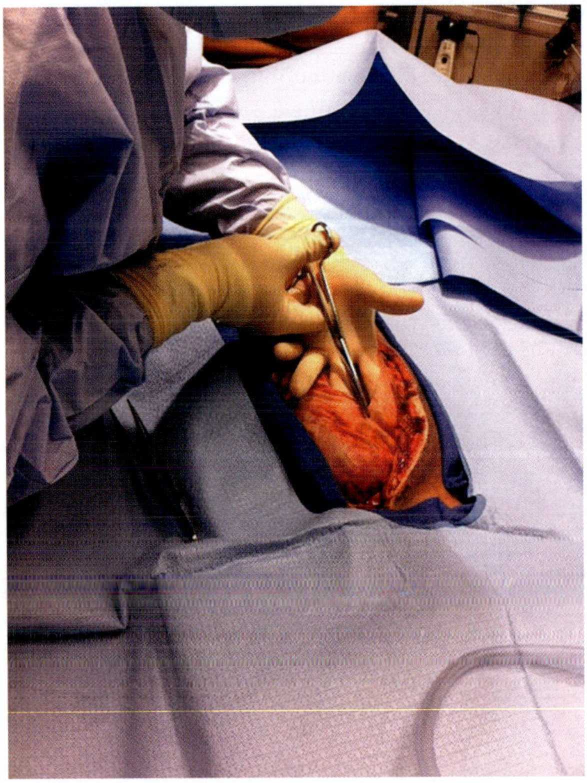

FIGURE 19.9 ▌ At subsequent operation, the mesh is cut in its center.

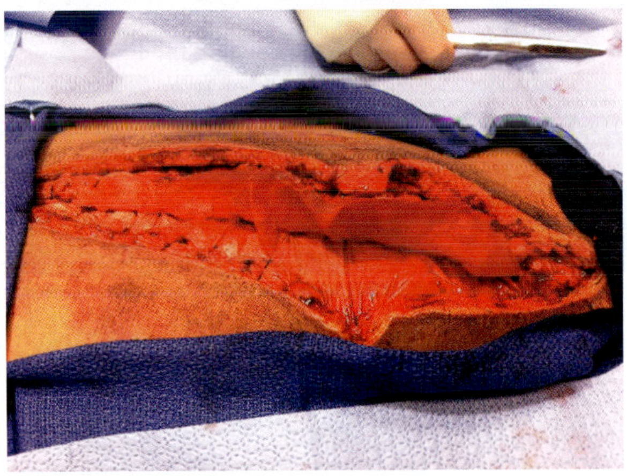

FIGURE 19.10 ▌ The cut center edges of the mesh are then drawn together and sutured to progressively close the abdomen.

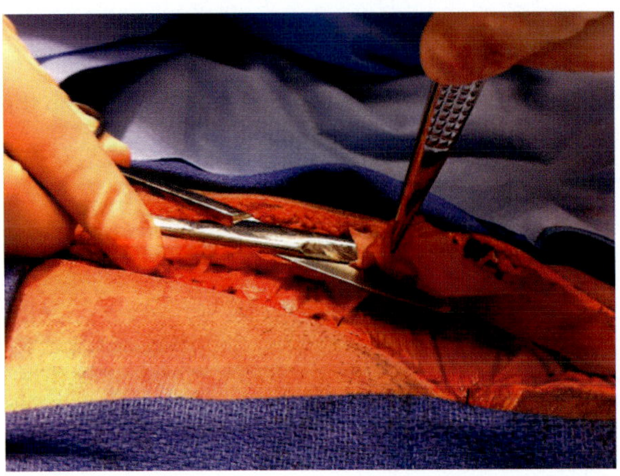

FIGURE 19.11 ▌ Excess center mesh is trimmed.

TIP

This step may be performed in the ICU and does not require replacement of the fenestrated drape below the mesh.

- When the fascia is easily approximated without tension, the Vicryl mesh is released from the fascia, the fenestrated drape removed, and the fascia primarily closed.
- Ryder open abdomen retention (ROAR) (Figs. 19.12, 19.13, and 19.14)

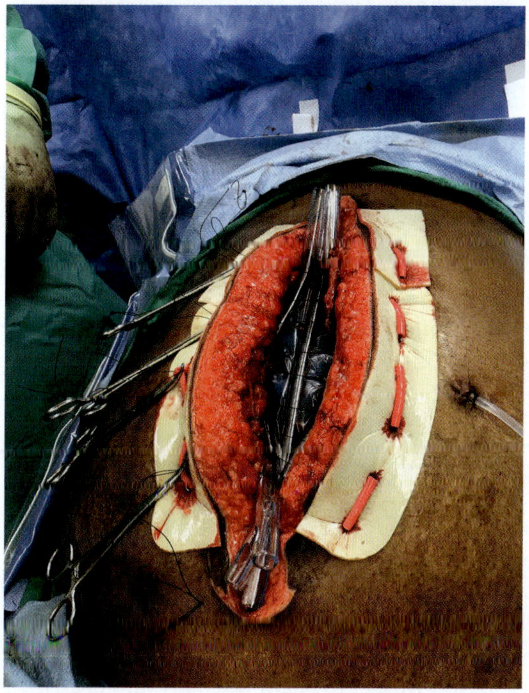

FIGURE 19.12 ▍ Full-thickness transabdominal retention sutures secured with clamps are used to progressively close the abdomen.

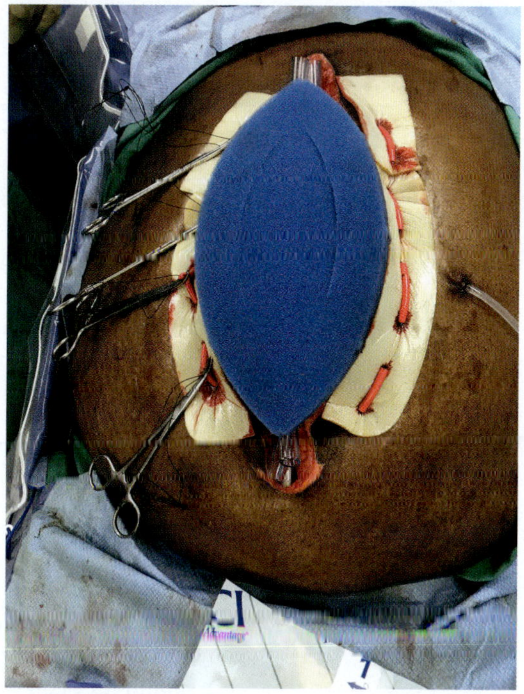

FIGURE 19.13 ▍ Chest tubes are used as bumpers to protect the underlying viscera from the retention sutures and red rubber catheters are used to protect the skin.

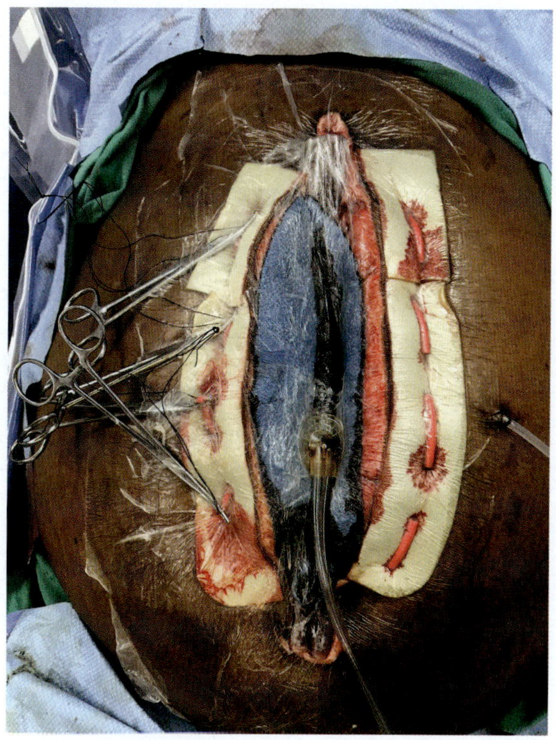

FIGURE 19.14 ▍ Occlusive dressing and suction are applied as the final step of the ROAR.

- The abdominal viscera are protected using a fenestrated drape (as above) or with an AbThera™ sponge.
- Full-thickness transabdominal retention sutures are placed using red rubber catheter segments and DuoDerm® (ConvaTec, Reading, United Kingdom) padding to protect the underlying skin.
- Large-bore chest tubes are placed beneath the retention sutures as bumpers to prevent injury to the underlying viscera.
- Fluid egress can be achieved using closed-suction drains or SENSAT.R.A.C. suction pad (3M, St. Paul, MN).
- Tension is applied to these retention sutures and maintained using surgical clamps.
- The tension is tightened every 24 to 48 hours.

TIP

This step may be performed in the ICU and does not require replacement of the chest tubes or drapes.

- Direct Peritoneal Resuscitation
  - Consider performing direct peritoneal resuscitation (DPR) in patients with viscera edema. DPR can help reduce bowel edema, improve perfusion of the abdominal viscera, and may prevent intestinal adhesions from forming before the fascia is closed.

POSTOPERATIVE CARE

- The closed-suction drains should be connected to wall suction in order to accommodate high-volume abdominal fluid drainage.
- Abdominal effluent volume should be carefully recorded and accounted for in ICU care. There is evidence to support early vasopressin as the preferred inotrope to minimize crystalloid loading. In general, once physiologic resuscitation is complete and the patient is no longer hypovolemic, ICU care should focus on de-resuscitation with equivalent intensity and priority. Positive fluid balance is a predictor for inability to close an open abdomen.
- Enteral nutrition in open abdomen patients is associated with higher rates of abdominal closure rate and higher survival compared to patients kept nil per os (NPO, nothing by mouth). Once GI continuity (or ostomy) has been restored, tube feeding should be initiated at a trophic rate and increasing to goal as tolerated. Although these patients are hypermetabolic, professional society (SCCM/ASPEN and ESPEN) recommends to target only 80% of estimated caloric needs in the first week of critical illness, but meeting protein demands.
- Prophylactic antibiotics are not recommended for the sole indication of open abdomen.
- Although rare, ACS can occur in the setting of an open abdomen (tertiary ACS) and bladder pressures should be measured in patients with clinical suspicion; for example, declining urinary output with PAP >25 mm Hg.

Suggested Readings

Acosta S, Bjarnason T, Petersson U, et al. Multicentre prospective study of fascial closure rate after open abdomen with vacuum and mesh-mediated fascial traction. *Br J Surg*. 2011;98(5):735–743.

Barker DE, Kaufman HJ, Smith LA, Ciraulo DL, Richart CL, Burns RP. Vacuum pack technique of temporary abdominal closure: a 7-year experience with 112 patients. *J Trauma*. 2000,48(2):201–206; discussion 206–207.

Cothren CC, Moore EE, Johnson JL, Moore JB, Burch JM. One hundred percent fascial approximation with sequential abdominal closure of the open abdomen. *Am J Surg*. 2006;192(2):238–242.

Fox N, Crutchfield M, LaChant M, Ross SE, Seamon MJ. Early abdominal closure improves long-term outcomes after damage-control laparotomy. *J Trauma Acute Care Surg*. 2013;75(5):854–858.

Miller PR, Meredith JW, Johnson JC, Chang MC. Prospective evaluation of vacuum-assisted fascial closure after open abdomen: planned ventral hernia rate is substantially reduced. *Ann Surg*. 2004;239(5):608–614; discussion 614–616.

Petersson U, Acosta S, Björck M. Vacuum-assisted wound closure and mesh-mediated fascial traction–a novel technique for late closure of the open abdomen. *World J Surg*. 2007;31(11):2133–2137.

Rasilainen S, Mentula P, Salminen P, et al. Superior primary fascial closure rate and lower mortality after open abdomen using negative pressure wound therapy with continuous fascial traction. *J Trauma Acute Care Surg*. 2020;89(6):1136–1142.

Sava J, Alam HB, Vercruysse G, et al. Western Trauma Association critical decisions in trauma: management of the open abdomen after damage control surgery. *J Trauma Acute Care Surg*. 2019;87(5):1232–1238.

Smith JW, Garrison NR, Matheson PJ, Franklin GA, Harbrecht BG, Richardson DJ. Direct peritoneal resuscitation accelerates primary abdominal wall closure after damage control surgery. *J Am Coll Surg*. 2010;210(5):658–664, 664–667.

Suliburk JW, Ware DN, Balogh Z, et al. Vacuum-assisted wound closure achieves early fascial closure of open abdomens after severe trauma. *J Trauma*. 2003;55(6):1155–1160; discussion 1160–1161.

SECTION V Pelvic Injuries

Chapter 20

Preperitoneal Pelvic Packing and Postpacking Arteriography

ERNEST E. MOORE AND CHARLES J. FOX

PERIOPERATIVE CONSIDERATIONS

Procedure Rationale

The mortality for patients arriving in shock with an unstable pelvic fracture continues to exceed 30% in major trauma centers throughout the United States. The pelvic vasculature is abundant with extensive collateral blood flow, and limited capacity for tamponade (Fig. 20.1). Initial management in the emergency department consists of pelvic compression to reduce pelvic volume with Zone III resuscitative endovascular balloon occlusion of the aorta (REBOA) for refractory shock (Fig. 20.1). Life threatening hemorrhage from pelvic fractures is believed to the venous in origin in >85% of patients. Consequently, packing of the pelvis is a logical early operative technique to prevent exsanguination. While used in Europe for decades, preperitoneal pelvic packing (PPP) has only been accepted widely in the United States over the past 15 years. The reticence to employ pelvic packing was largely based on a suboptimal technique of packing done previously via a laparotomy. PPP should be viewed as a complimentary approach to selective angioembolization (AE) for pelvic bleeding and AE may be required in 10% to 15% of patients following PPP. The advantages of PPP in conjunction with REBOA and pelvic external fixation, however, are rapid achievement of pelvic hemostasis and the ability to manage associated injuries while in the operating room (OR). The increasing availability of the hybrid OR has further emphasized the potential use of PPP followed by selective AE when there is angiographic evidence of continued arterial bleeding.

Our current practice is to perform pelvic angiography for all severely displaced (anteroposterior compression [APC] III, lateral compression [LC] III, and vertical shear) fracture patterns as well as in those patients with a blush evident on prepacking computed tomography (CT) scanning or altered lower extremity perfusion.

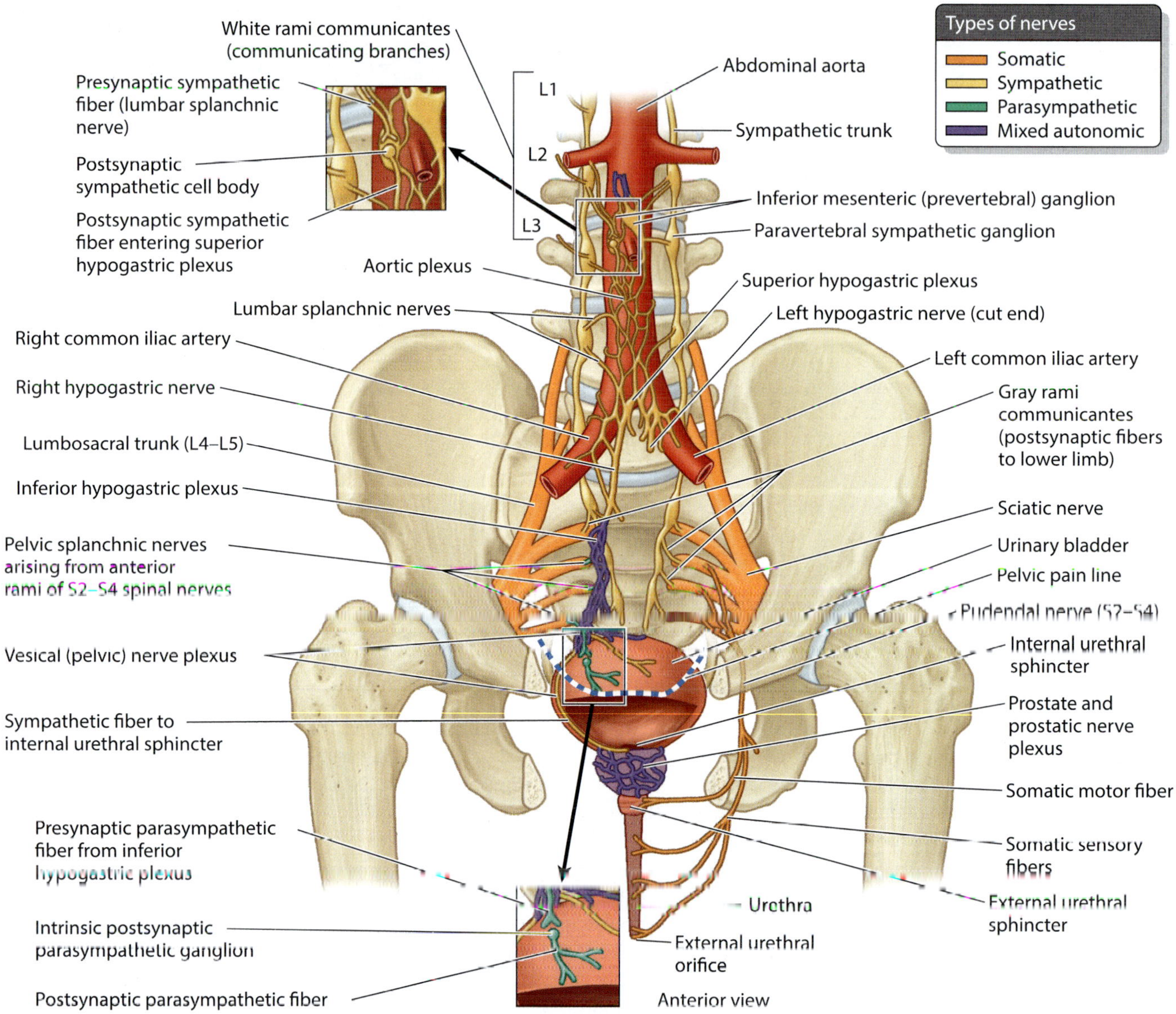

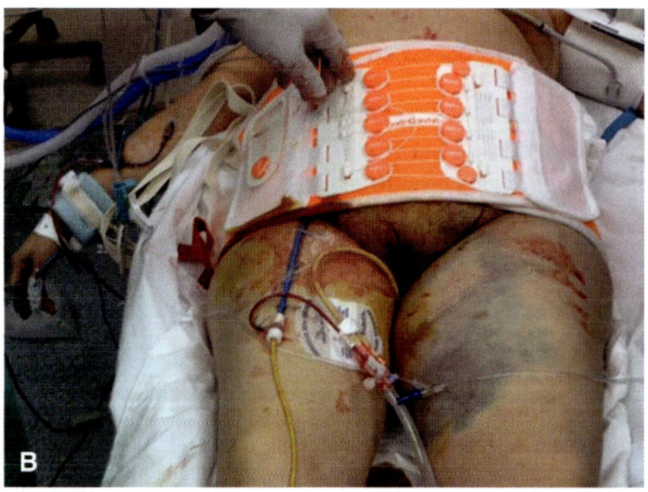

FIGURE 20.1 ▌ Major pelvic fractures can provoke life-threatening bleeding due to the extensive blood supply to the pelvis (**A**). (From Pelvis and Perineum. In: Dalley AF II, Agur AMR, eds. *Moore's Clinically Oriented Anatomy.* 9th ed. Wolters Kluwer; 2023:559–671. Figure 6.29.) Initial management in the ED consists of pelvic compression and Zone III REBOA for refractory shock (**B**).

TIP

PPP is done in conjunction with external fixation of the pelvis by the orthopedic trauma team (Fig. 20.2). External skeletal fixation reduces the pelvic volume and thus facilitates PPP tamponade of bleeding. Further, the trauma team can assist with apposition of the pubic rami anteriorly while adjusting the pelvic frame.

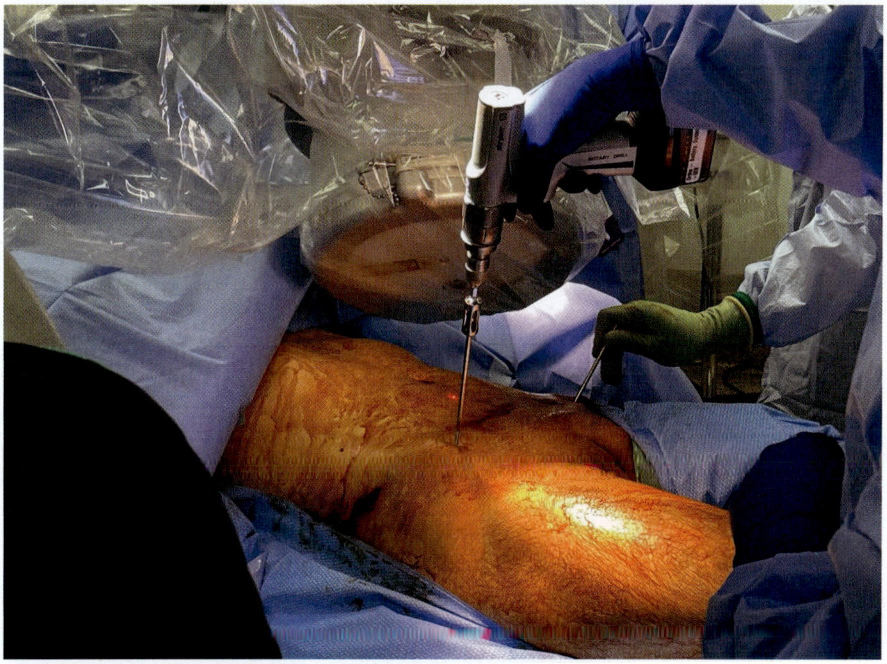

FIGURE 20.2 | PPP tamponade of pelvic fracture bleeding requires external fixation of the pelvis, optimally performed by the orthopedic trauma team prior to the incision.

Essential Equipment

- 10-blade scalpel
- Medium Richardson retractor
- Laparotomy pads × 6
- Ringed forceps
- Thrombin spray
- Cephalexin 2 gram
- Standard needle holder
- # 1 PDS suture
- Skin stapler

Transfemoral Pelvic Angiography

- Micropuncture access kit, 5 Fr
- 5-Fr sheath, 11 cm
- Omni flush catheter
- 0.035-inch angled glide wire, 180 cm
- 0.035-inch angled glide catheter, 65 cm
- Radiopaque contrast agent in 10- and 20-mL syringes

Positioning and Prepping

TIP

Unstable pelvic fractures are often associated with additional life- or limb-threatening injuries. Consequently, wide skin preparation should be done in the event of the need for thoracotomy, laparotomy, or lower extremity vascular access. The lower leg on the side of a REBOA should be prepped for vascular assessment prior to leaving the OR.

- Supine with both arms extended out.
- The REBOA sheath and catheter should be prepared for direct access (see Chapter 2).
- The contralateral inguinal region should be prepared for angiography access.
- Radial arterial line is placed on the side opposite of the REBOA.
- Anticipate blood loss and have blood products available.

SURGICAL APPROACH

TIP

The skin incision and fascial opening should be limited to permit a separate midline laparotomy if necessary for intraperitoneal injuries, while maintaining pelvic tamponade.

The Zone III ER REBOA should remain fully inflated during packing; the pREBOA can be used to maintain a proximal systolic pressure >100 mm Hg with a distal systolic pressure targeted to 60 mm Hg (see Chapter 2). The skin incision extends from the pubis cephalad approximately one-half the distance to the umbilicus. The fascia is opened in the midline until the pelvic hematoma is observed or entered with the fascial incision (Fig. 20.3). If the hematoma remains intact, the overlying peritoneum should be separated with a finger.

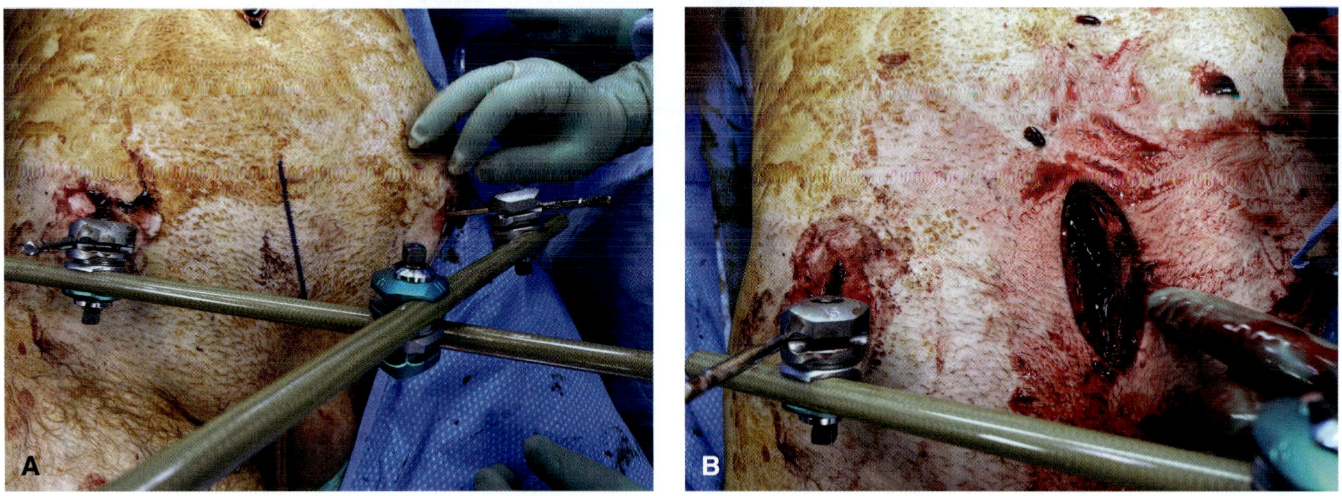

FIGURE 20.3 ▌The skin incision extends from the pubis cephalad approximately one-half the distance to the umbilicus (**A**). A finger should be used to open the hematoma if remains intact after the fascial separation (**B**).

- Often vigorous bleeding occurs with unroofing the hematoma (Fig. 20.4). There is no benefit in evacuating the hematoma.
- Packing is initiated with standard laparotomy pads on the side with the most severe fracture. If time permits, we spray thrombin onto the lap pad to enhance clot formation. Alternatively, kaolin-impregnated gauze can be used for the same purpose. To reduce the infection rate, we add powdered cephalexin to the surface of the lap pad. Alternatively, antibiotic beads can be placed.

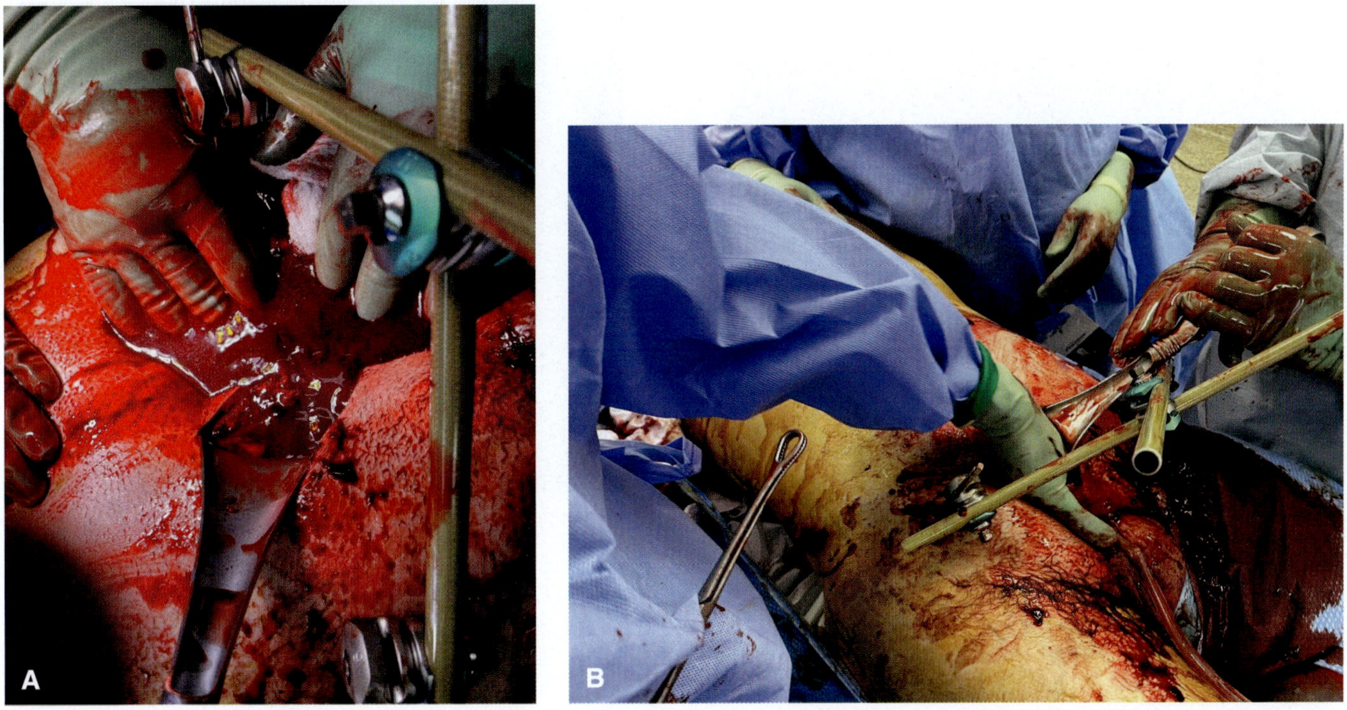

FIGURE 20.4 ▌ Vigorous bleeding is often encountered when the pelvic hematoma is entered (**A**). A medium-sized Richardson retractor is used to elevate the abdominopelvic wall to facilitate placement of laparotomy pads with the bladder retracted to the opposite side (**B**).

- A medium-sized Richardson retractor is used to elevate the abdominopelvic wall (Fig. 20.4), with the bladder retracted to the opposite side. Packs are introduced unrolled with ringed forceps into the side with the most severe pelvic fractures. It is critical to place the first lap pad deep into the pelvis (Fig. 20.5), with two additional lap pads placed on top of the first. Following packing of the most severely injured side, the same procedure is pursued on the contralateral side.

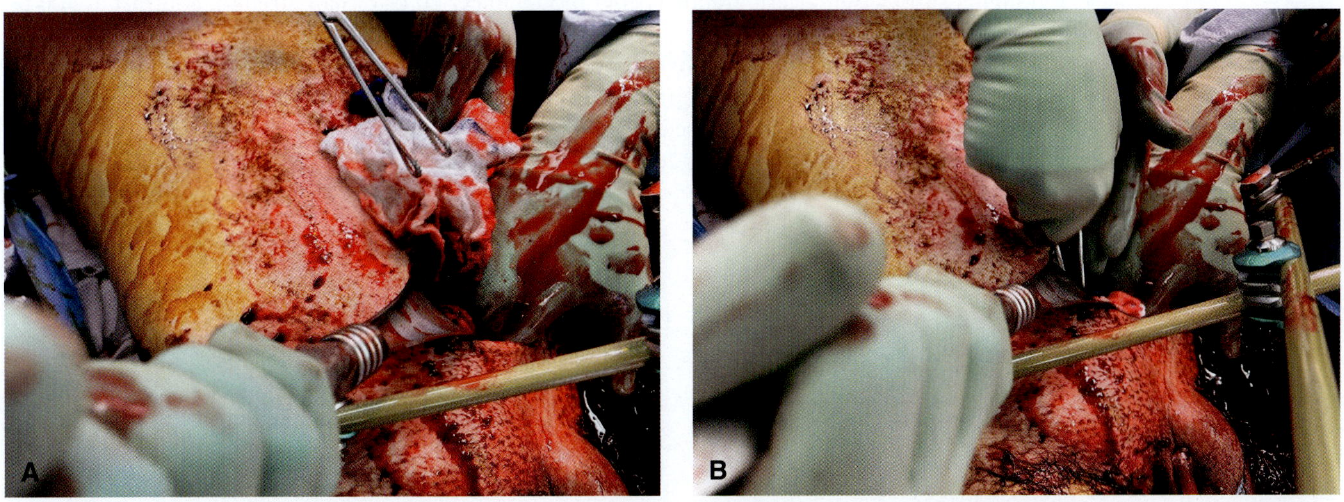

FIGURE 20.5 ▌ Unrolled laparotomy pads are inserted with ringed forceps (**A**). It is critical to place the first pad deep into the pelvis (**B**).

- Typically three lap pads are positioned on each side of the pelvis (Fig. 20.6). Packing with more pads increases compression of the iliac veins, enhancing the risk of venous thrombosis.
- The midline fascia is reapproximated with continuous #1 PDS suture to maximize tamponade. The skin is stapled anticipating early pack removal.

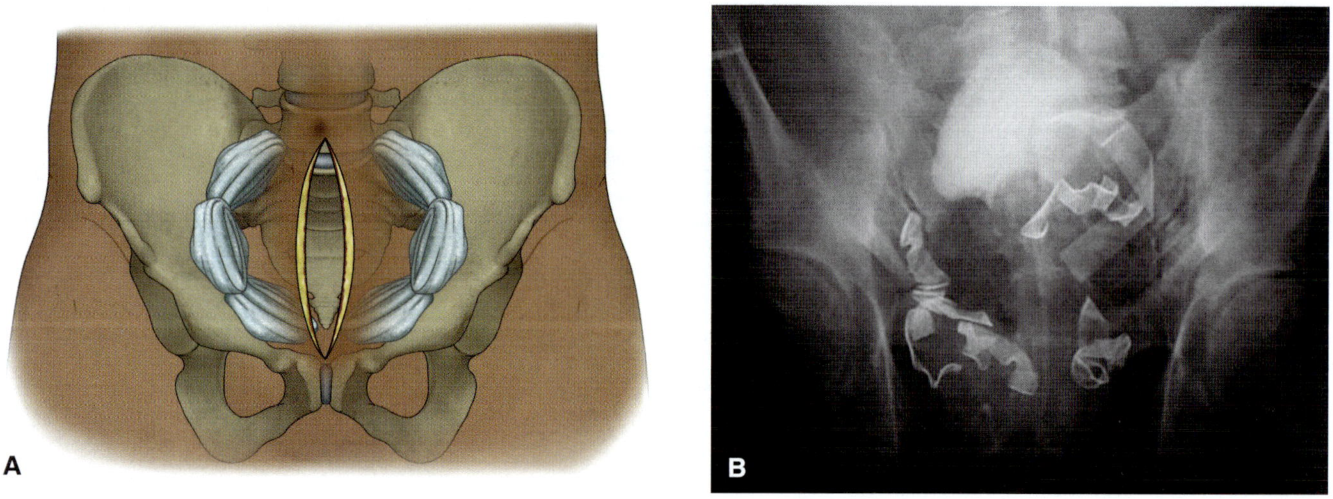

FIGURE 20.6 ❙ Typically three lap pads are placed on each side (**A**). a plain radiograph illustrates the proper position of the lap pads (**B**).

Post-Packing Arteriography

TIP

If the REBOA can be removed, pelvic angiography is performed through the existing 7-Fr sheath. If the REBOA is inflated or left in position for possible reinflation, a 5-Fr femoral sheath is placed in the contralateral common femoral artery for pelvic angiography. Alternatively, transradial access can be used when there is concern for an iliofemoral arterial injury.

While post-packing angiography is optimally done in a hybrid OR, an acceptable quality angiogram can be accomplished with a C-arm in a standard OR.

- Advance the glide wire fluoroscopically into the infrarenal aorta.
- Advance the Omni flush catheter over the glide wire to the third lumbar vertebrae (L3).
- Remove the glide wire and connect high pressure tubing.
- On digital subtraction arteriography (DSA) mode, inject 20 cc of half-strength contrast at 300 psi at 10 cc/sec (Fig. 20.7A).
- When a power injector is not available, a hand injection can be performed with the REBOA inflated.
- Reference the image and using roadmap feature, pull the flush catheter into the ipsilateral common iliac artery and use a glide wire to select the internal iliac artery.
- Exchange the flush catheter for a glide catheter over the wire (Fig. 20.7B).

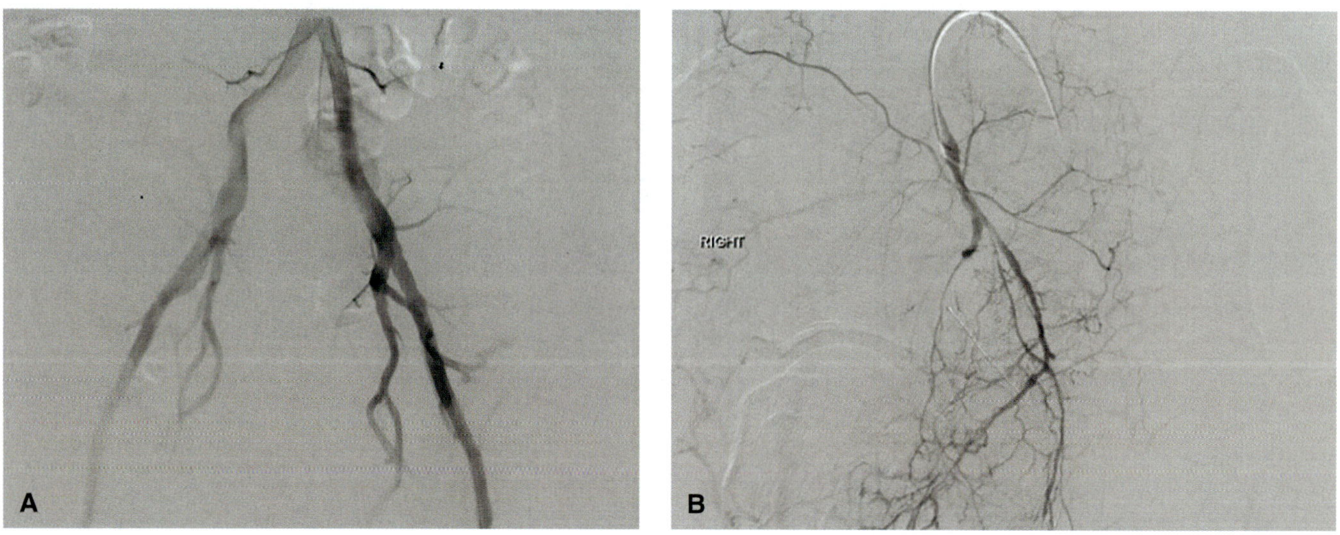

FIGURE 20.7 ❙ Post-packing pelvic angiography is done via an Omni flush catheter (**A**). Selective internal iliac arteriography is accomplished through an angled glide catheter (**B**).

- Hand inject 5 to 10 mL of contrast and continue to hold the DSA pedal for 10 to 20 seconds (venous phase) to look for signs of bleeding from the anterior and posterior divisions.
- If further selective angiography is warranted, repeat these steps with an angled glide wire and catheter slowly advancing into the distal branch vessels (Fig. 20.8).
- For contralateral iliac arterial images, position the flush catheter at the aortic bifurcation and select the common iliac artery with a glide wire, followed by a glide catheter and advance as desired.
- For transradial pelvic angiography, use a 5-Fr slender radial artery sheath and navigate the preferred long catheters and wires beyond the REBOA balloon to the abdominal aortic bifurcation.
- Post-packing angiography may identify major arterial injuries that require reconstruction. An example is a right external iliac artery injury that we reconstructed at the initial operation for packing (Fig. 20.9).

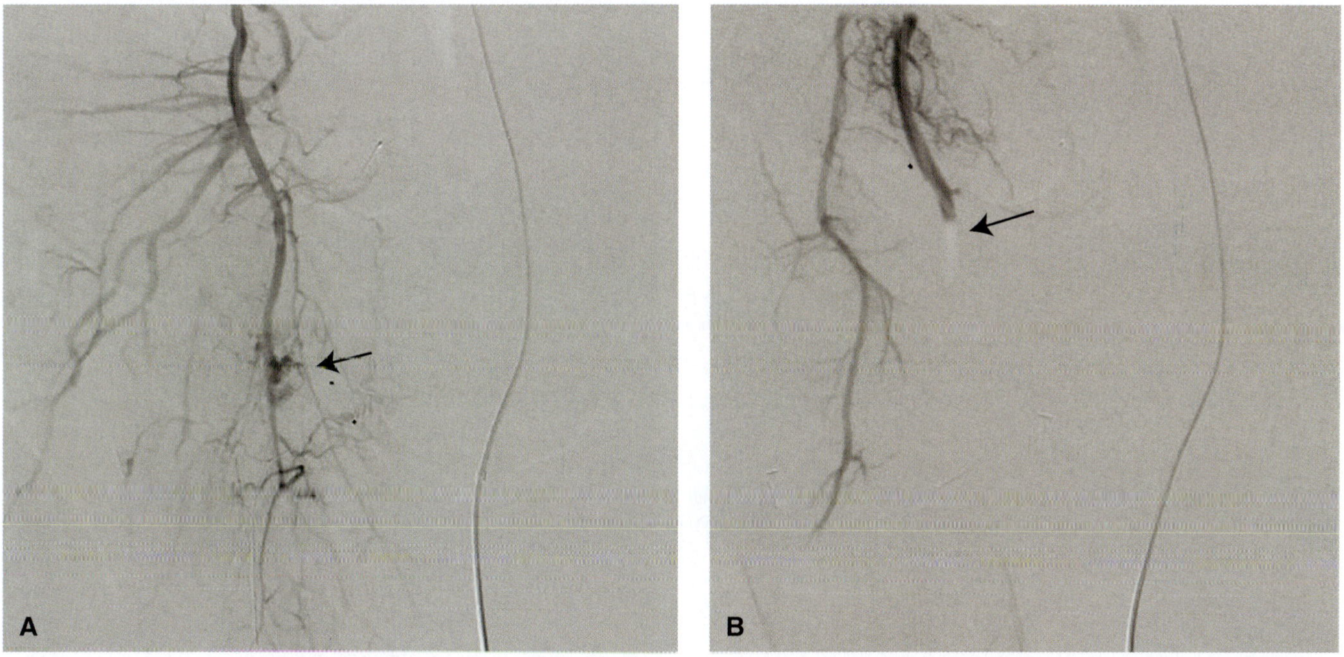

FIGURE 20.8 ▌ Selective iliac angiography identified multiple bleeding sites (**A**, *arrow*). Selective gel foam embolization (*arrow*) of the anterior segment of the internal iliac artery controlled active bleeding (**B**).

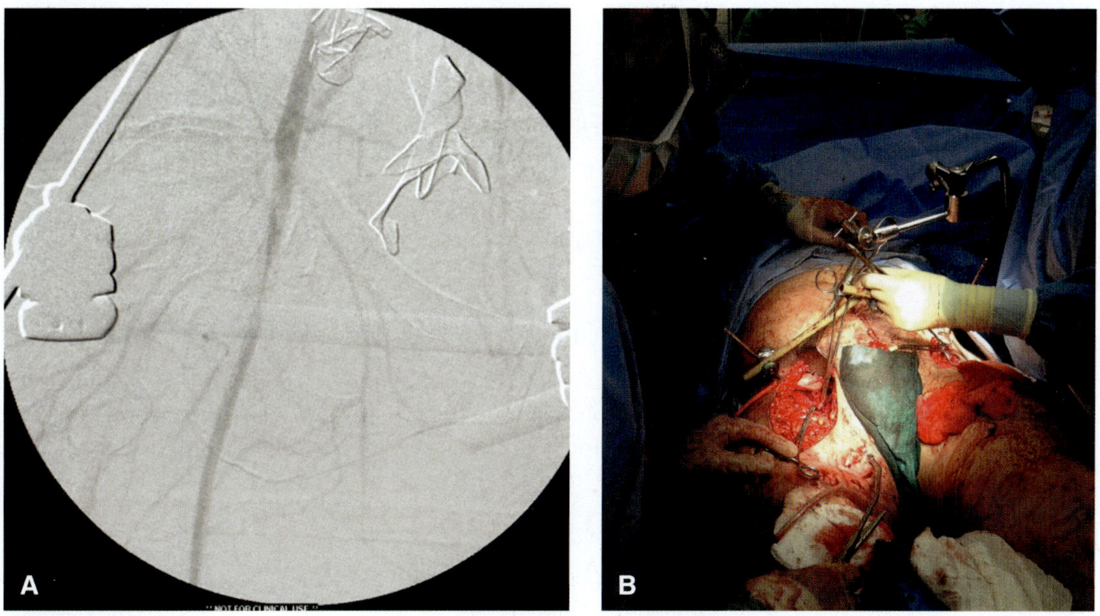

FIGURE 20.9 ▌ Post-packing angiography identified a right external iliac artery (**A**), which was repaired at the initial operation for packing (**B**).

Associated Injuries

Pelvic Venous Injuries

PPP is very effective in controlling pelvic venous bleeding. We recently managed a patient with a 3.5-cm perforation of the left common iliac vein (Fig. 20.10), discovered at the time of unpacking 18 hours later. The vein was suture repaired without sequela.

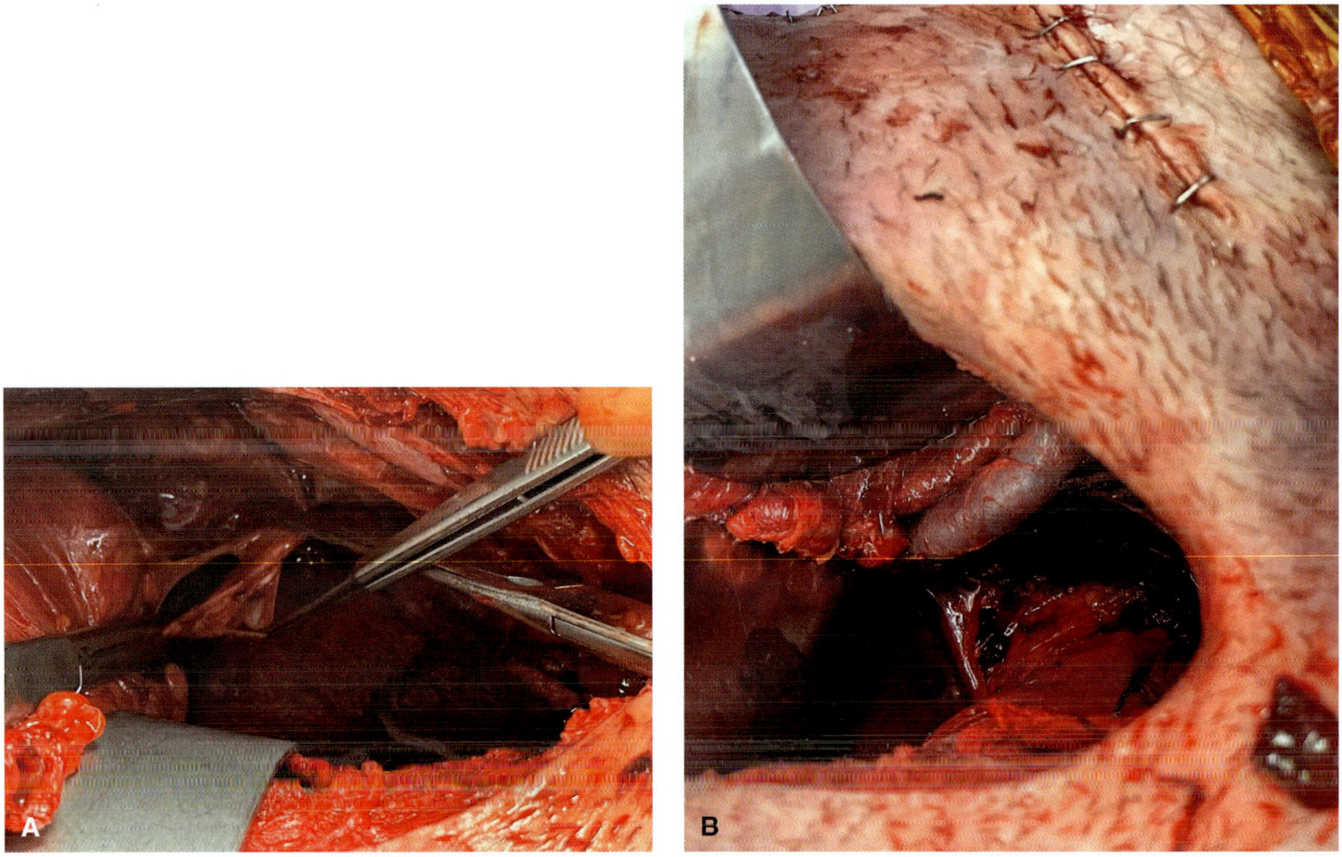

FIGURE 20.10 This 3.5-cm perforation of the left common iliac vein was managed successfully with PPP (**A**). The injury was found at unpacking 18 hours later and suture repaired (**B**).

Bladder Injuries

If there is pelvic fracture fragmentation adjacent to the bladder or hematuria exists, the bladder is filled with saline-diluted methylene blue dye to evaluate for a perforation.

Urethral Injuries

A transected urethral may preclude Foley catheter placement, necessitating insertion of a suprapubic catheter.

Rectal and Vaginal Injuries

Pelvic bone fragments may penetrate the rectum or vagina, producing the environment for an advanced pelvic soft tissue infection. Rigid sigmoidoscopy and a vaginal examination should be done at the time of pack removal for fracture patterns at risk for thee injuries.

POSTOPERATIVE CARE

- Patients requiring PPP for pelvic fracture bleeding are managed in the surgical intensive care unit (SICU) with ongoing resuscitation to reverse metabolic acidosis and restore normal coagulation.

- Total body CT scanning should be completed as soon as possible due to the high risk of associated injuries, including traumatic brain injury (TBI), torn descending thoracic aorta, and abdominal solid organ injuries.
- The REBOA sheath should be removed as soon as the hypocoagulable phenotype of trauma-induced coagulopathy (TIC) is eliminated to avoid thrombosis, and the involved extremity should undergo duplex scanning.
- Recurrent pelvic bleeding from occluded arteries may occur with restoration of normal perfusion, and this may require delayed secondary selective AE. This scenario occurs in approximately 10% of our patients, and reinforces the role of post-packing pelvic angiography at the time of initial PPP.
- The major risks of PPP are pelvic infections and venous thromboembolism. We believe early removal of the pelvic packs is important to minimize these risks and, therefore, return the patient to the OR as soon as physiologically safe. In general, we target pack removal for 12 hours and attempt to accomplish this within 24 hours in all patients.

Suggested Readings

Burlew CC, Moore EE, Stahel PF, et al. Preperitoneal pelvic packing reduces mortality in patients with life-threatening hemorrhage due to unstable pelvic fractures. *J Trauma Acute Care Surg*. 2017;82:233–242.

Heelan AA, Freedberg M, Moore EE, et al. Worth looking! venous thromboembolism in patients who undergo preperitoneal pelvic packing warrants screening duplex. *Am J Surg*. 2020;220:1395–1399.

Magee GA, Fox CJ, Moore EE. Resuscitative endovascular balloon occlusion of the aorta in pelvic ring fractures: The Denver Health protocol. *Injury*. 2021;52:2702–2706.

Parry JA, Smith WR, Moore EE, et al. The past, present, and future management of hemodynamic instability in patients with unstable pelvic ring injuries. *Injury*. 2020;22:2693–2698.

Smith WR, Moore EE, Osborn P, et al. Retroperitoneal packing as a resuscitation technique for hemodynamically unstable patients with pelvic fractures: report of two representative cases and a description of technique. *J Trauma*. 2005;59:1510–1514.

Suzuki T, Smith WR, Moore EE. Pelvic packing or angiography: competitive or complementary? *Injury*. 2009;40:343–353.

Tesoriero RB, Bruns BR, Narayan M, et al. Angiographic embolization for hemorrhage following pelvic fracture: is it "time" for a paradigm shift? *J Trauma Acute Care Surg*. 2017;82:18–26.

Chapter 21
Lumbar Spine Exposure

CHARLES J. FOX

PERIOPERATIVE CONSIDERATIONS

TIP

Review the conduct of the operation with the scrub technician to ensure the technical challenges of the operation can be met. There is no time for a "learning curve" during lumbar bleeding that could be encountered during the exposure.

- Anticipate blood loss and have products with rapid infuser in the operating room.
- Use a Cell Saver for reoperative cases.
- Have a major vascular set in the room
- Review MR, CT, and plain radiographs for the bony and vascular anatomy.
- Perform a well-documented preoperative neurovascular exam.
- Morbid obesity (BMI >35) is a risk for vascular injury.

Procedure Rationale

- Advances in spinal instrumentation have increased demand for anterior retroperitoneal spine exposure for lumbar interbody fusion and corpectomy for the trauma patient.
- Although vascular injury remains the most dreaded complication, the anterior approach is also associated with potential injury to the bowel, ureter, and adjacent nerves. The following overview focuses on sufficient exposure to minimize injury. A team approach to anterior lumbar spine surgery can reduce complications while offering technical benefits and a durable reconstruction of the spine.

Anatomy

TIP

The diaphragm can be divided with a linear stapler. The staples will provide additional strength for the sutures. Alternating colored sutures will allow for easier approximation of the muscle at the time of closure.

- L1–L2 levels are best approached laterally from the retroperitoneum (Fig. 21.1A).
- The diaphragm is occasionally divided (circumferentially) for the L1 exposure, but the left crus of the diaphragm will require division for L1–L2.
- A lumbar tributary to the left renal vein should be identified and ligated during L1–L2 exposures to avoid bleeding during left kidney rotation.
- L3–L5 levels are best approached anteriorly from the retroperitoneum (Fig. 21.1B).
- The L3 level may require ligation of a few lumbar vessels before attempting aortoiliac mobilization.

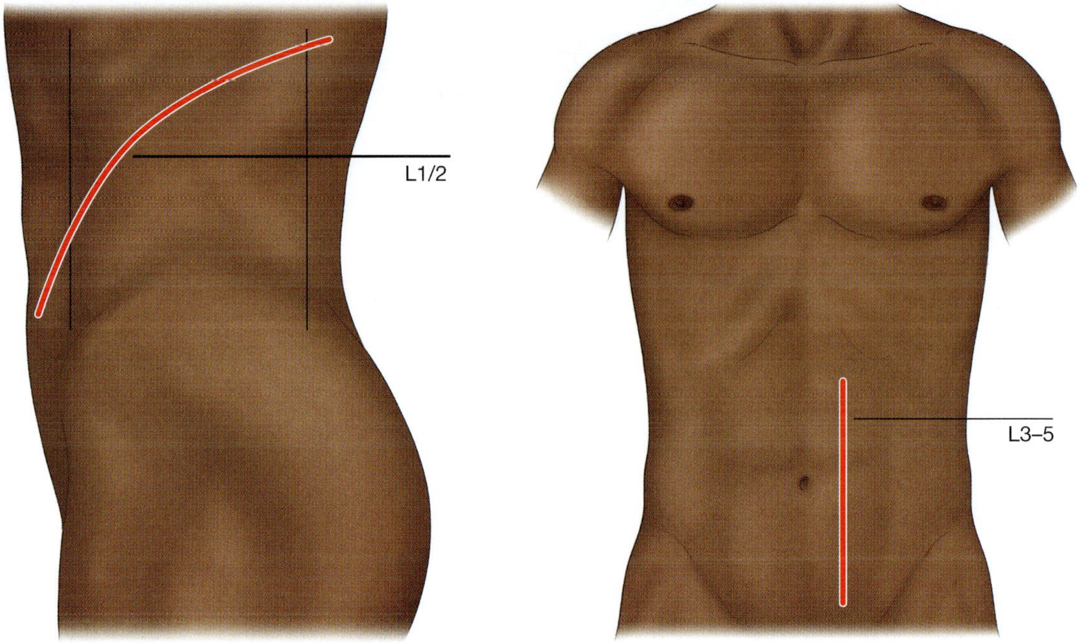

A B

FIGURE 21.1 ❙ Illustrations show the oblique (L1–L2, **A**) and paramedian (L3–L5, **B**) surgical incisions.

- The peritoneal contents and the ureter are reflected medially during the anterior retroperitoneal lumbosacral spine exposure avoiding injury to adjacent nerves (Fig. 21.2).

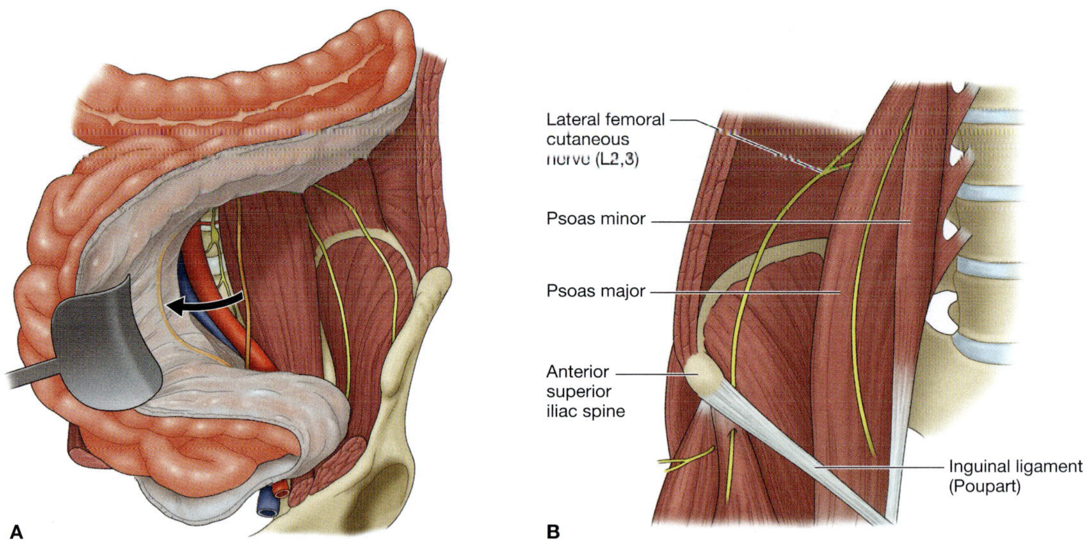

A B

FIGURE 21.2 ❙ The abdominal contents with ureter are reflected medially during the anterior retroperitoneal lumbosacral spine exposure (**A**). It is important to recognize the genitofemoral nerve and remain anterior to the psoas muscle on the initial approach (**B**).

- The left common iliac vein (CIV) is reflected medially for L4 exposures to avoid tension on the vena cava bifurcation (Fig. 21.3A).
- The left iliac artery is mobilized as needed but usually can remain lateral for an L5 exposure (Fig. 21.3B).
- The posterior rectus sheath terminates at the semilunar line.

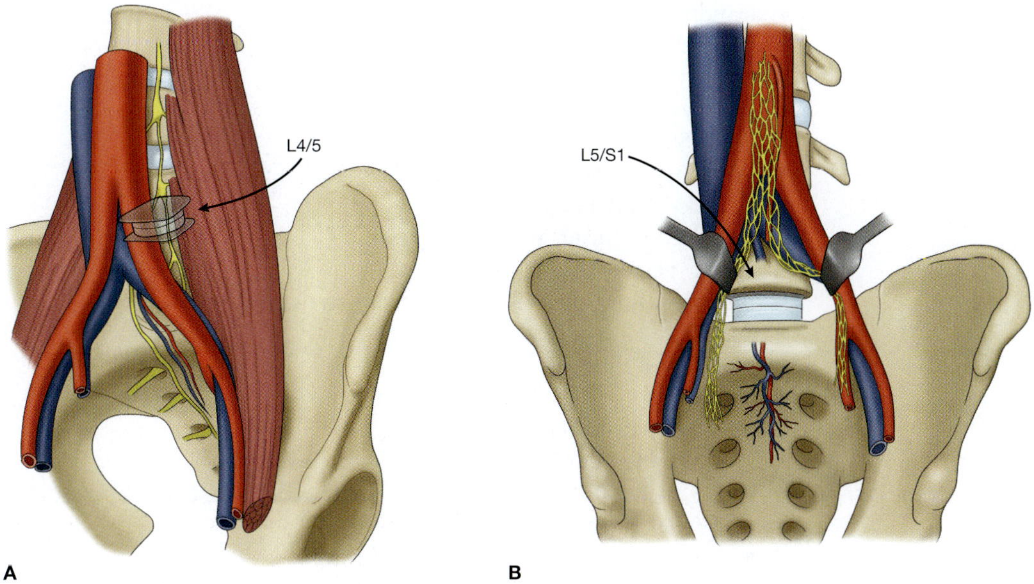

FIGURE 21.3 ❚ The L4–L5 exposure requires mobilization of the left common iliac vein to avoid injury at the iliocaval bifurcation (**A**). The Iliac vein and artery are not separated and reflected laterally during the L5–S1 exposure (**B**).

Essential Equipment

TIP

Inform the surgical team to always pass double armed sutures and have all suture sizes readily available and loaded on vascular instruments.

- Headlight
- Loupe magnification 2.5
- Table-attached Omni-Tract, EndoRing, or SynFrame Retractor Systems (Fig. 21.4)

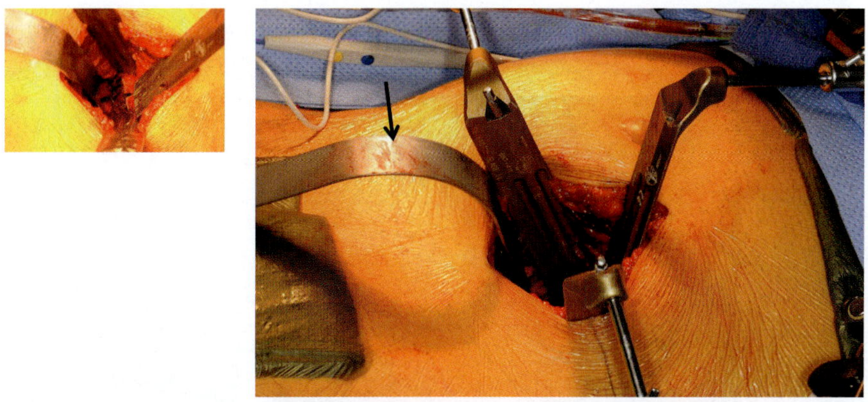

FIGURE 21.4 ❚ The table-attached radiolucent EndoRing retractor system (Medtronic, Minneapolis, MN) along with a handheld renal vein retractor (*arrow*) provides good exposure for this L4–L5 lumbosacral spine exposure (*inset*).

- Bladder, splanchnic, renal vein blades for Omni-Tract
- DeBakey forceps
- Metzenbaum scissors
- Yankauer suction, bulb tip
- Richardson retractor
- Deaver retractor
- Sponge sticks
- Hemoclip and Hemoclip appliers (manual loads)
- Kittner dissectors and peanut sponges

- Handheld renal vein retractor
- Cobb elevator
- Castroviejo and Ryder needle drivers (long)
- Microvascular Gerald forceps
- Potts–Smith scissors
- Wiley hypogastric or Henley subclavian clamps
- Satinsky–DeBakey clamp
- DeBakey–Bahnson aortic clamp
- Silastic vessel Loops
- Rummel Tourniquet (Red rubber catheter and umbilical tape)
- Teflon or felt pledgets
- 28-Fr chest tubes
- Sutures
  - 2-0 Polypropylene (diaphragm)
  - No. 1 Vicryl or Ethibond (Pericostal closure)
  - 3-0, 4-0, 5-0 Prolene on a C1 & RB1 needles (vascular repair)
  - 3-0 Silk plain and stick ties (long)
  - 0 & 2-0 Absorbable sutures for closing
  - 4-0 Monocryl sutures or skin stapler
- Sterile 8- to 10-MHz Doppler probe
- Thrombin 1,000 U/mL, 20-mL vial
- Gelfoam
- Fibrin sealant
- Cell saver autologous blood recovery system
- C-Arm fluoroscopy machine
- Mayo stand & Bean bag immobilizer (L1–L2)
- Ioban antimicrobial drape (Large)
- Bovie and bipolar electrocautery
- Spinal needle

Patient Positioning

Positioning for L1–L2

- Right lateral decubitus on bean bag without spinal rotation (Fig. 21.5A & B).

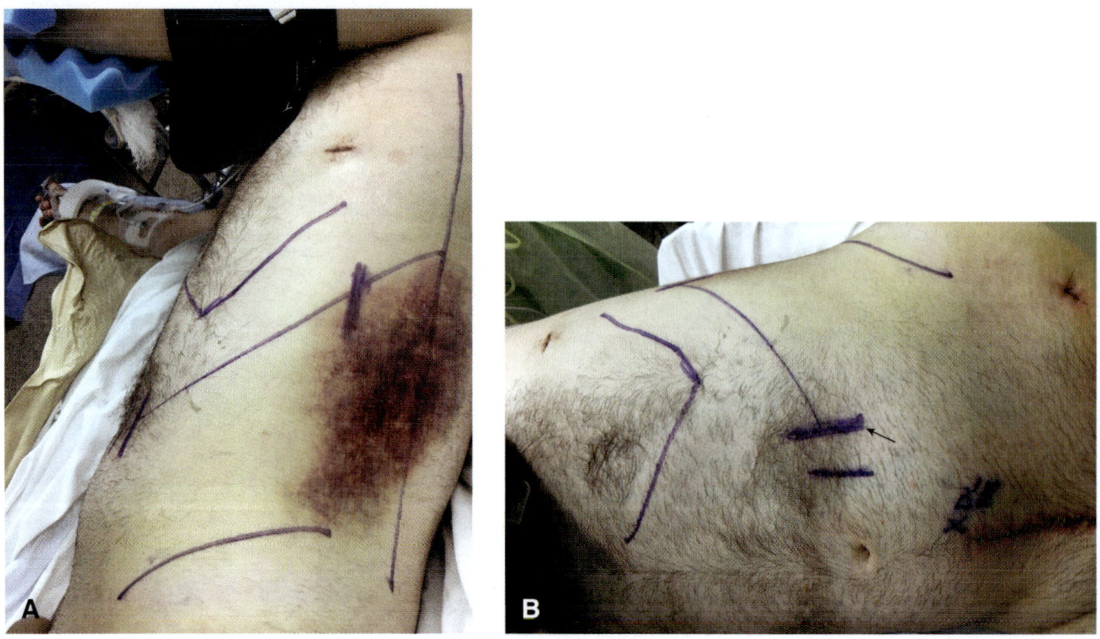

FIGURE 21.5 ▌ Lateral decubitus positioning of a trauma patient on a bean bag for L2 corpectomy (**A**). Surgical markings display the costal margin, anterior superior iliac spine, the posterior axillary line, and the incision beginning at the lateral border of the rectus muscle (**B**, *arrow*). A spine exposure unlike the dissection for an abdominal aortic aneurysm needs to stay more posterior.

- Left arm padded over Mayo stand.
- Radial arterial line.
- Neurologic monitoring of evoked potentials.
- Lower body warmer.
- Protect all pressure points with egg crate padding and tape.
- Make surgical markings on anterior superior iliac spine, lateral border of rectus muscle, axillary line, and scapula tip.
- Anterior and lateral fluoroscopic images are recommended before incision.

Positioning for L3–L5

- Supine with arms padded across chest resting on pillow (ease of C-Arm movements).
- Padding and monitoring remains the same as L1–L2 positioning.
- Apply an oxygen monitor sensor on the left great toe to monitor return of circulation.
- Make vertical surgical marking along the lateral border of rectus muscle.

TIP

Needle confirmation of the correct vertebral level is advisable.

TECHNIQUE

Exposure: Retroperitoneal Approach to L1-L2

- Oblique left flank skin incision from lateral border of rectus at umbilicus to axillary line (Fig. 21.6A).
- Extend incision across 10th intercostal space (suprarenal) or 11th (infrarenal) as desired.
- A subperiosteal division of the 10th or 11th rib aids the exposure and is well tolerated (Fig. 21.6B).

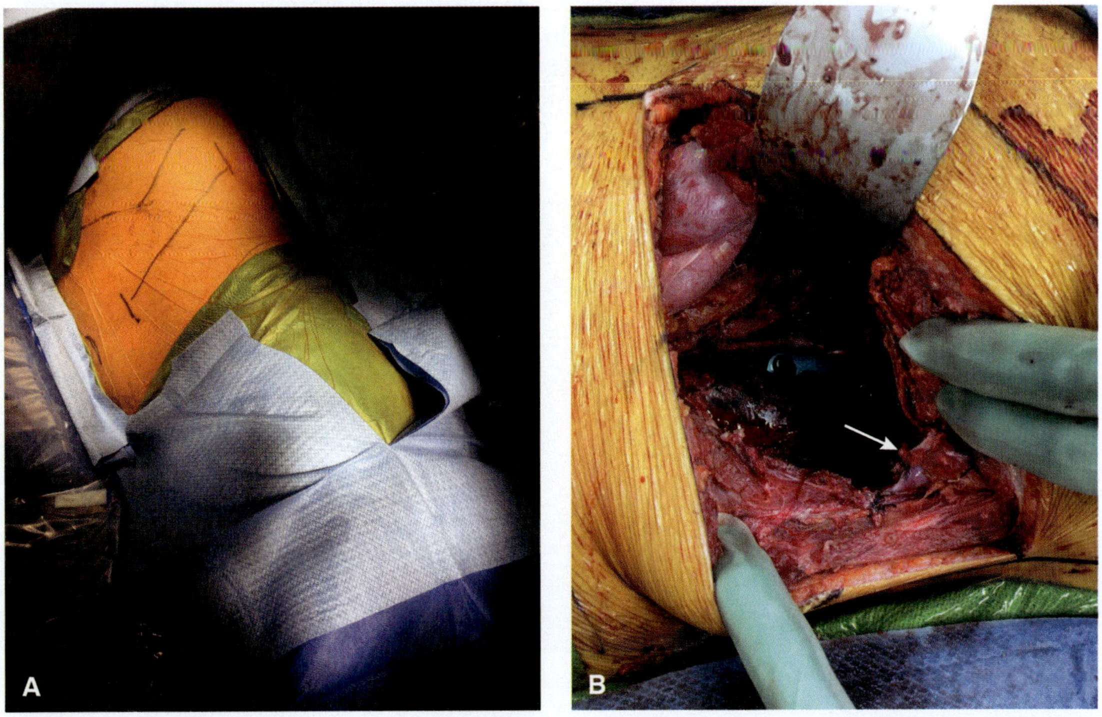

FIGURE 21.6 ▌ Surgical markings are placed before the Ioban draping (**A**) to easily identify the anatomic landmarks without ink smudging for accurate exposure across the proper rib interspace. The 10th rib was partially resected during this exposure without sequelae (**B**, *arrow*).

- Extend incision 5 cm below umbilicus to improve the visualization of the iliac vessels (Fig. 21.7).

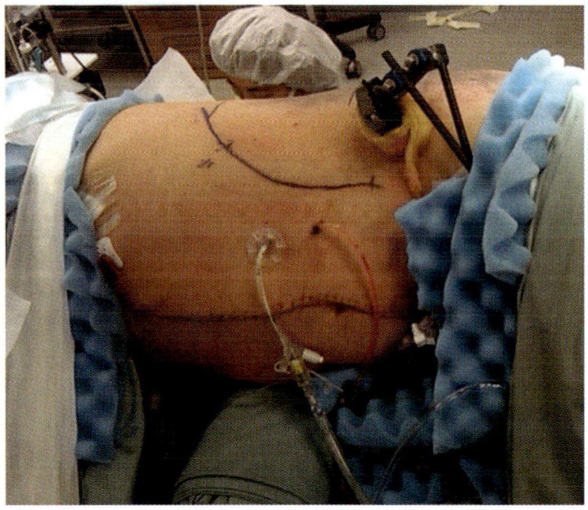

FIGURE 21.7 ▌ The retroperitoneal exposure for an L2 and L3 burst fracture is done in the right lateral decubitus position without rotating the spine. Consider extending the incision below the umbilicus when a dissection near the iliac vessels is anticipated.

- Underlying muscle including crus fibers are cauterized to avoid bleeding.
- The peritoneum and left kidney are swept medially and cephalad after dividing any veins.
- Small peritoneal rents are more likely to occur medially and should be repaired with absorbable sutures.
- Omni-Tract splanchnic (2), bladder and renal vein blades afford excellent exposure.
- A few lumbar vessels are often sacrificed but aortic mobilization is rarely necessary.
- A Cobb elevator is used to clean the longitudinal ligament and vertebral body.
- A bent spinal needle is placed in the desired disc space for a quality fluoroscopic image.
- Burst fractures are a common indication for lumbar exposure and require a wide surgical field for corpectomy and implants (Fig. 21.8).

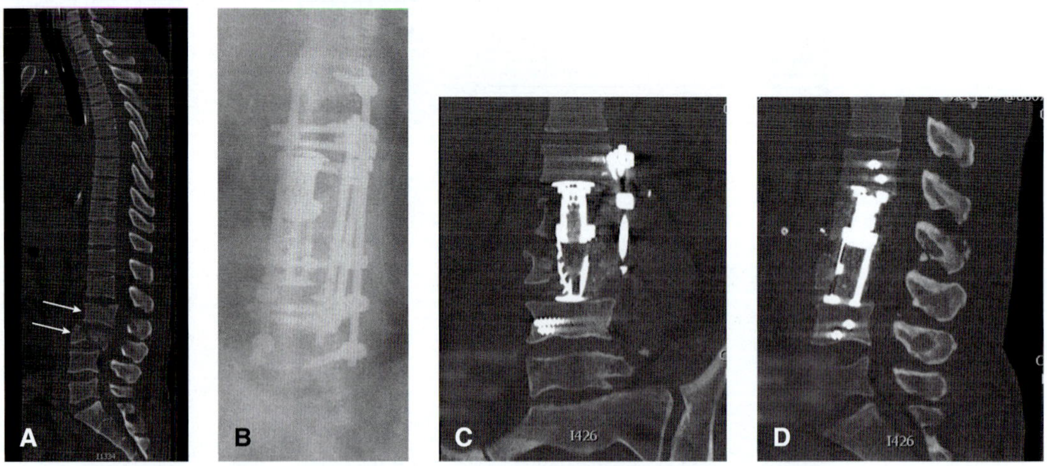

FIGURE 21.8 ▌ Sagittal computed tomography (CT) scan of thoracolumbar spine with burst fractures (**A**, *arrows*) and plain radiograph (**B**) with corresponding coronal and sagittal views (**C, D**) after L1–L4 exposure and two-level corpectomy.

Exposure: Retroperitoneal Approach to L3-L5

TIP

The paramedian incision should be the approximate length of the surgeon's hand, oriented at the umbilicus for L4 and incising above or below depending on the exact level of the exposure.

- 6-cm left paramedian incision above (L3) or below (L5) the umbilicus using fluoroscopy.
- Divide the anterior rectus fascia and dissect in a lateral plane taking down perforators.
- Perform a deeper fingertip retroperitoneal dissection into loose areolar tissue.
- Start the peritoneal separation laterally and continue medially to avoid tears.
- Identify the genitofemoral nerve and remain anterior to the psoas muscle.
- Palpate the pulsatile common iliac artery while sweeping medial.
- Use a Deaver to pull the peritoneal contents and ureter to the midline.
- Divide transversalis fibers to relax tension and aid in the L3–L4 exposures.
- Safely mobilize the CIV by ligating/dividing its venous tributaries.
- Retrograde ejaculation is prevented by using bipolar cautery and minimizing dissection.
- The iliolumbar vein, near the hypogastric artery, is routinely ligated for L4 exposures.
- Ligate the middle sacral artery with silk ties and Hemoclips.
- A few well-placed interrupted sutures will not stenose the CIV.
- Sweep fatty tissue off the anterior longitudinal ligament with Peanuts and Sponge sticks.
- It is crucial to expose and easily visualize the end plates of the vertebral body above and below the intended level (Fig. 21.9).

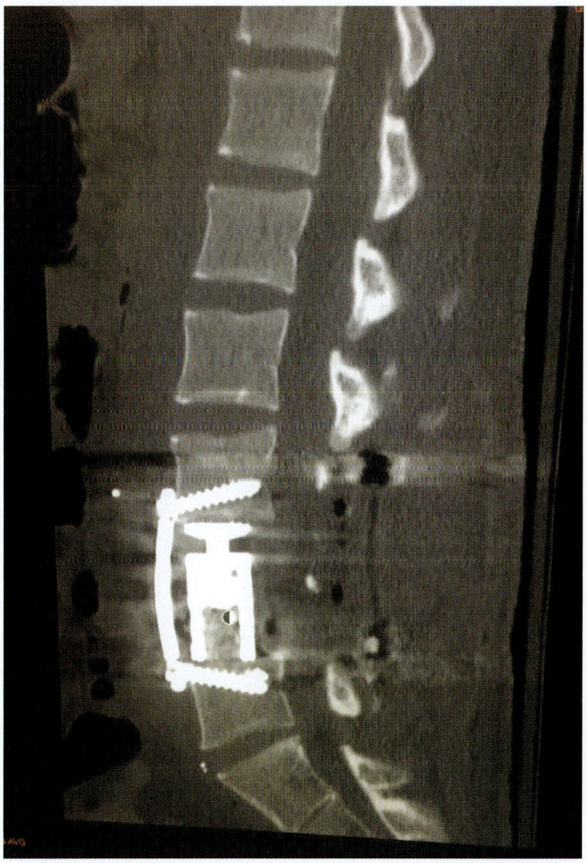

FIGURE 21.9 ▌ The lateral radiograph following L4 corpectomy depicts the need for a wide exposure (L3–L5) for adequate prosthesis implantation and proper screw placements.

- A bent spinal needle is placed in the desired disc and fluoroscopic images are taken.
- Remain attentive during the spine procedure and replace disturbed retractors.
- The anterior rectus fascia is closed with 0 absorbable suture.
- Scarpa fascia is closed with 2-0 absorbable suture.

POSTOPERATIVE CARE

- 24-hour ICU admission for pulse comparison and hemodynamic monitoring.
- Monitor for limb swelling and potential for deep venous thrombosis (DVT).

- Early ambulation and DVT chemoprophylaxis is encouraged.
- Ileus is uncommon and early refeeding is recommended.
- Hernia, retrograde ejaculation, lymphocele, and abdominal bulges are anticipated complications.

Suggested Readings

Ballard JL, Carlson G, Chen J, et al. Anterior thoracolumbar spine exposure: critical review and analysis. *Ann Vasc Surg*. 2014; 28(2):465–469.

Bianchi C, Ballard JL, Abou-Zamzam AM, et al. Anterior retroperitoneal lumbosacral spine exposure: operative technique and results. *Ann Vasc Surg*. 2003;17(2):137–142.

Dua A, Fox J, Patel B, et al. A team approach to anterior lumbar spine surgery in the military. *Vascular*. 2014;22(4):246–251.

SECTION VII Extremity Vascular Injuries

Chapter 22
Axillary Artery

ERNEST E. MOORE AND CHARLES J. FOX

PERIOPERATIVE CONSIDERATIONS

Procedure Rationale

- The axillary artery is a relatively deep structure in the anterior chest wall, and is typically injured due to penetrating wounds. Anterior shoulder dislocation is the most common blunt mechanism (Fig. 22.1).

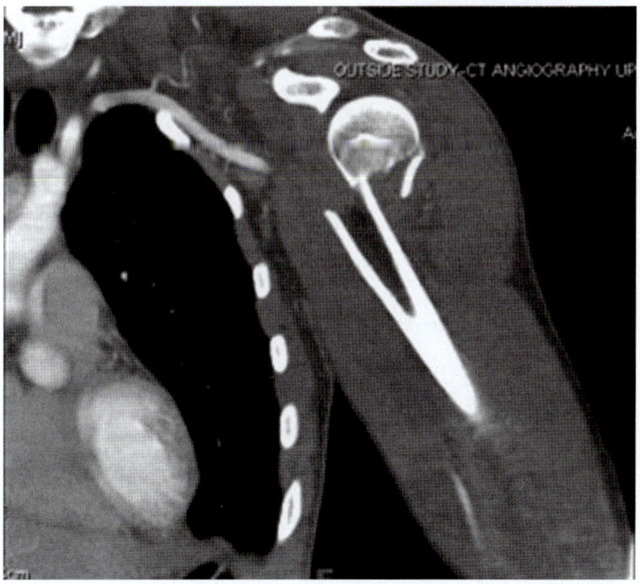

FIGURE 22.1 | Should dislocations or fractures can result in a blunt injury with occlusion of the axillary artery.

The brachial plexus is intertwined with the axillary vessels (Fig. 22.2) and, thus, a frequent associated injury.

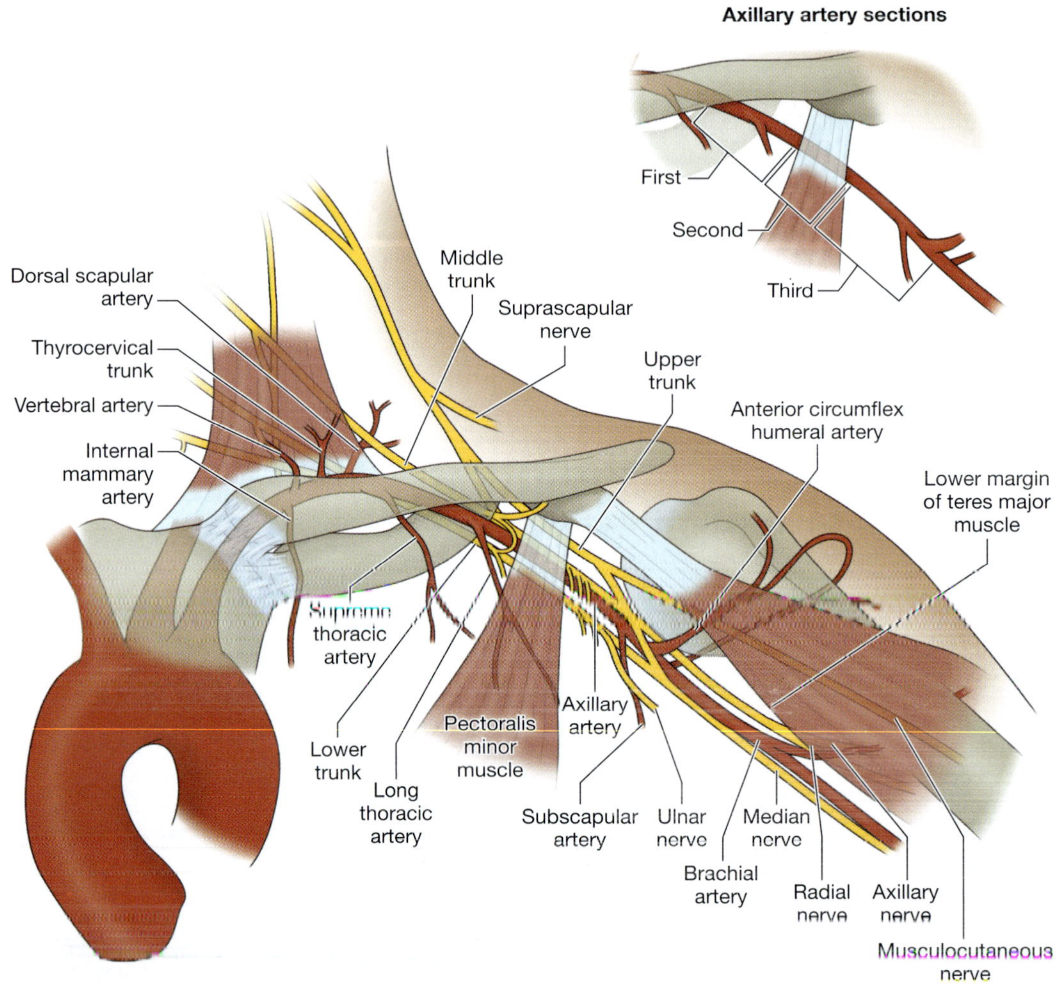

FIGURE 22.2 ▮ The multiple structures of the axillary neurovascular bundle mandate careful dissection and clamping.

While there are major branches (thoracoacromial, lateral thoracic, and subscapular) from the axillary artery, these generally do not provide sufficient collateral perfusion to the arm and thus the axillary artery, unlike the subclavian, warrants prompt reconstruction. The axillary artery is divided into three segments with the second segment deep to the pectoralis minor muscle. The first portion begins at the subclavius muscle and the third portion ends at the teres major. Due to the deep positon and surrounding musculature, injuries of the axillary artery infrequently bleed externally or into the thorax, but instead manifest as a sizable hematoma.

- Because injuries of the proximal axillary artery may necessitate proximal control of the distal subclavian artery, a CTA is usually done for stable patients to confirm the site of injury. While endovascular stenting has become more common, delayed thrombosis is frequent and stenting is suboptimal in the third portion due to motion in the shoulder.

Essential Equipment

TIP

The precise location of junctional vascular injuries can be challenging and, thus, essential equipment for proximal control should be immediately available.

- Headlight
- Loupe magnification 2.5 glasses

- Adson–Beckman retractors
- Gigli saw
- Castroviejo and Ryder needle driver
- Microvascular Gerald forceps
- Potts–Smith scissors
- Angled vascular clamps
- Satinsky clamp
- Silastic vessel loops, red for vessels, and yellow for nerves
- Rummel tourniquet (red rubber catheter and umbilical tape)
- Teflon or felt pledgets
- Profunda vascular clamps (angled and straight)
- 1 pack of 6-inch Argyle shunts (8, 10, 12, 14 Fr)
- 15-cm Pruitt–Inahara shunt with T port (9 Fr)
- Sutures
  - 6-0 Prolene on a C1 or BV1 needle
  - 3-0 Silk plain and stick ties
- Sterile 8- to 10-MHz Doppler probe
- Heparinized saline 50 to 100 units in 1,000 mL saline
- Papaverine 30 mg/mL, 10-mL vials
- Tissue plasminogen activator 5-mg vial
- Fogarty embolectomy catheters #2, #3, #4
- Bulldog vascular clamps
- 3-Way stopcock and A line extension tubing
- 10-, 20-cc syringes of heparin saline on 18-gauge IV catheter with blunt needle (Olive) tip
- 19- or 21-gauge butterfly needle or angiocatheter
- Contrast agent 50 mL (Omnipaque-240, GE Healthcare, Inc., Chicago, IL)
- Linear 8- to 10-MHz Doppler probe
- Ring reinforced 6- and 8-mm polytetrafluoroethylene (PTFE).
- Polyester or bovine pericardial patch
- Gel foam or Surgicel
- Fibrin sealant or Bioglue

Patient Positioning

TIP

Do not forget to prepare the groin for a potential greater saphenous vein harvest, although size mismatch may warrant a PTFE graft.

- Supine with ipsilateral arm extended out.
- Skin preparation should include the neck, chest, and ipsilateral upper extremity including the hand to assess perfusion.
- A shoulder roll may assist for exposure.
- Anticipate the need for a saphenous vein harvest by prepping the groin site.
- Radial arterial line is placed on the opposite side of the injury.
- Anticipate blood loss and have blood products available.
- Lower body Bair Hugger warmer.

TECHNIQUE

Surgical Approach

TIP

The skin incision should be generous because of the deep location of the axillary artery surrounded by the brachial plexus and axillary vein. Injuries to the proximal axillary artery may require access to the distal subclavian artery (see Chapter 8).

- The skin incision is located 2 cm below the clavicle, extending from the mid clavicle across the deltopectoral groove into the upper arm (Fig. 22.3).
- Divide the subcutaneous tissue using the Bovie electrocautery to identify the pectoralis major.
- Split the fibers of the pectoralis major along their length to access the axillary vessels (Fig. 22.4).

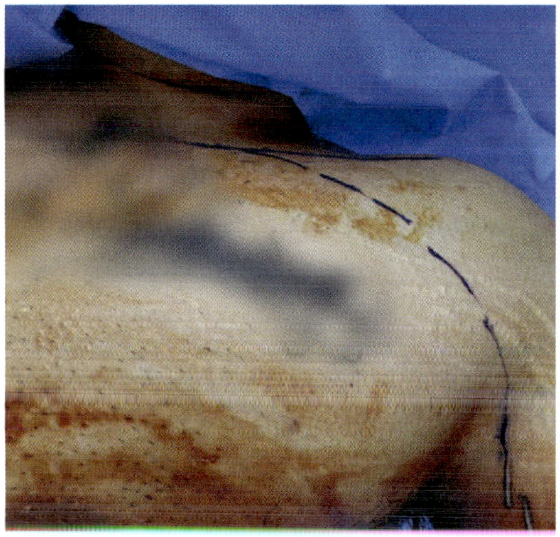

FIGURE 22.3 ▮ The skin incision courses 2 cm below the clavicle and is extended via the deltopectoral groove.

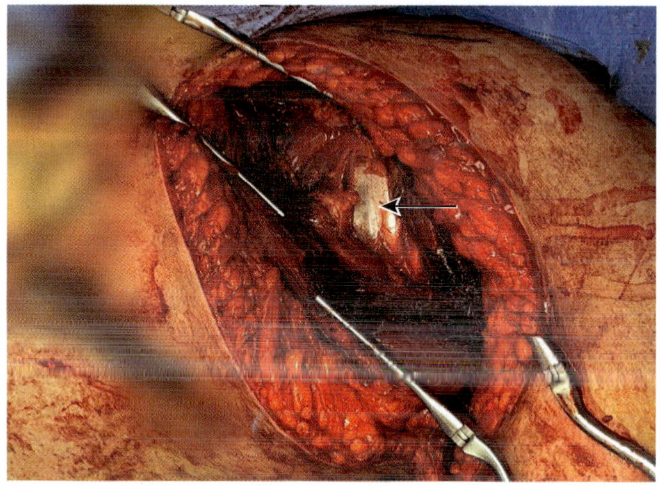

FIGURE 22.4 ▮ The fibers of the pectoralis muscle are separated, exposing the deeper pectoralis minor (*arrow*) which overlies the second portion of the axillary artery.

  - If there is a large arterial defect with active bleeding, an alternative is to divide the pectoralis major 2 cm proximal to its insertion onto the humerus for later reconstruction.
  - Adson–Beckman retractors provide retraction of the musculature.
- Divide the pectoralis minor muscle close to the coracoid process. Open the neurovascular envelope to expose the axillary artery and vein and intertwining brachial plexus (Fig. 22.5)

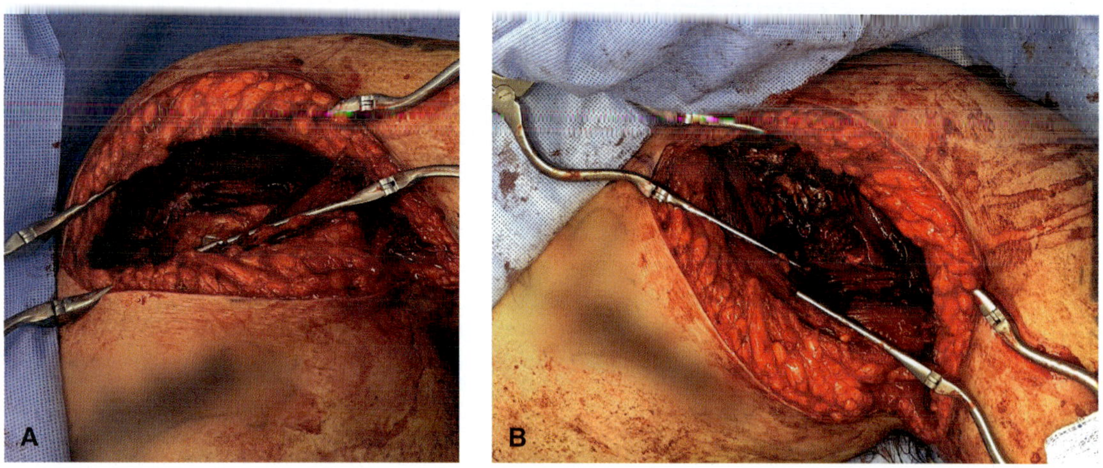

FIGURE 22.5 ▮ Following division of the pectoralis minor muscle (**A**), the neurovascular envelop is entered to isolate the axillary vessels (**B**).

  - Isolate the axillary structures. Multiple venous tributaries may require ligation.
  - The axillary artery should be isolated first to facilitate proximal vascular control (Fig. 22.6).
  - The regional trunks of the brachial plexus should be identified and isolated with color-coded vascular loops prior to formal exploration for axillary reconstruction.

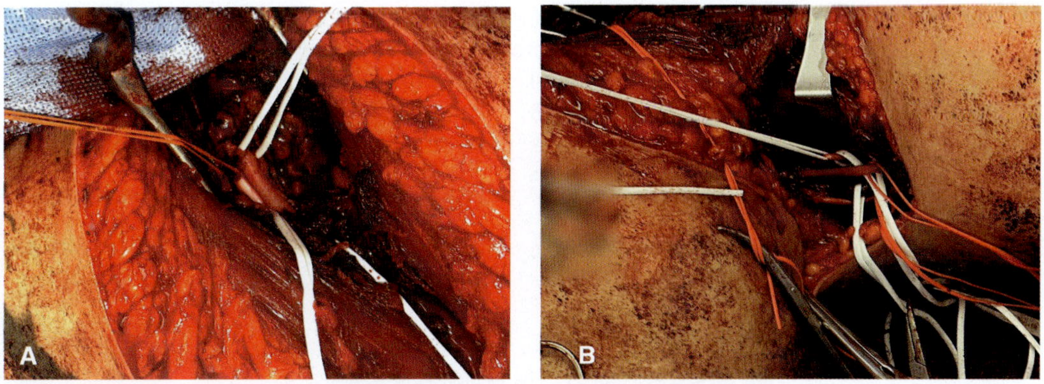

FIGURE 22.6 ▌ The axillary artery and cords of the brachial plexus should be identified (**A**) and isolated with vascular loops (**B**).

- Due to the risk of arm ischemia, a temporary intravascular shunt is recommended. We prefer the Pruitt–Inahara shunt (Fig. 22.7) because it allows for monitoring perfusion, access for arteriography, and administration of papaverine for distal vasospasm or tPA for residual small thrombi.
- Reconstruct the axillary artery. Autologous greater saphenous vein (GSV) is preferred when adequate sized vein is available. However, the diameter of the axillary artery in adults may match best with an 8-mm PTFE (Fig. 22.8).

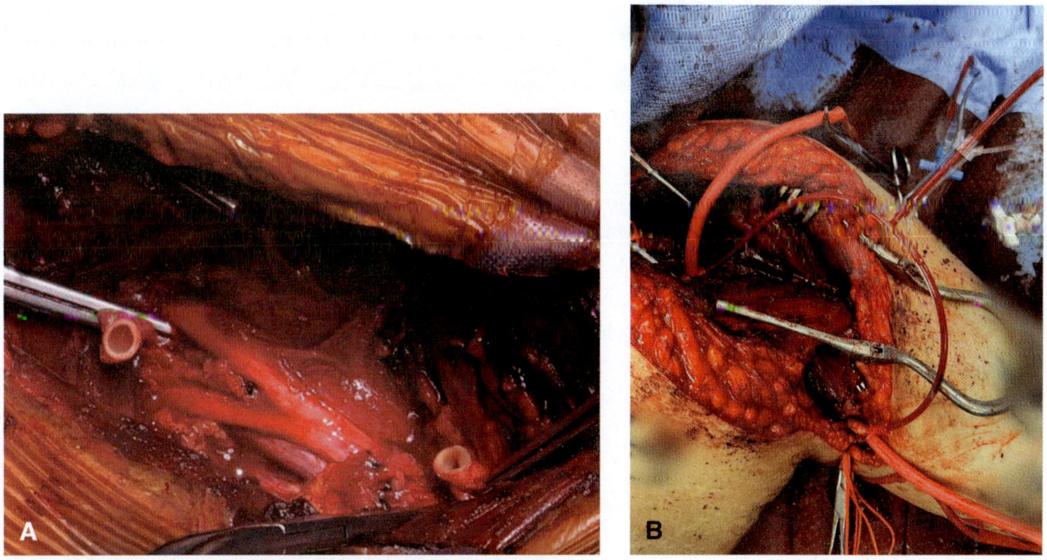

FIGURE 22.7 ▌ Due to the risk of arm ischemia an intravascular shunt is placed into the proximal and distal limbs of the transected artery (**A**). A 9-Fr Pruitt–Inahara shunt has the advantage of a T for monitoring flow, arteriography, or infusion of a fibrinolytic (**B**).

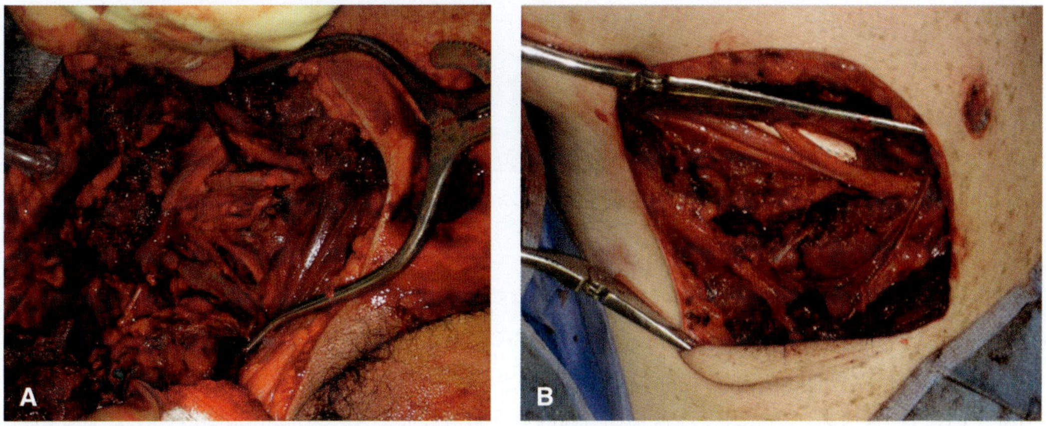

FIGURE 22.8 ▌ Autologous vein is preferred for reconstruction when there is an adequate sized greater saphenous vein (**A**). However, an 8-mm PTFE may be the best matched for a large adult (**B**).

- Ring-enforced PTFE is not necessary for the first and second portions of the axillary artery, but should be used if crossing the shoulder joint (Fig. 22.9A).
- If the injury extends into the brachial artery, GSV is preferred but a 7- to 4-mm PTFE bridge can be used (Fig. 22.9B).
- Completion Duplex ultrasound or angiography is recommended following the reconstruction.

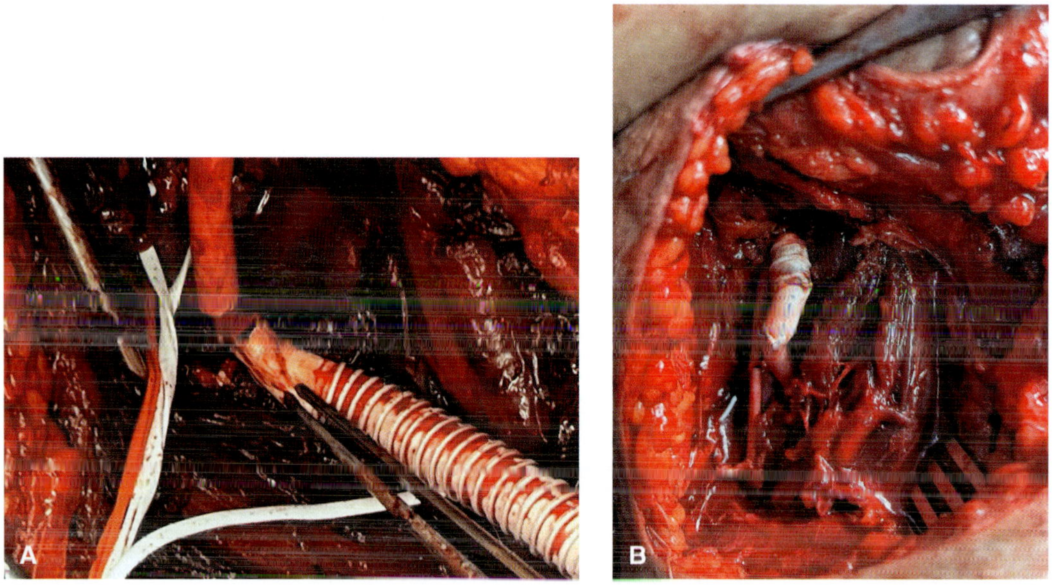

FIGURE 22.9 ❙ Ring-enforced PTFE should be used when crossing the shoulder joint. A 7- to 4-mm heparin-bonded PTFE can be used to bridge to the brachial artery. The proximal anastomosis is shown in (**A**) and distal in (**B**).

- Due to limited collateral blood flow, reperfusion compartment syndrome of the forearm is a significant risk following axillary reconstruction (Fig. 22.10).
- Moreover, arm swelling is expected when the axillary vein is ligated. The technical details of compartment release are reviewed in Chapter 26

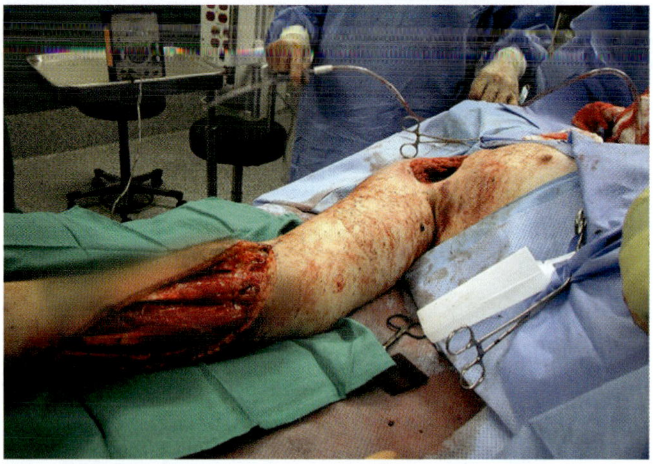

FIGURE 22.10 ❙ Forearm compartment release may be warranted for compartment hypertension secondary to reperfusion or extensive swelling.

Endovascular Techniques

TIP

An endovascular repair is best reserved for the hemodynamically stable patient with a focal injury.

- An endovascular approach allows treatment of an injury that may be surgically challenging, but has a significant risk of thrombosis.
- CTA directs preoperative endovascular plans as covered stents are frequently used to treat pseudoaneurysms or arteriovenous fistulae (Fig. 22.11).
- A transfemoral approach allows for proximal balloon occlusion. In some cases, a retrograde (transbrachial) approach can revascularize a difficult transection.
- Coils are useful for occluding a branch vessel.

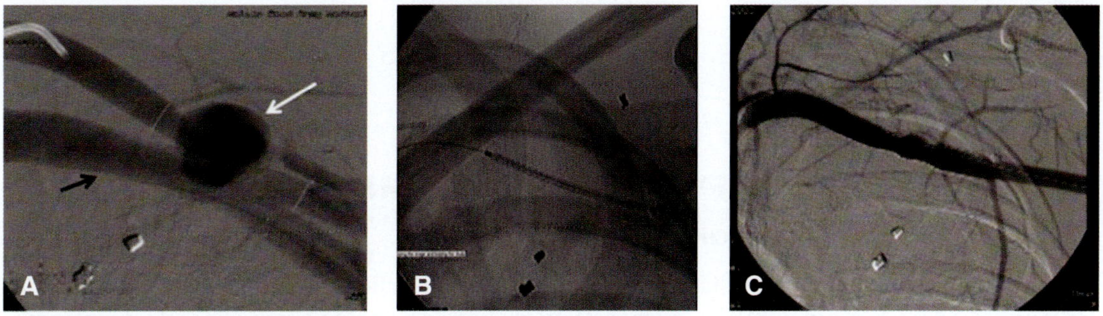

FIGURE 22.11 ▮ An endovascular stent is an alternative approach for delayed presentations or occult vascular injuries: (**A**) depicts an axillary pseudoaneurysm, (**B**) illustrates the wire and stent across the injury, (**C**) shows the axillary artery with stent covering the injury.

POSTOPERATIVE CARE

TIP

Brachial plexus injuries are common and early involvement of the Hand team is recommended.

- Admit the patient to the surgical intensive care unit for 24-hour pulse evaluation.
- Monitor for pain and neurologic findings suggestive of forearm compartment syndrome.
- Initiate antiplatelet therapy when hemostasis is ensured and coagulation status is normalized.
- Due to the possibility of late thrombosis, Duplex assessment should be done annually for at least 3 years.

Suggested Readings

Angus LDG, Gerber N, Munnangi S, Wallace R, Singh S, Digiacomo J. Management and outcomes of isolated axillary artery injury: a five-year national trauma data bank analysis. *Ann Vasc Surg*. 2020;65:113–123.

Chopra A, Modrall JG, Knowles M, Phelan HA, Valentine RJ, Chung J. Uncertain patency of covered stents placed for traumatic axillosubclavian artery injury. *J Am Coll Surg*. 2016;223(1):174–183.

Waller CJ, Cogbill TH, Kallies KJ, et al. Contemporary management of subclavian and axillary artery injuries-a western trauma association multicenter review. *J Trauma Acute Care Surg*. 2017;83(6):1023–1031.

Chapter 23
Brachial Artery

ERNEST E. MOORE AND CHARLES J. FOX

PERIOPERATIVE CONSIDERATIONS

Procedure Rationale

- The brachial artery is a relatively superficial structure in the medial upper arm and is typically injured due to penetrating wounds. The noted exception is the supracondylar fracture in children where brachial arterial injury occurs in 5% to 10%.
- The brachial artery is the continuation of the axillary artery beyond the lower margin of teres major muscle. It continues down the medial surface of the arm until it reaches the cubital fossa at the elbow, and then divides into the radial and ulnar arteries which run down the forearm. In 10% of individuals, the bifurcation occurs much earlier and the ulnar and radial arteries extend through the upper arm, and there may be duplicate brachial arteries in 5%.
- Fortunately, there is a robust collateral arterial system through the profunda brachii as well as radial and ulnar collateral systems (Fig. 23.1). However, this collateral system may be disrupted by shotgun

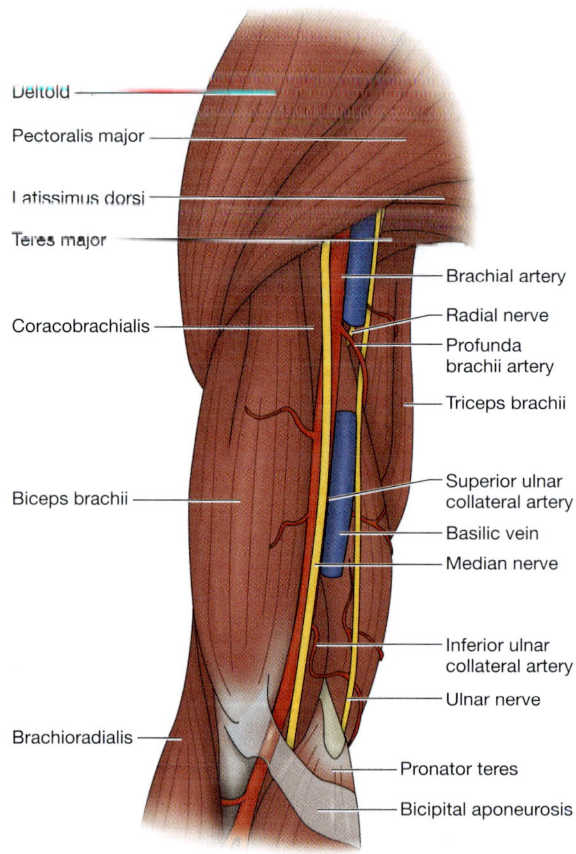

FIGURE 23.1 ❙ Anatomy of the brachial artery and adjacent nerves.

wounds or crush injuries. There is generally abundant venous drainage of the arm via the basilic, cephalic, and brachial veins with numerous interconnections. The brachial artery is in proximity to the radial and ulnar arteries in the proximal upper arm and the median nerve is closely associated with the brachial artery throughout its course (Fig. 23.1). Thus, these nerves need to be carefully protected during dissection, particularly when obtaining proximal control in a hematoma with active bleeding.

Essential Equipment

- Headlight
- Loupe magnification 2.5 glasses
- Adson–Beckman retractors
- Castroviejo and Ryder needle driver
- Microvascular Gerald forceps
- Potts–Smith scissors
- Angled vascular clamps
- Silastic vessel loops, red for vessels, and yellow for nerves
- Rummel tourniquet (red rubber catheter and umbilical tape)
- Profunda vascular clamps (angled and straight)
- 1 pack of 6-inch Argyle shunts (8 Fr)
- 15-cm Pruitt–Inahara shunt with T port (7 Fr)
- Sutures
  - 6-0 Prolene on a C1 or BV1 needle
  - 3-0 silk plain and stick ties
- Sterile 8- to 10-MHz Doppler probe
- Heparinized saline 50 to 100 units in 1,000 mL saline
- Papaverine 30-mg/mL vial
- Tissue plasminogen activator 2-mg/mL vial
- Fogarty embolectomy catheters #2, #3
- Bulldog vascular clamps
- 3-Way stopcock and A-line extension tubing
- 10-, 20-cc syringes of heparin saline on 18-gauge IV catheter with blunt needle (Olive) tip
- 19 or 21-gauge butterfly needle or angiocatheter
- Contrast agent 50 mL (Omnipaque-240, GE Healthcare, Inc., Chicago, IL)
- Linear 8- to 10-MHz Doppler probe
- Gel foam or Surgicel

Patient Positioning

TIP

Do not forget to prepare the upper thigh for a potential greater saphenous vein harvest (Fig. 23.2), although the basilic vein is ideal for a short interposition graft.

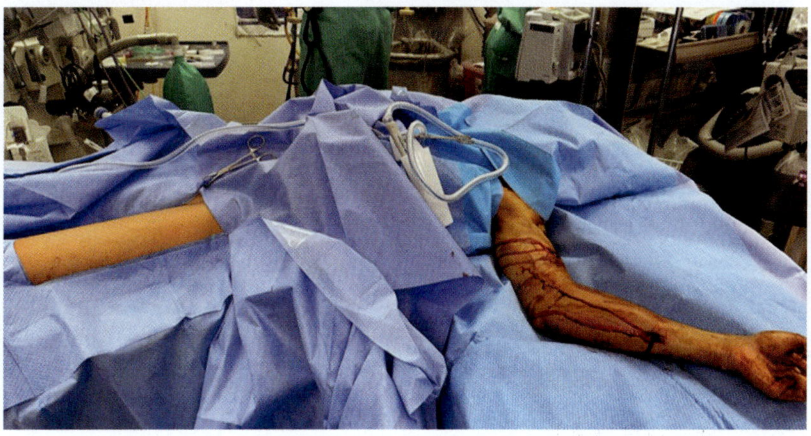

FIGURE 23.2 | Operative planning should include the possible need for a greater saphenous vein conduit.

- Supine with ipsilateral arm extended (Fig. 23.2).
- Skin preparation should include the upper chest, ipsilateral upper arm, and hand to assess perfusion.
- Anticipate the need for a greater saphenous vein harvest by prepping the upper thigh.
- Radial arterial line is placed on the opposite side of the injury.
- Anticipate blood loss and have blood products available.
- Lower body Bair Hugger warmer.

SURGICAL APPROACH

TIP

Angiography is infrequently required for the diagnosis of a brachial injury; intraoperative ultrasound can be helpful to localize the injury.

- The location of the skin incision is based on the anticipated site of injury. The incision should be generous to facilitate exposure of the brachial artery without injuring the median nerve (Fig. 23.3).
- If brachial exposure is anticipated below the elbow crease the skin incision should purse an S course with the crease opened in a horizontal direction to avoid a skin stricture across the joint space (Fig. 23.4).

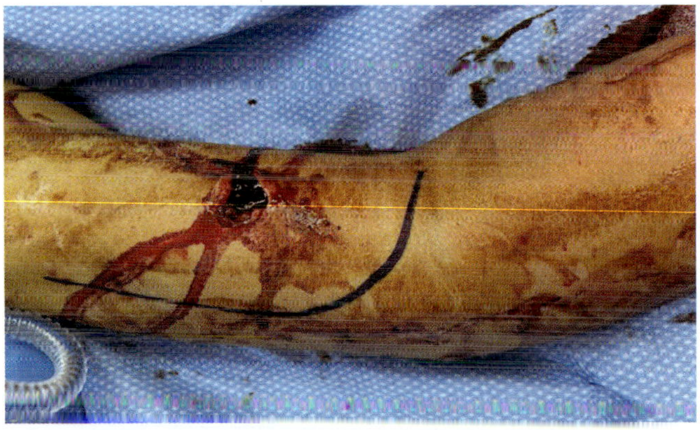

FIGURE 23.3 | Exploration of the brachial artery is in the medial arm, and the incision should be ample to provide prompt access for proximal arterial control.

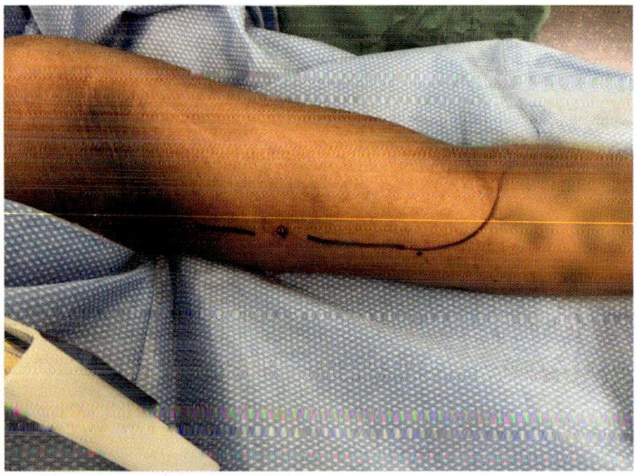

FIGURE 23.4 | The incision should follow an S configuration if exploration is anticipated beyond the elbow crease.

- Divide the subcutaneous tissue using the Bovie electrocautery to identify the deep fascia of the arm (Fig. 23.5), and identify the neurovascular bundle posterior to the biceps muscle.
- Open the neurovascular bundle to expose the brachial artery, paired brachial veins, and the median nerve (Fig. 23.6).

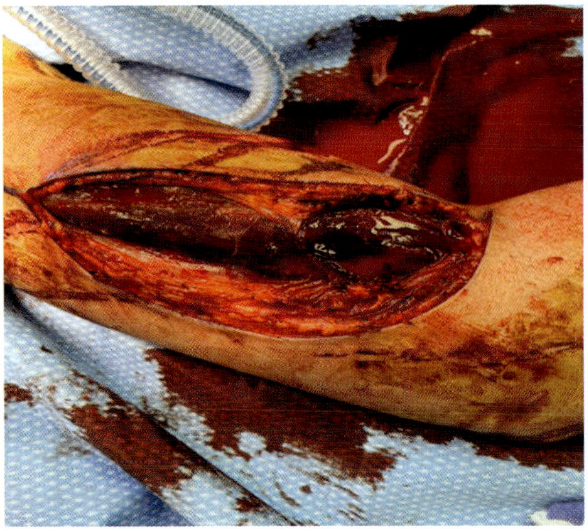

FIGURE 23.5 | The neurovascular bundle, containing the brachial artery, paired brachial veins, and median nerve, is posterior to the biceps muscle.

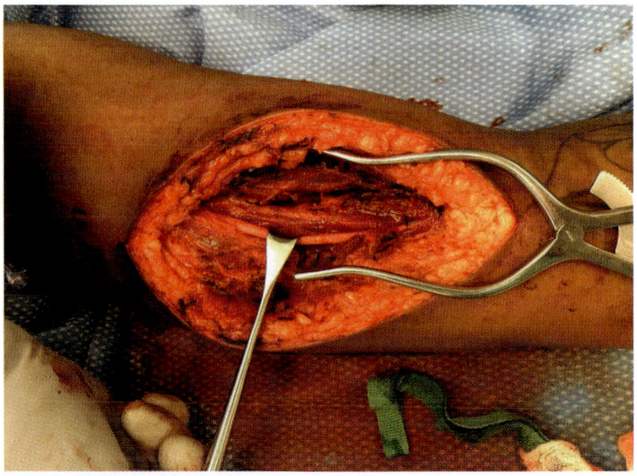

FIGURE 23.6 | The median nerve is in close proximity to the brachial artery throughout the upper arm.

- Reconstruction of the brachial artery is conducted similar to other extremity vascular injuries: (1) obtain proximal control, (2) Fogarty exploration of proximal artery to remove clot and heparin flus, and (3) Fogarty exploration of the distal artery for clot removal and heparin flush. While not essential for most brachial injuries due to extensive collateral blood flow, we often place a Pruitt–Inahara shunt to limit ischemic time. As mentioned in the Techniques chapter, the T arm permits infusing of antispasm therapy and fibrinolytics as well as access for an arteriogram.
- Repair of a laceration of the brachial can be accomplished with simple wound closure or reconstruction of the brachial artery with a vein interposition graft.
- A gunshot wound or blunt injury generally requires debridement and, thus, a short interposition graft. The basilic vein is usually a good size match for this purpose (Fig. 23.7). The greater saphenous vein is more suitable for longer interposition grafts (Fig. 23.8).

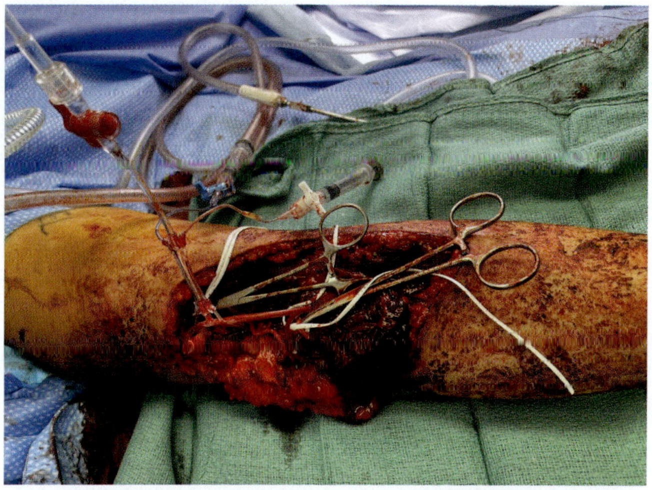

FIGURE 23.7 | An 8-Fr Pruitt–Inahara can be inserted and tPA infused via the T arm when there is prolonged ischemia.

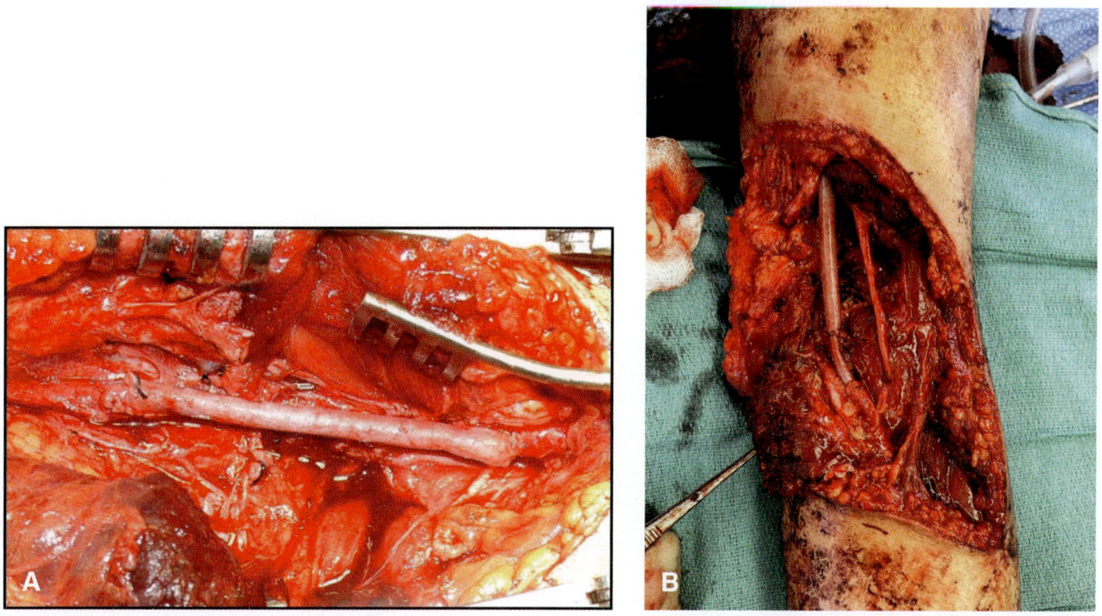

FIGURE 23.8 | A reversed greater saphenous vein graft (**A**) is employed for longer segment injuries, or alternatively a Humacyte graft (**B**) particularly with high risk of infection.

- The skin incision is usually closed with staples to permit local wound exploration if required (Fig. 23.9).
- Following brachial repair, a Doppler study or preferably a Duplex examination is done to ensure return of adequate blood flow (Fig. 23.9). Forearm compartment syndrome is rare following a brachial arterial injury because of collateral blood flow. The procedure is covered in the Chapter 26.

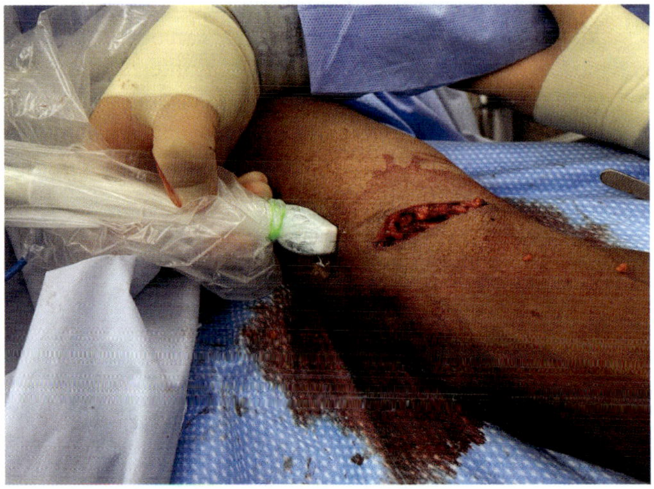

FIGURE 23.9 ▌ Duplex scanning is excellent for ensuring distal perfusion after brachial artery repair.

POSTOPERATIVE MANAGEMENT

TIP

Median nerve injuries are common and early involvement of the Hand team is recommended if any neurologic symptoms.

- Admit to the surgical intensive care unit for 2-hour pulse evaluation for 24 hours.
- Monitor for neurologic symptoms suggestive of forearm compartment syndrome.
- Initiate antiplatelet therapy when hemostasis is ensured and coagulation status is normalized.

Suggested Readings

Asensio JA, Kessler JJ II, Miljkovic SS, et al. Brachial artery injuries operative management and predictors of outcome. *Ann Vasc Surg*. 2020;69:146–157.

Franz RW, Skytta CK, Shah KJ, Hartman JF, Wright ML. A five-year review of management of upper-extremity arterial injuries at an urban level I trauma center. *Ann Vasc Surg*. 2012;26(5):655–664.

Chapter 24
Iliofemoral Artery Injury

CHARLES J. FOX AND ERNEST E. MOORE

PERIOPERATIVE CONSIDERATIONS

Procedure Rationale

- Trauma to the iliofemoral vessels remains a challenging problem to manage and, compared to other extremity vascular injuries, is frequently associated with complications because of the importance of the blood supply to the pelvis and lower extremity (Fig. 24.1) and the potential for wound complications.

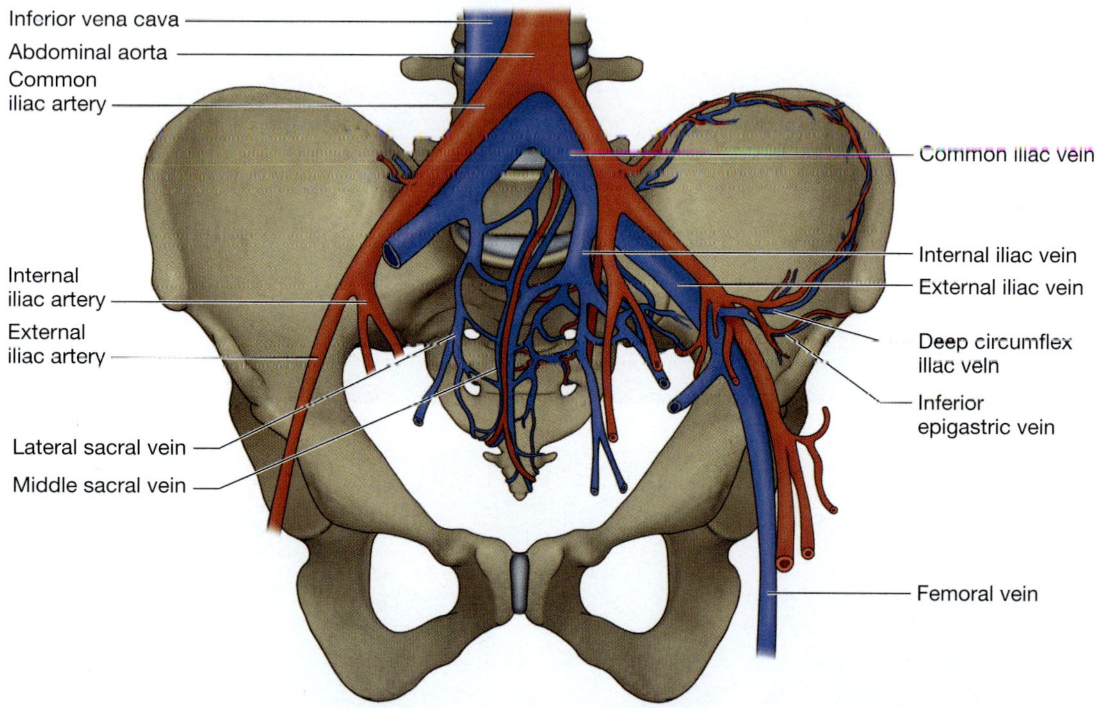

FIGURE 24.1 ❙ Cartoon illustration of the iliac artery and venous anatomy.

- Penetrating wounds to the iliofemoral vessels can bleed severely and have a high rate of amputation when associated with prolonged ischemic time, infection, and associated soft tissue damage. The increased incidence of arterial injury with the use of computed tomography angiography (CTA) has been appreciated and many of these intimal defects and small pseudoaneurysms can be managed medically and will improve over time.

Perioperative Considerations

TIP

It is important to know the preoperative pulse examination and confirm that examination with continuous wave Doppler.

- A Doppler assessment and ankle brachial index (ABI) of the injured extremity is an essential component of the assessment.
- Hard signs of injury require prompt operative intervention and there is little utility in obtaining additional imaging for a penetrating wound to the thigh or pelvis.
  - A pulseless extremity should go directly to the operating room for revascularization to minimize ischemic time.
  - Active bleeding or an expanding hematoma requires immediate control by tourniquet or digital compression.
  - Bruits and thrills may represent occult injuries such as an arteriovenous fistula and additional imaging is useful for preoperative planning.
  - Stable patients with an abnormal ABI should undergo further diagnostic imaging for assessment and preoperative planning.
- Tourniquets are not generally helpful in junctional regions but should not be removed until the patient is hemodynamically stable and blood is available (Fig. 24.2).
- A hasty betadine or chlorhexidine splash prep is the most expeditious way to get started (Fig. 24.3).

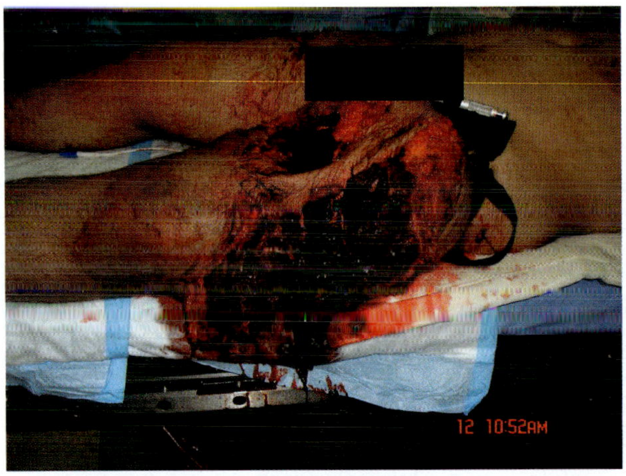

FIGURE 24.2 ▌A tourniquet may be ineffective in junctional areas.

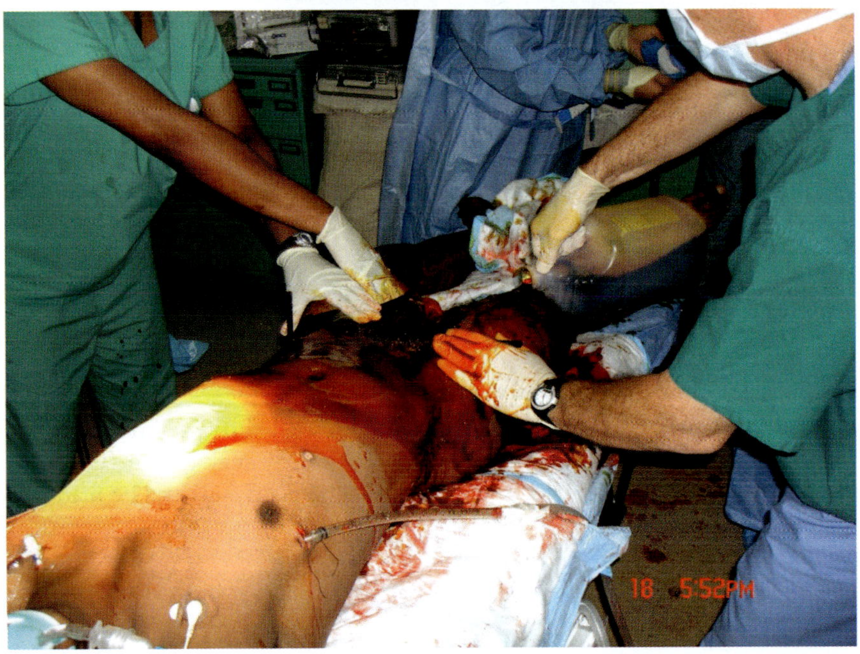

FIGURE 24.3 ▌A betadine splash prep may be the most expedient in urgent situations.

- Examine plain radiographs for patterns associated with arterial injury.
- CTA is useful for evaluating the precise location of a vascular injury but should not delay operative intervention if there is threat of limb loss due to ischemic time.
- Although a contralateral saphenous vein harvest should be anticipated, the vein is not a good size match for the iliac or common femoral artery (8 to 10 mm).
- Prosthetic materials are appropriate for traumatic uncontaminated iliofemoral wounds.
- Consider an intravascular shunt to re-establish distal perfusion if delayed revascularization is being considered.

Essential Equipment

TIP

Communicate early to the anesthesia and operating room staff important details such as need for a wide surgical preparation (nipples to knees), positioning instructions, major vascular instruments, graft materials, and the potential for fluoroscopic imaging. A urinary catheter, arterial line, and large-bore intravenous access is mandatory. Blood products should be available.

- Headlight
- Loupe magnification 2.5
- Beckman, Weitlaner, and Bookwalter retractors
- Castroviejo and Ryder needle drivers
- Microvascular forceps
- DeBakey aortic clamp
- Profunda vascular clamps (angled and straight)
- Wiley hypogastric vascular clamps
- Sponge sticks
- Vascular shunt
  - 15- or 31-cm Pruitt-Inahara shunt (with T port) 8 to 14 mm balloon diameter
  - One pack of 6- or 11-inch Argyle (8-, 10-, 12-, 14-French) shunts
- Sutures
  - 3-0 Prolene suture on an SH needle (common iliac)
  - 4-0 Prolene suture on an RBI needle (hypogastric)
  - 5-0 on a C1 needle (external, femoral)
  - 3-0 silk plain and stick ties
  - 2-0 Ethibond sutures (inguinal ligament)
  - 2-0 and 3-0 Vicryl sutures (groin closure)
- Grafts
  - 8-mm ringed ePTFE (femoral)
  - 10-mm Dacron (iliac)
  - Cryopreserved artery if contamination
- Sterile 8- to 10-MHz Doppler probe
- Heparinized saline 50 to 100 units/mL saline
- Papaverine 60 mg in 20 cc of saline for topical use
- Fogarty embolectomy catheters no. 2 and no. 3
- Bulldog soft vascular clamps
- Three-way stopcock and A-line extension tubing
- 10-cc syringes of heparinized saline on 18-gauge IV catheter
- Portable ultrasound machine

Patient Positioning

TIP

Do not underestimate the potential for blood loss and massive transfusion.

- Place upper body Bair warmer and radial arterial line.
- Prep both legs nipples to knees.
- A supine position using a longitudinal incision is best for a femoral injury.
- An iliac injury can be reached by division of the inguinal ligament, or a midline laparotomy or, in selective cases, a retroperitoneal dissection using a curvilinear incision.

TECHNIQUE

Surgical Approach: Iliac

TIP

Have all necessary equipment in the room before making an incision to explore an iliac vessel. Hasty control of the entire iliac segment is best done with a midline laparotomy incision.

- Following a midline laparotomy, reflect the small bowel and palpate the distal abdominal aorta for the purpose of setting a DeBakey aortic clamp if needed.
- The table-mounted Omni tract retractor has specialized retractor blades that provides excellent exposure and flexibility.
- Open the avascular plane of Toldt and reflect the left colon medially.
- Identify the psoas muscle and avoid harm to the overlying genitofemoral nerve.
- Identify the ureter coursing caudally and medial over the hypogastric artery.
- The hypogastric artery and vein can be ligated if needed.
- Reflect all structures medially and dissect the common iliac artery staying close to the adventitia, avoiding injury to the vein medially or nerves laterally.
- Isolate the iliac artery, taking precautions to avoid venous injury (Fig. 24.4).

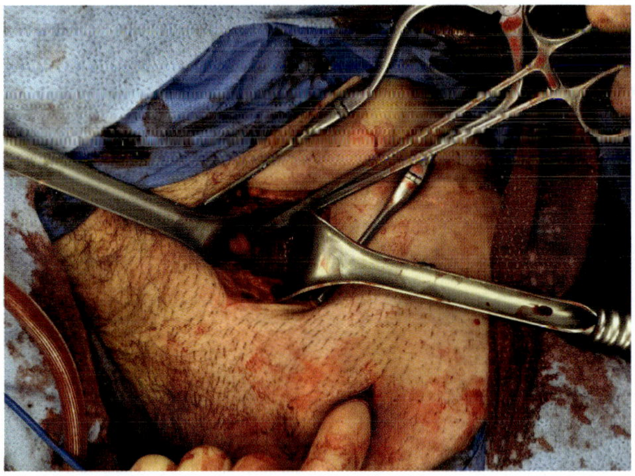

FIGURE 24.4 ▮ External iliac artery control through a retroperitoneal approach.

- Venous injury may require hasty division of the common iliac artery.
- A deep pelvic dissection may result in venous plexus bleeding or spermatic cord injury in an attempt to reach the distal external iliac artery.
- The far distal external iliac injury can be controlled by partial division of the inguinal ligament as approached from the groin or complete division in an emergency.
- An occlusion balloon should be considered when the situation dictates.

Surgical Approach: Femoral

TIP

Plan for the worst-case scenario. The dissection can be challenging. Use assistants for exposure. It is better to make an incision too large rather than too small. Plan for the exposure to eventually go well above and below the originally intended dissection.

- Two fingers lateral to the public tubercle make a longitudinal line with one-third going proximal to the inguinal ligament (anterior–superior iliac spine to tubercle) (Fig. 24.5).
- It is crucial to start with gaining proximal and distal control (Fig. 24.6).

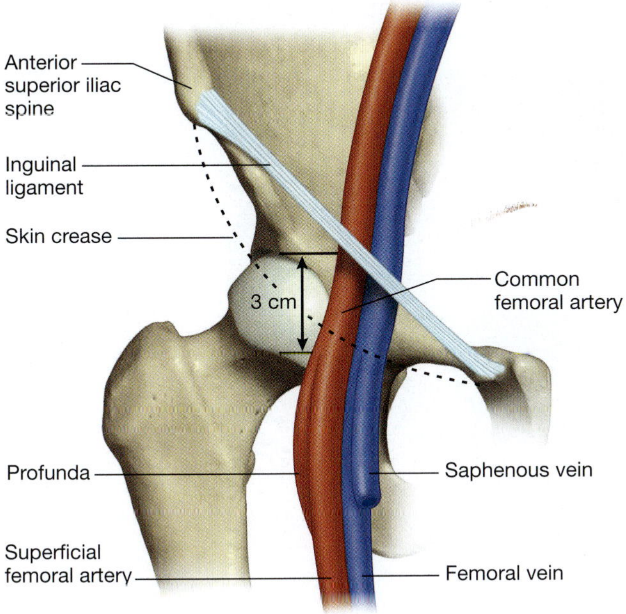

FIGURE 24.5 ▌ Cartoon illustration of the femoral artery and venous anatomy. Note the skin crease is often a deceptive landmark to the common femoral artery.

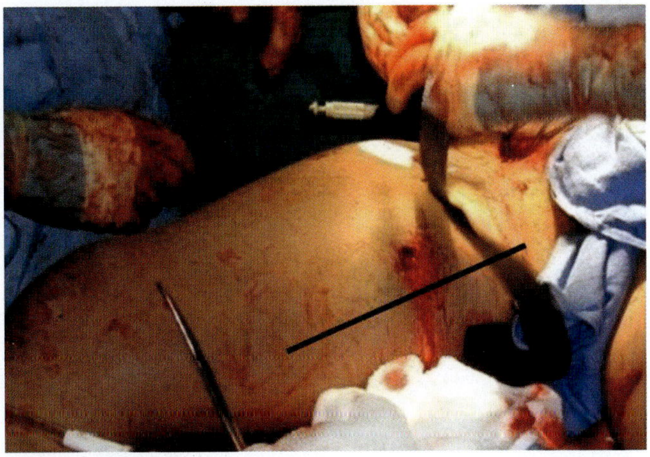

FIGURE 24.6 ▌ The size of the medial incision (*black line*) should not be underestimated to obtain control of femoral hemorrhage.

- Care should be taken to avoid injury to the saphenous or femoral vein during the incision and deep dissection. Watch for sharp Weitlaner retractors that can cause iatrogenic injury.
- The distal portion of the inguinal ligament is a good landmark to find the proximal common femoral artery in obese patients. Dissect the ligament a few centimeters medial and lateral for some mobility and set a hand-held retractor.
- Divide the inguinal ligament if proximal control of the distal external iliac artery is needed.
- Identify the proximal SFA, and profunda femoral branches before repairing the common femoral artery. This will minimize back bleeding during the arteriotomy.
- The profunda femoral artery and vein are easily torn if the dissection is too aggressive.
- There is a prominent circumflex femoral vein crossing under the inguinal ligament that should be ligated and divided before attempting to control the external iliac artery.
- A Pruitt-Inahara shunt is useful because of its flexibility and length and the benefit of having a T port for infusion of medications and contrast.
  - Heparin saline can be intermittently instilled to confirm forward flow rather than a stagnant column of blood
  - A shunt angiogram may be performed via the T port to demonstrate outflow to the foot. If the angiogram demonstrates clot or vasospasm, early intervention is performed.
- The femoral or iliac vein is repaired after the arterial repair when possible.
- Anticipate a calf fasciotomy if a reperfusion injury is expected or if the common femoral or iliac veins are ligated.
- Thigh fasciotomy is rare and can be very morbid.

Vascular Reconstruction: Iliac

TIP

Always ensure that the graft is properly matched to the size of the native artery.

- Repair options include suture for small lacerations, a patch for larger lacerations, or an interposition graft.
- When the segmental defect is large (>2 cm) then an interposition graft is preferred.
- The internal iliac can be ligated for hemorrhage control or additional mobility.
- A tensionless end-to-end repair is preferable if there is fecal contamination (Fig. 24.7).

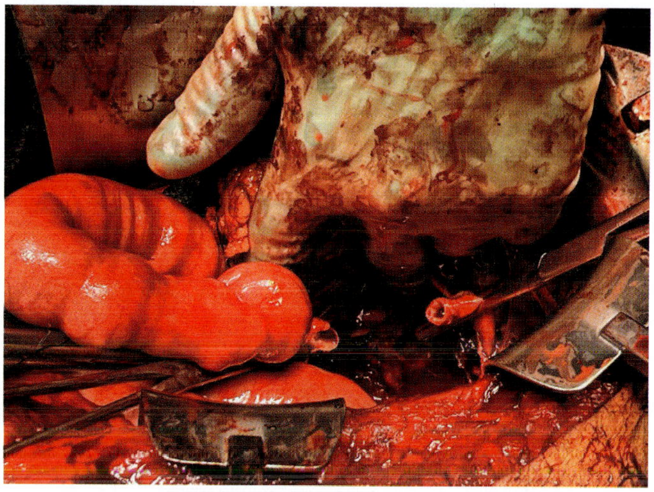

FIGURE 24.7 ▮ The right iliac artery is transected to expose a venous injury.

- Vein grafts do poorly in this location due to size mismatch and kinking.
- Remove fresh thrombus and intimal debris by flushing and Fogarty catheters.
- Give systemic IV heparin at 80 units/kg if no contraindications.
- Always inspect the outflow tract, flush liberally and gently pass a Fogarty thrombectomy catheter to remove any fresh arterial thrombus if the back bleeding is not profuse.
- Use caution to not overinflate (hub shows max liquid capacity) the balloon catheter. If any resistance is encountered, carefully deflate some saline and withdrawal.
- When a patch is desired, a Dacron or Bovine pericardial patch is typically used (Fig. 24.8).

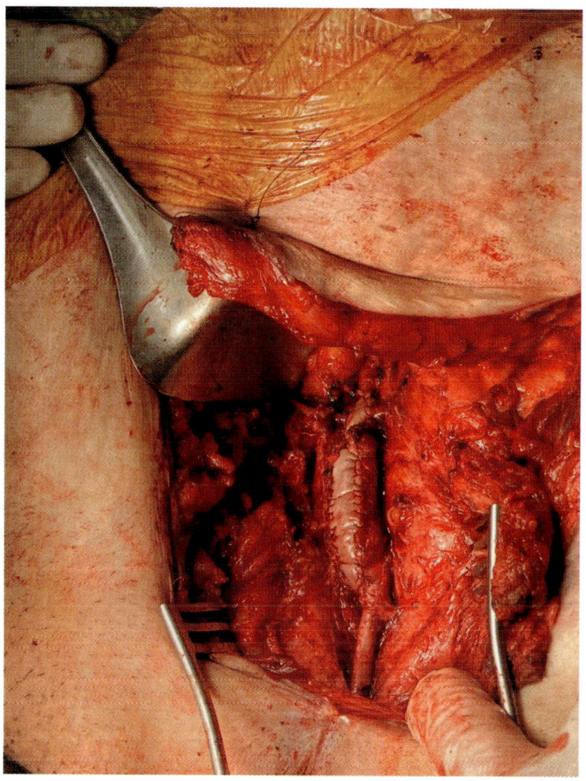

FIGURE 24.8 ▮ A bovine pericardial patch is placed over the common femoral artery defect preserving the deep and superficial femoral branches.

- An 8- to 10-mm prosthetic interposition graft with ringed ePTFE or Dacron is appropriate.
  - The proximal anastomosis is performed with a 3-0 or 4-0 double-armed Prolene suture.
  - For interposition grafts, leave an intact posterior wall and parachute the anastomosis using 36-inch sutures if the pelvic cavity is deep.
  - Confirm inflow after the proximal anastomosis.
  - Complete the distal anastomosis but flush the graft (retrograde and then forward) before the final suture is tied.
- Completion angiograms are seldom after iliac artery repair.
- The wound is closed in several interrupted layers without drains.
- A triphasic Doppler signal may not be appreciate after hypovolemic shock without a period of rewarming but vigilant reassessment is important.
- A fasciotomy is highly recommended after venous ligation or prolonged ischemic time.

Vascular Reconstruction: Femoral

TIP

Always ensure that a graft is covered entirely in layers with healthy and viable muscle tissue.

- A tensionless end-to-end primary repair of an arterial injury is favored when the defect is too large for a lateral suture or a patch (>1/3 circumference).
- When the segmental defect is large (>2 cm), then an interposition graft is preferred (Fig. 24.9).

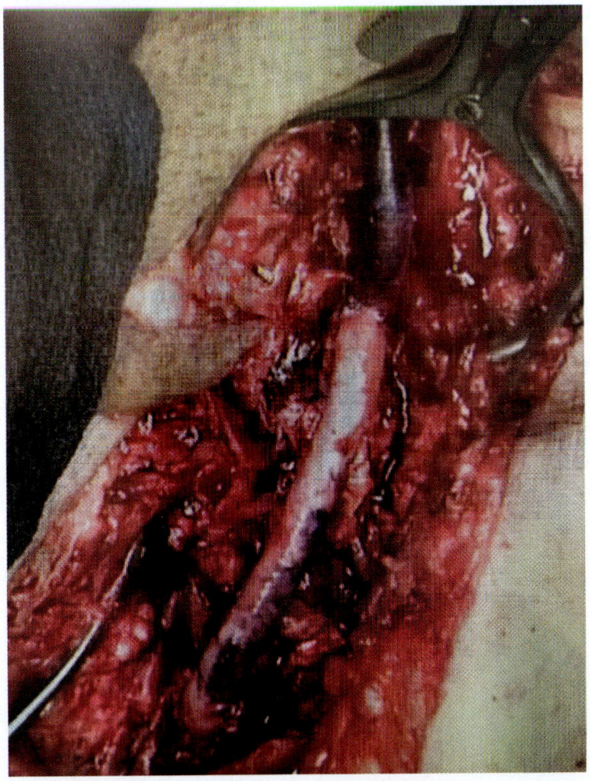

FIGURE 24.9 ▮ A cryopreserved artery is used for an end-to-end iliofemoral reconstruction of the common femoral artery routing the external iliac to the profunda femoral artery followed by a jump graft to the superficial femoral artery. This is important for deep femoral artery preservation.

- Adequate debridement of all intimal damage is essential to fully evaluate the reconstructive options.
- Leaving some posterior attachments will prevent too much recoil of the vessel ends into the deep thigh or pelvis.
- Always inspect the outflow tract, flush liberally, and gently pass a Fogarty thrombectomy catheter to remove any fresh arterial thrombus if the back bleeding is not profuse.

- Use caution to not overinflate (hub shows max liquid capacity) the balloon catheter. If any resistance is encountered, carefully deflate some saline and withdrawal.
- Determine the size of conduit needed. The saphenous vein from the contralateral groin is generally too small for a common femoral reconstruction but excellent for the superficial femoral artery (Fig. 24.10).

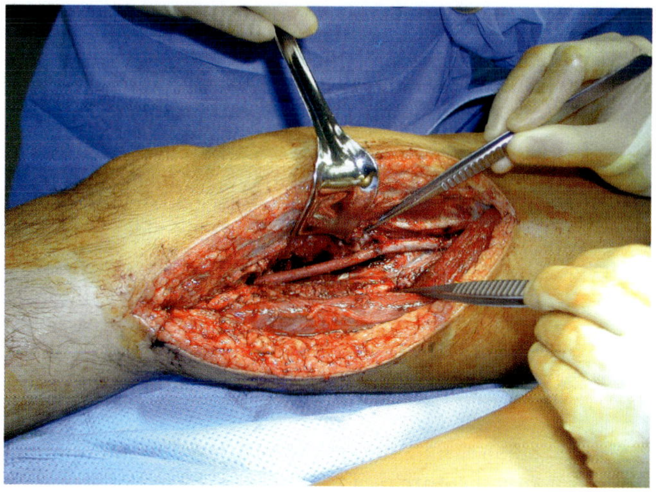

FIGURE 24.10 ▌ The reversed saphenous interposition graft is the preferred conduit for the superficial femoral artery.

- When a patch is desired, a Dacron or Bovine pericardial patch is typically used.
- A prosthetic interposition graft with ringed ePTFE or Dacron is appropriate.
  - Inflow should strike the palm forcibly.
  - Back bleeding from the distal vessel should be visible and steady.
  - The proximal anastomosis is performed with a 5-0 or 6-0 double-armed Prolene suture.
    - A parachute or four-quadrant heel-to-toe anastomosis technique may be employed.
    - Alternatively, a single posterior fixation suture (with three knots) followed by a running suture 180 degrees each direction with anterior completion tie can be performed.
  - Confirm inflow after the proximal anastomosis.
  - Complete the distal anastomosis but flush the graft (retrograde and then forward) before the final suture is tied.
- Completion angiogram can be done selectively using a hand injected 20-cc volume of contrast through a butterfly needle or intravenous 18-gauge angiocatheter placed into the proximal artery.
- Ensure the graft is covered with Sartorius muscle and the fascia closed.
- The wound is closed in several interrupted layers of absorbable suture without drains.
- A triphasic Doppler signal may not be appreciate after hypovolemic shock without a period of rewarming.
- A fasciotomy is highly recommended after venous ligation, 4 hours of ischemic time, or if the patient will be transported to another facility.

POSTOPERATIVE CARE

TIP

Patients should be recovered in an intensive care unit with hourly monitoring of pedal pulses and verification using Doppler signals.

- A completion angiogram is rarely necessary if there is a reliable Doppler examination.
- Obtain a baseline postrevascularization ABI to recognize early failures.
- Anticipate bleeding and gently correct coagulopathy guided by thromboelastography.
- Monitor for calf compartment syndrome.
- Avoid vasoactive agents in the resuscitative period.
- Prescribe 81- to 325-mg oral aspirin and DVT prophylaxis.

- Systemic anticoagulants are not necessary.
- If fasciotomies were performed, return to OR in 24 to 48 hours.

Suggested Readings

Feliciano DV, Moore EE, West MA, et al. Western Trauma Association critical decisions in trauma: evaluation and management of peripheral vascular injury, part II. *J Trauma Acute Care Surg*. 2013;75(3):391–397.

Feliciano DV, Moore FA, Moore EE, et al. Evaluation and management of peripheral vascular injury. Part 1. Western Trauma Association/critical decisions in trauma. *J Trauma*. 2011;70(6):1551–1556.

Inaba K, Aksoy H, Seamon MJ, et al; Multicenter Shunt Study Group. Multicenter evaluation of temporary intravascular shunt use in vascular trauma. *J Trauma Acute Care Surg*. 2016;80(3):359–364; discussion 364–365.

Magee GA, Cho J, Matsushima K, et al. Isolated iliac vascular injuries, and outcome of repair versus ligation of isolated iliac vein injury. *J Vasc Surg*. 2018;67(1):254–261.

Chapter 25
Popliteal Vascular Injury

CHARLES J. FOX AND ERNEST E. MOORE

PERIOPERATIVE CONSIDERATIONS

TIP

Communicate early to the operating room staff important details such as need for external fixation, vein harvest, preparation and positioning instructions, and a fluoroscopic imaging table. Unnecessary delays prolong the ischemic time and jeopardize limb salvage.

- A Doppler assessment and Ankle Brachial Index (ABI) are essential.
- Bleeding and pulselessness require prompt operative intervention.
- Tourniquets are removed when the patient is stable, and blood is available (Figure 25.1).

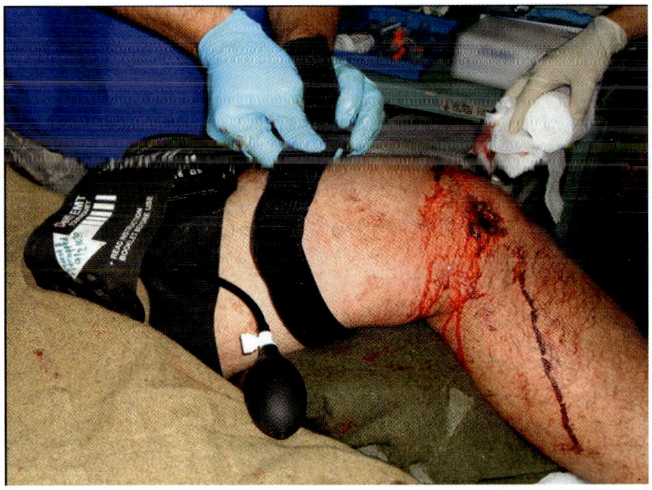

FIGURE 25.1 ❙ Removing the tourniquet from a stable patient in the emergency department. (Reproduced from Fox CJ, Starnes BW. Vascular surgery on the modern battlefield. *Surg Clin North Am*. 2007;87(5):1193–1211, xi.)

- Examine plain radiographs for patterns associated with arterial injury (Fig. 25.2).
  - Supracondylar femur fracture

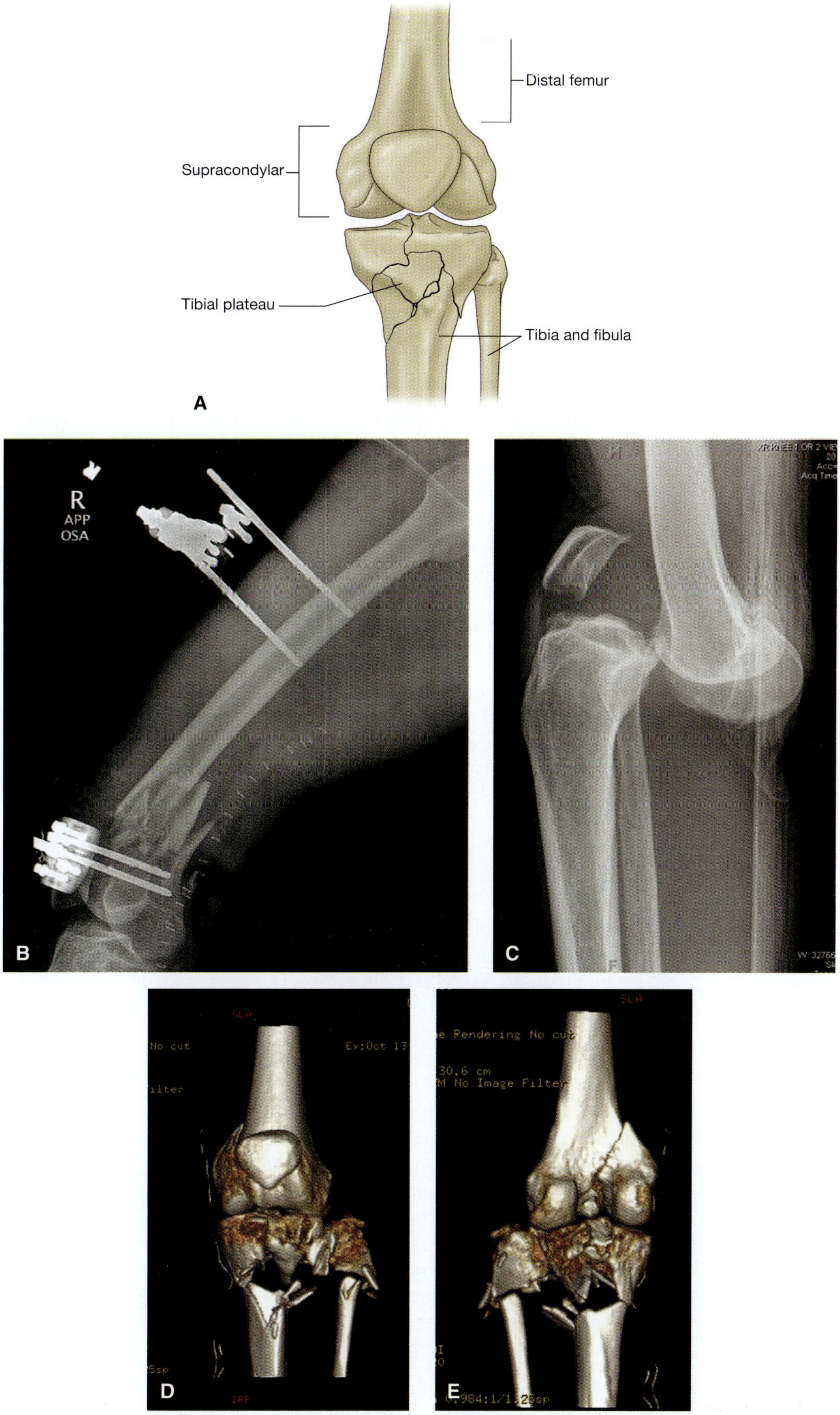

FIGURE 25.2 ▌ Typical fractures that are associated with popliteal arterial injury (**A**) with corresponding plain radiographs of a supracondylar femur fracture (**B**) and a posterior knee dislocation (**C**). A three-dimensional computed tomography shows an anterior (**D**) and posterior views (**E**) of a tibial plateau fracture. All had injury to the popliteal artery. (**B** from Fox CJ, Starnes, BW. Vascular surgery on the modern battlefield. *Surg Clin North Am*. 2007;87(5):1193–1211, xi.)

    - Knee dislocation
    - Tibial plateau fracture
- Computed tomography angiography (CTA) is useful for evaluating a blunt injury, particularly if considering the posterior approach. However, CTA should not delay intervention for an ischemic limb.
- Anticipate the need for a contralateral saphenous vein harvest.
- Consider an intravascular shunt before external fixation when delay in revascularization is anticipated or when ischemic time has been long.
- Apply external fixation prior to vascular reconstruction if unstable fracture/dislocation to ensure a tensionless anastomosis.
- Request a digital subtraction capable C-arm for completion angiography.
- Mangled extremities require a consensus opinion of trauma, vascular, and orthopedic teams to determine salvagability. Scoring systems are no substitute for clinical judgment.

Procedure Rationale

- Trauma to the popliteal artery remains a challenging problem to manage and, compared to other extremity vascular injuries, is frequently associated with complications.
- These wounds when open can bleed severely and have a high rate of amputation that is compounded by pre-existing vascular disease, hypoperfusion, ischemic time, and associated soft tissue damage.
- Many times, resuscitation becomes the Achilles heel of the intended limb salvage and these efforts are further compounded by the need for interfacility patient transfer. Early recognition of this injury and prompt treatment are crucial to success, and expectations need to be communicated clearly to the patient and family.

Essential Equipment

- Headlight
- Loupe magnification 2.5
- Beckman retractors
- Castroviejo needle driver
- Microvascular forceps
- Profunda vascular clamps (angled and straight)
- Shunts
    - 1 pack of 6- or 11-inch Argyle (8-, 10-, 12-, 14-Fr) shunts
    - 15- or 31-cm Pruitt–Inahara shunt (with T-port) 8- to 10-mm balloon diameter
- Sutures
    - 5-0 and 6-0 Prolene on a C1 or BV1 needle
    - 3-0 Silk plain and stick ties
    - 2-0 Ethibond, Vicryl and silk sutures (for tendon identification)
    - 3-0 Vicryl or PDS sutures
- Sterile 8- to 10-MHz Doppler probe
- Heparinized saline 50 to 100 units/mL saline
- Papaverine 60 mg in 20 cc of saline
- Fogarty embolectomy catheters #2 & #3
- Bulldog soft vascular clamps
- 3-Way stopcock and A-line extension tubing
- 10-cc syringes of heparinized saline on 18-gauge IV catheter
- Portable ultrasound machine

Patient Positioning

TIP

Prep the field tourniquet into the sterile field when there is open external bleeding, and take the tourniquet down after obtaining proximal control.

- Place upper body Bair warmer and radial arterial line.
- A medial approach in supine position is the standard exposure for multisystem injured patients.
- For an isolated knee injury, a posterior approach should be considered particularly if the patient is morbidly obese.
  - When an interposition graft is necessary, the conduit length will be short (5-8 cm).
  - Pad all pressure points and apply a thigh tourniquet before prone positioning.
  - Maintain the ability to bend knee joint by prepping the foot into the surgical field.
  - May require turning the patient from supine to prone unless a vein harvest is performed empirically.
  - External fixation can be applied in the prone position.
  - Injuries that extend proximal to the adductor hiatus should be repaired medially.
- A sterile pneumatic tourniquet can replace the prehospital tourniquet.
- Prep both legs from umbilicus to feet circumferentially.
- Orient external fixation to allow for ease of the medial exposure (Fig. 25.3).

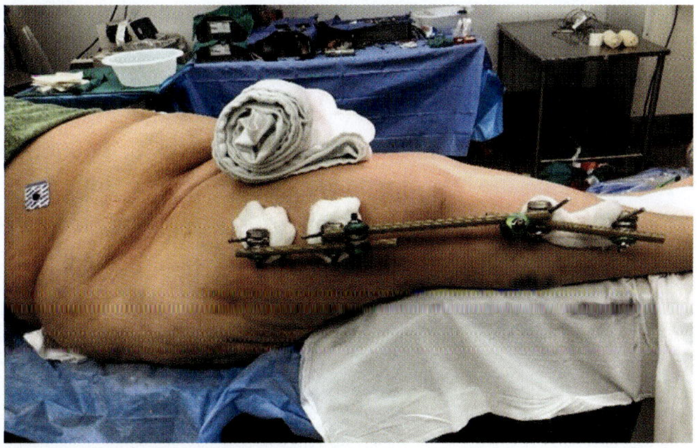

FIGURE 25.3 ▌ An external fixator can be easily adjusted when needed to accommodate a challenging medial approach.

TECHNIQUE

Surgical Approach-Medial

TIP

When limb threat exists, it is better to make an incision too large rather than too small.

- A large medial incision across the knee joint is made to control active hemorrhage (Fig. 25.4).

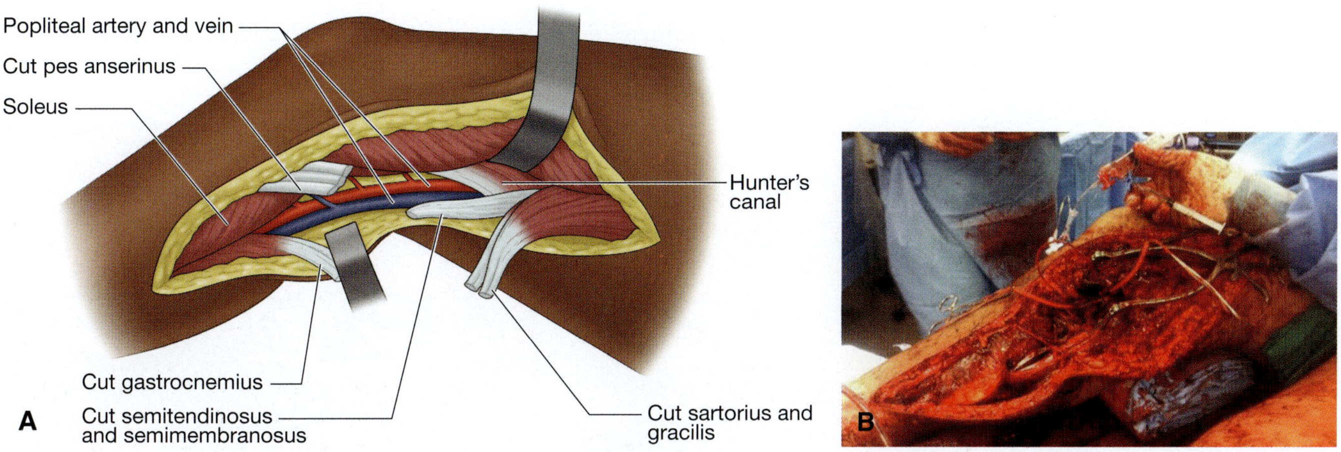

FIGURE 25.4 ▌ The medial approach (**A**) is the recommended exposure for patients with multisystem trauma. An extensive medial incision may be necessary to control bleeding (**B**).

- Potential for bleeding should not be underestimated, and enough exposure is crucial to gain proximal and distal control.
- Care should be taken to avoid injury to the saphenous vein during the incision (Fig. 25.5).

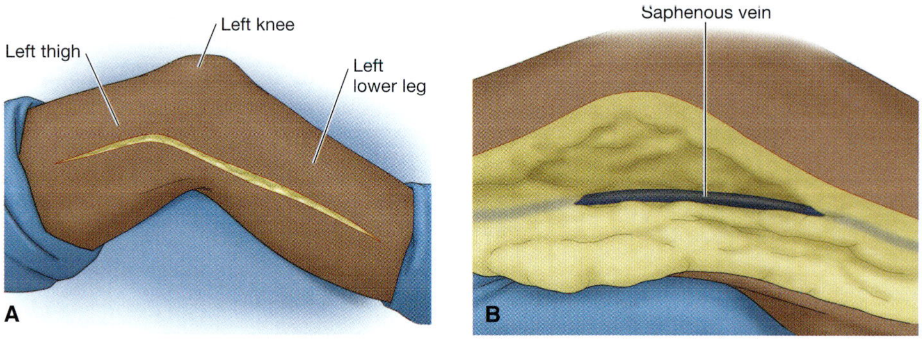

FIGURE 25.5 ❙ The initial incision for the medial approach to the popliteal artery (**A**) is determined by the injury location. Care is taken to avoid injury to the saphenous vein (**B**).

  - A saphenous can also be taken from an amputated extremity.
- Anticipate the fasciotomy incision during the initial exposure.
- While avoiding the saphenous vein, dissect into the crural fascia between the vastus medialis superiorly and sartorius posteriorly (Fig. 25.6).

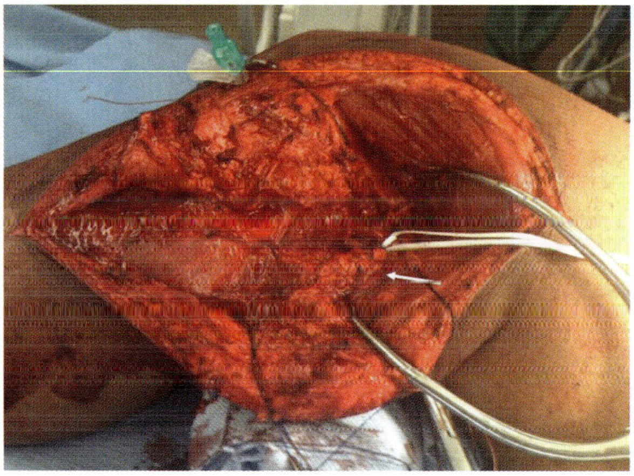

FIGURE 25.6 ❙ The dissection into the crural fascia is made between the vastus medialis superiorly and the sartorius muscle (*arrow*) is reflected posteriorly.

- Divide the sartorius, gracilis, and semitendinosus if needed and mark the cut margins of the tendon with stick ties of different colors for later identification (Fig. 25.7).

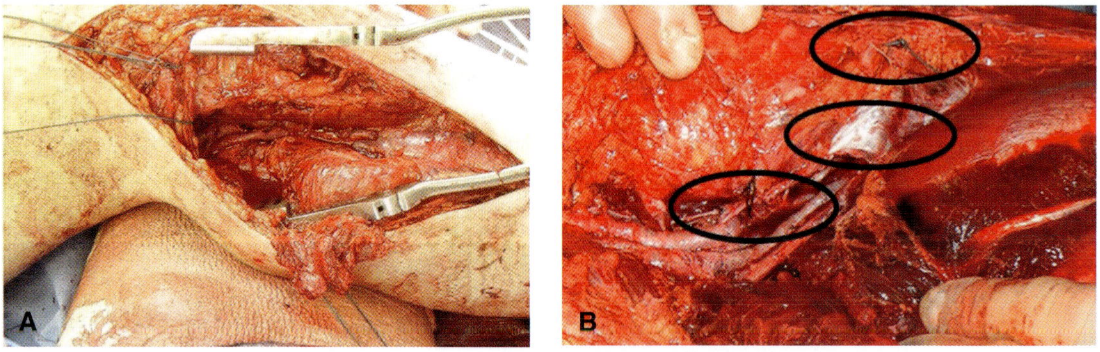

FIGURE 25.7 ❙ Divide the sartorius, gracilis, and semitendinosus if needed (**A**) and mark the cut margins of the tendon with stick ties of different colors for later identification (**B**).

- Probe the loose areolar fatty tissue of the popliteal fossa to isolate the artery and vein.
- The tibioperoneal trunk is just distal and posterior to the anterior tibial vein (Fig. 25.8).

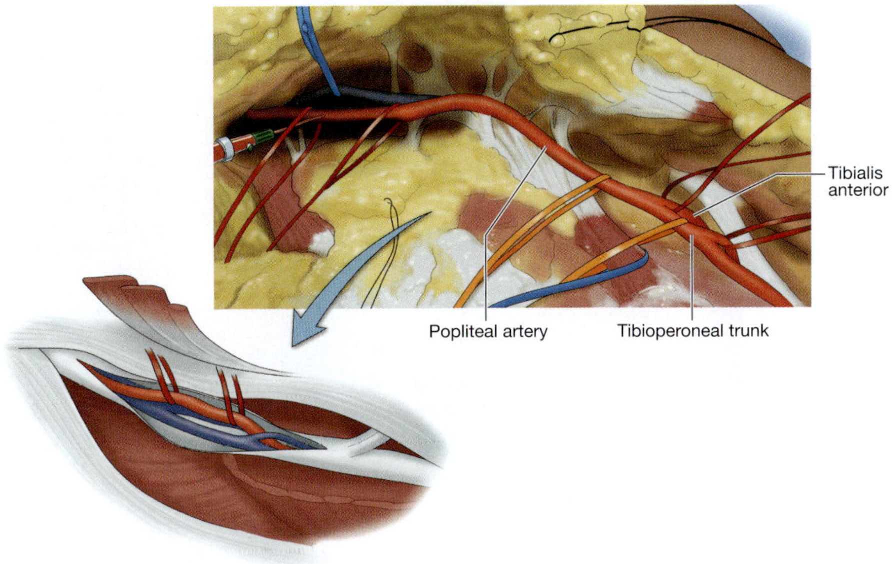

FIGURE 25.8 ▮ The tibioperoneal trunk is just distal and posterior to the anterior tibial vein.

- A transected distal arterial end of a mangled limb can be found by passing a Fogarty retrograde from the posterior tibial artery if necessary.
- Profunda clamps are placed well beyond the injury.
- A Pruitt–Inahara shunt (Fig. 25.9) is preferred because the T-port has the following advantages:

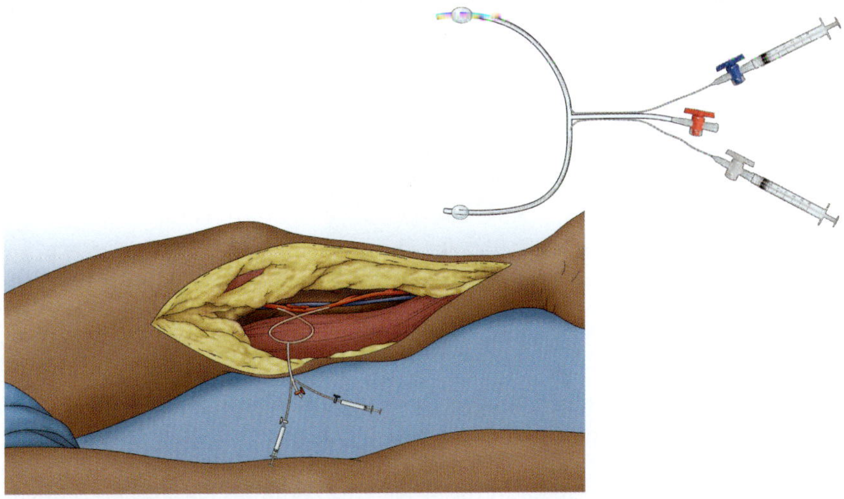

FIGURE 25.9 ▮ A Pruitt–Inahara shunt is preferred because the T port allows intermittent confirmation of flow and TPA infusion or contrast administration for completion angiography.

  - Intermittent confirmation of flow
  - Contrast administration for completion angiography
  - Tissue plasminogen activator(tPA) can be infused when there is prolonged ischemic time
- The vein is repaired when time and patient condition allows.
- For blunt injuries with both popliteal artery and vein transection, we prefer to repair the vein with a ring reinforced 6-mm polytetrafluoroethylene (PTFE) interposition graft.

Surgical Approach-Posterior

- The S-shaped incision superomedial to inferolateral (Fig. 25.10).

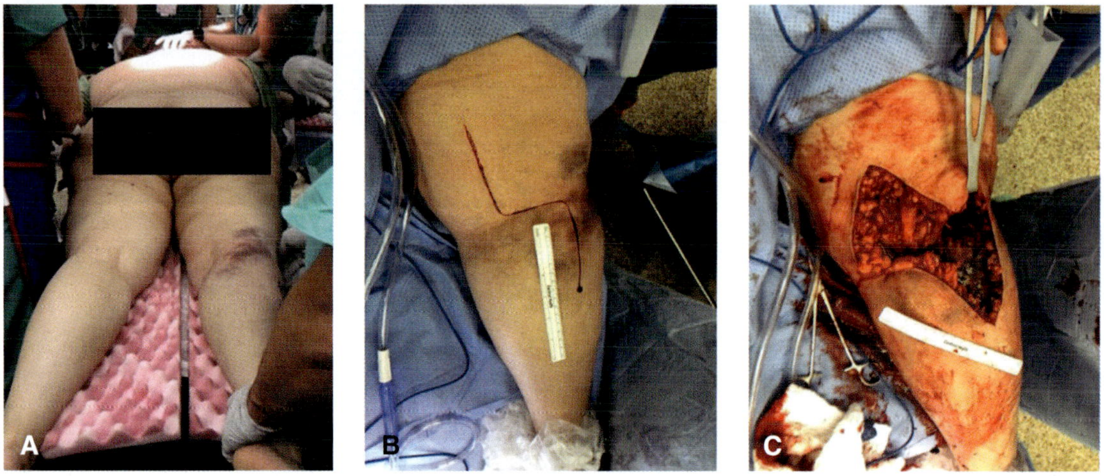

FIGURE 25.10 ▌ A posterior approach should be considered for an isolated traumatic injury and allows for a short interposition graft. A morbidly obese patient with a right knee dislocation is placed prone (**A**). The posterior approach begins with a superomedial to inferolateral incision across the knee joint (**B**). The small saphenous is followed into the popliteal fossa guiding one to the popliteal vein, artery, and adjacent nerves (**C**).

- Identify and protect the sural nerve and lesser saphenous vein (LSV).
- Open the deep fascia and trace the LSV into the saphenopopliteal junction (SPJ) (Fig. 25.11).

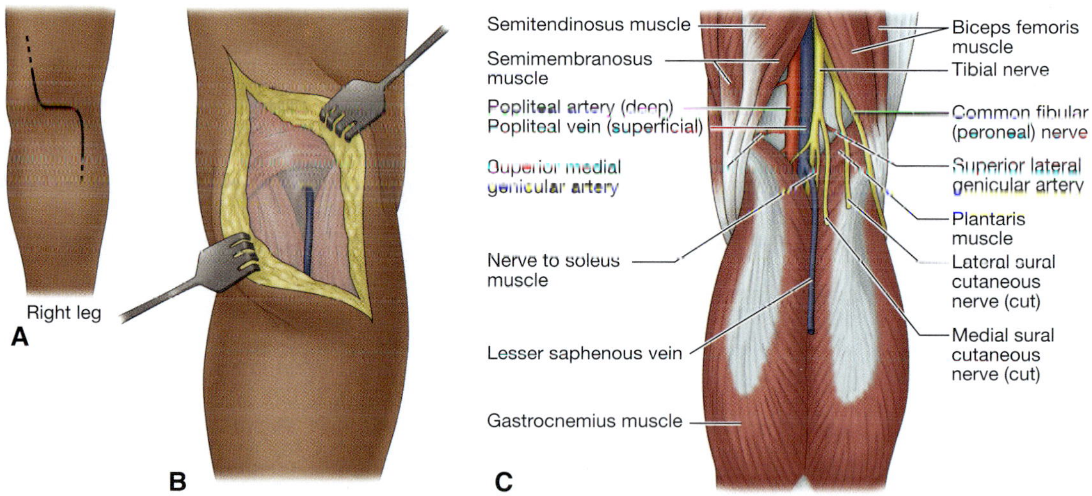

FIGURE 25.11 ▌ An S-shaped incision is made over the saphenopopliteal junction (**A**) for using the lesser saphenous vein (**B**) as a guide to the neurovascular bundle (**C**).

- The vein is lateral to the artery; the common peroneal and tibial nerves are the most lateral structures (Fig. 25.12).

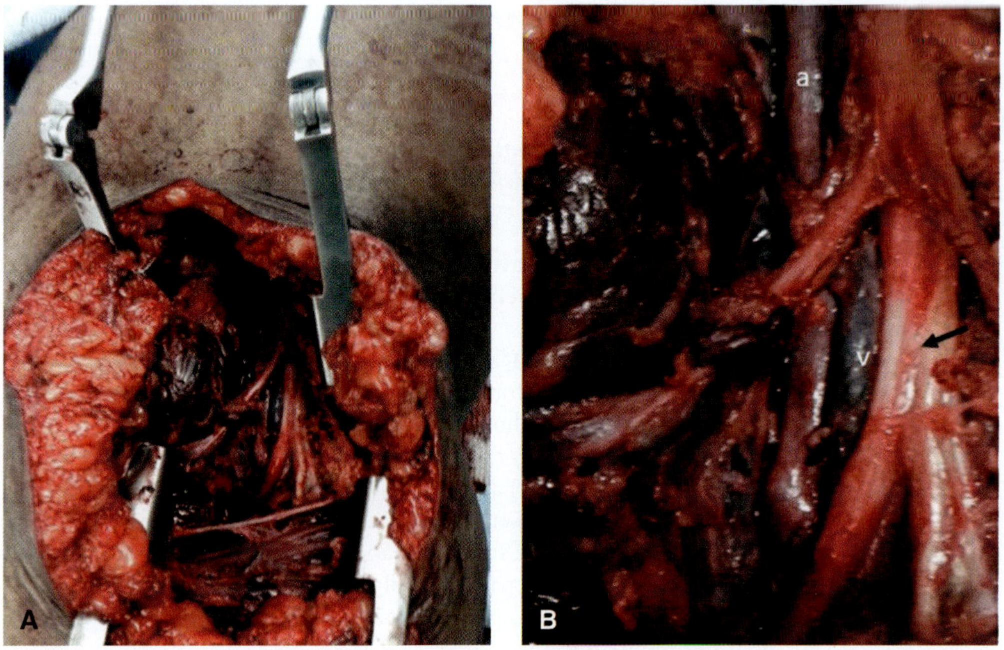

FIGURE 25.12 ❙ Exposure of the neurovascular bundle in the right popliteal fossa (**A**). The vein (v) is lateral to the artery (*a*) used for arterial repair and the common peroneal and tibial nerves are the most lateral structures (*arrow*, **B**).

- More distal dissection will expose the proximal anterior tibial and tibioperoneal trunk.
- Perform a 15-cm greater saphenous vein harvest in the supine position and flip the patient into the prone or consider the LSV or a bioprosthetic graft when alternative conduits are necessary (Fig. 25.13).

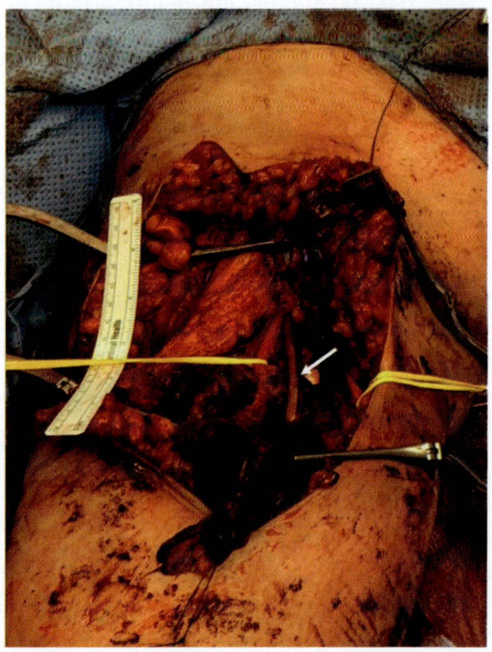

FIGURE 25.13 ❙ A 5-cm Human Acellular Vessel (Humacyte, Inc., Durham, NC) made an excellent bioprosthetic conduit for this revascularization (*white arrow*). Note the line drawn down the top to maintain orientation and avoid twisting of the anastomosis. *Yellow silastic loops* are holding the tibial nerve and a slip of muscle tissue.

Vascular Reconstruction

TIP

Always ensure that the graft, autologous or prosthetic, is covered entirely with healthy and viable muscle tissue. When the defect is large and cannot be covered route the bypass graft around the zone of injury.

- An end anastomosis is favored when lateral suture cannot repair without stenosis.
- A reversed saphenous vein interposition graft is favored when end anastomosis would have any tension.
- Adequate debridement of all intimal damage is essential.
- Shunts may allow time for fasciotomy or vein harvest. Furthermore, much of the anastomosis can be performed with the shunt in place to minimize ischemic time.
- A number 2 or 3 Fogarty embolectomy catheter should be done prior to shunt placement to ensure all proximal (#3 Fogarty) and distal (#2 Fogarty) thrombus is removed.
- Ensure smooth shunt insertion and careful balloon dilation to avoid further injury.
- Saphenous vein ends are spatulated and the graft is dilated with heparinized saline.
- Inflow should strike the palm forcibly. Back bleeding should be visible and steady.
- Confirm inflow after the proximal anastomosis. Complete distal anastomosis and flush before the final sutures are tied.
- A parachute or four-quadrant heel to toe anastomosis technique should be employed.
- Mark one side of the vein with a marking pen to maintain meticulous orientation.
- If the vein is sewn in a non-reversed configuration, pass a valvulotome before finishing the distal anastomosis.
- A hand-injected 10-cc volume of contrast through a butterfly needle or intravenous 18-gauge angiocatheter placed into the artery will allow confirmation of graft patency and tibial run off.
- Liberally flush with heparinized saline and apply topical papaverine as needed.
- Consider 200-400 micrograms of intraarterial nitroglycerine to relieve vasospasm or 5-10 mg Tissue plasminogen activator (tPA) if distal embolization is suspected.
- Ensure the graft is covered with muscle and the fascia closed.
- The wound is closed in several interrupted layers of absorbable suture without drains.
- A triphasic Doppler signal may not be appreciated after hypovolemic shock without a period of rewarming. Optimally, resistance and flow should be determined by Duplex.
- A fasciotomy should be highly considered after venous ligation, 4 hours of ischemic time, or if the patient will be transported to another facility.

POSTOPERATIVE CARE

TIP

The amount of postoperative bleeding after concomitant vein injury and fasciotomy cannot be overemphasized. Expect postoperative bleeding and treat any underlying coagulopathy using thromboelastography (TEG) as a guide.

- Continuous hourly reassessment with Doppler examination is important.
- Obtain a baseline post-revascularization ABI to recognize early failures.
- Anticipate bleeding and correct coagulopathy guided by thromboelastography.
- Monitor for compartment syndrome.
- Avoid vasoactive agents in the resuscitative period.
- Prescribe 81-325 mg oral Aspirin and DVT prophylaxis.
- Systemic anticoagulants are not necessary for patients who do not have occlusive disease.
- Weight bearing as tolerated.
- Return to OR in 24 to 48 hours for wound inspection and partial/complete fasciotomy closure.
- Negative pressure wound therapy is useful for closing deep cavitary wounds.

Suggested Readings

Feliciano DV, Moore EE, West MA, et al. Western trauma association critical decisions in trauma: evaluation and management of peripheral vascular injury, part II. *J Trauma Acute Care Surg*. 2013;75(3):391–397.

Feliciano DV, Moore FA, Moore EE, et al. Evaluation and management of peripheral vascular injury. Part 1. Western trauma association/critical decisions in trauma. *J Trauma*. 2011;70(6):1551–1556.

Fox CJ, Moore EE. The posterior approach to the mid-popliteal vessels is the preferred approach for an isolated knee injury. *J Trauma Acute Care Surg*. 2020;89(4):e101–e105.

Fox CJ, Perkins JG, Kragh JF Jr, Singh NN, Patel B, Ficke JR. Popliteal artery repair in massively transfused military trauma casualties: a pursuit to save life and limb. *J Trauma*. 2010;69(Suppl 1):S123–S134.

Inaba K, Aksoy H, Seamon MJ, et al. Multicenter evaluation of temporary intravascular shunt use in vascular trauma. *J Trauma Acute Care Surg*. 2016;80(3):359–364; discussion 364–365.

Chapter 26

Compartment Syndrome of the Upper Extremity

KRYSTLE R. TUAÑO, THOMAS J. FRANCE, AND MERYL SINGER

PERIOPERATIVE CONSIDERATIONS

Procedure Rationale

- Acute compartment syndrome (ACS) is defined as a limb-threatening condition caused by increased pressure within the confined spaces of a fascial or osteofascial anatomic compartment. If this is left untreated, irreversible damage can occur, resulting in fibrosis and contracture. This occurs when tissue pressure exceeds perfusion pressure, leading to inadequate oxygenation, circulatory impairment, ischemia, and cellular anoxia. Volkmann ischemic contracture is a term that is used to describe the varying degrees of the end-stage manifestations of tissue ischemia following compartment syndrome. Systemic manifestations can also arise from a severe local compartment syndrome called crush syndrome, which can lead to renal, cardiac, and respiratory failure, as well as intravascular coagulation, due to the rapid return of toxic muscle products into the circulatory system.
- Skeletal muscle may partially recover after 6 hours of compression. However, permanent damage can occur after 8 hours. Peripheral nerves are more sensitive to ischemic change. Nerve function is affected after 1 hour of ischemia and may undergo irreversible damage after 4 to 6 hours.
- Due to the variety of conditions that can result in upper extremity ACS, it is difficult to determine the true incidence. Similarly, it is difficult to determine the overall debility and patient impact that results from the long-term sequelae of missed, undiagnosed/untreated, or mismanaged ACS. According to the National Trauma Data Bank, 1.22% of forearm fractures and 3.79% of tibial fractures underwent fasciotomy for compartment syndrome, with a 1% estimated incidence in pediatric upper extremity fractures. ACS is more prevalent in young patients, with a mean age of 32 years in males and 44 years in females, and in patients suffering from penetrating trauma, open fractures, vascular injuries, and elbow dislocations. Branco and colleagues found a 0.41% incidence of fasciotomies associated with all upper extremity traumas in a large series of trauma patients, with a 6.7 to 16% rate associated with traumatic arterial injuries.

TIP

The surgeon in charge should review all relevant imaging and perform a complete history and physical examination. There are many potential causes of ACS, and treatment of the underlying condition will prevent potential postoperative persistence of increased intracompartmental pressures.

Pathophysiology

- Several theories and models have been developed to describe the complex pathophysiology of ACS. The final common pathway is cellular anoxia.
- Increased pressure within the osteofascial compartment affects venous return and results in decreased arterial pressure with increased venous pressure, ultimately leading to cellular anoxia.
- Muscle degeneration generally occurs in the center of the muscle belly, as vascularity in this area is most compromised. The most commonly affected muscles are supplied by the anterior interosseous artery, beginning with the deep compartments.

TIP

Treatment within the critical window of reversible changes is paramount. A missed compartment syndrome can result in irreversible damage with significant morbidity for the patient. Clinicians should have a high suspicion for ACS, despite the presumed severity of the inciting event, if there is significant pain out of proportion to examination. Definitive diagnosis and treatment should not be delayed until additional findings are present.

Etiology, Pathophysiology, and Epidemiology

- Trauma is often reported as the most common cause of forearm ACS, which is commonly associated with fractures, crush injuries, burns, and head injuries. It is often a result of high-energy limb injury, but can also be associated with atraumatic or iatrogenic causes, such as intravenous infiltration, transradial coronary catheterization, and neuromonitoring electrodes. Relatively uncommon causes described in the literature include carbon monoxide poisoning, recreational activities including push-up golf, or henna application.
- As described by Jones et al., there are two major categories that the many conditions ACS is associated with can be sorted into: conditions that decrease compartment volume and conditions that increase compartment contents.

Conditions that decrease compartment volume: increased external pressure for a prolonged period of time, traction, limb lengthening, tight dressings or casts/splints, and burns (eschar).

Conditions that increase compartment contents: infiltration, snake bites, intensive use of muscles during exercise (chronic exertional compartment syndrome), seizures, eclampsia, tetany, reperfusion injury, edema, infection, bleeding disorders, high-pressure injections, vascular injuries, anticoagulation, and trauma.

Pediatric Considerations

- Supracondylar fracture of the humerus is the most common cause of ACS in children.
- A special consideration is the emphasis on bivalving of casts placed on acute fractures to allow for pressure release, thereby decreasing the possibility of ACS.

Literature has shown that there is no significant difference in loss of reduction after closed reduction in patients with univalve versus bivalve casts.

RELEVANT ANATOMY

Compartments

Arm

- The arm is divided into two compartments, anterior and posterior, which are separated by the medial and lateral intermuscular septa
  - Anterior contains: Biceps brachii, brachialis, and coracobrachialis
  - Posterior contains: Triceps brachii

Forearm

- The forearm is divided into three compartments, volar, dorsal, and mobile wad of three (mobile wad of Henry)
  - Volar contains: The flexor muscles (superficial, intermediate, and deep subdivisions)
    - Superficial: Flexor carpi ulnaris, palmaris longus, flexor carpi radialis, pronator teres
    - Intermediate: Flexor digitorum superficialis
    - Deep: Flexor digitorum profundus, flexor pollicis longus, pronator quadratus
  - Dorsal contains: The extensor muscles
    - Superficial: Extensor digitorum communis, extensor digiti minimi, extensor carpi ulnaris, anconeus
    - Deep: Supinator, abductor pollicis longus, extensor pollicis longus, extensor pollicis brevis, and extensor indicis proprius
  - Mobile wad of three (mobile wad of Henry) contains: Brachioradialis, extensor carpi radialis longus, and extensor carpi radialis brevis

Hand

- The hand is divided into 10 distinct compartments: dorsal interossei (4), palmar (volar) interossei (3), thenar, hypothenar, adductor
  - Seven compartments for the interossei
    - Four dorsal and three palmar
  - Adductor compartment: Adductor pollicis
  - Thenar compartment: Abductor pollicis brevis, opponens pollicis, and flexor pollicis brevis
  - Hypothenar compartment: Abductor digiti minimi, flexor digiti minimi, and opponens digiti minimi

Finger

- The fingers are divided into two distinct compartments, bounded by the skin, Grayson and Cleland ligaments
  - Grayson ligaments are volar to the neurovascular bundle
  - Cleland ligaments are dorsal to the neurovascular bundle

Clinical Signs and Diagnosis

- Diagnosis is primarily based on clinical examination.
- ACS is more prevalent in males younger than 35 years, penetrating trauma, elbow dislocations, and open fractures, with a dramatically increased need for surgical intervention when associated with vascular injuries. In contrast, compartment syndrome of the hand is most commonly associated with intravenous injections.
- The classical "six *P*s" have been described as hallmarks for the diagnosis of compartment syndrome: pain, pressure, paresthesias, pallor, paralysis, and pulselessness. Poikilothermia is sometimes substituted as one of the *P*s, which indicates that the affected extremity is cool relative to the body temperature.
- Pain can be an early finding; however, it peaks at around 2 to 6 hours and then gradually subsides as muscle necrosis progresses and nerve function declines.
- In pediatric patients, the "*A*s, not the *P*s" can be used as hallmarks for diagnosis: increasing requirement for analgesia, anxiety (restlessness), agitation (crying).
- Direct measurement of compartment pressures can assist in determining the diagnosis, particularly when a patient is obtunded or sedated, and clinical examination may be incomplete or unreliable.
  - ACS of the finger is a clinical diagnosis and is not determined through the use of pressure measurement.

Direct Compartment Pressure Measurements

- Normal intracompartmental pressures range from 0 to 8 mm Hg, and an absolute value above 30 mm Hg is considered critical.
- Delta P, which is the difference between diastolic blood pressure and measured compartment pressure, is often used as a more accurate assessment.
- A delta P value of less than or equal to 30 mm Hg is indicative of the need for fasciotomy.
- Pressure measurements are indicated in polytrauma patients, obtunded patients, or when physical examination findings are inconclusive. However, if there are positive clinical findings, urgent surgical intervention is recommended, foregoing formal pressure measurements..
- A variety of techniques exist for compartment pressure measurement.
- A recent systematic review, including 12 retrospective reviews of 84 cases of forearm compartment syndrome, found a variety of compartment measurement techniques, including a wick catheter, slit catheter, the Whitesides' infusion technique, and the Stryker brand Intra-Compartmental (STIC) Pressure Monitor Device.
- Wick catheter placement has been described by Gelberman et al., which involves insertion of a saline-filled catheter into the proximal volar and/or dorsal compartments. Proper placement into the muscle bellies was confirmed by a brisk rise in pressure reading while palpating the compartment or passive muscle contraction. Voluntary muscle contraction is, by default, not the recommended technique to ensure adequate positioning of the compartment pressure measuring device, as the patient undergoing invasive compartment measurement is likely unable to follow commands.

- Most compartment pressure measurements require a separate penetration into the volar, dorsal, and/or mobile wad, however, a technique using one entry site from the dorsal compartment, through the interosseous membrane, and into the volar compartment has been described.
- The STIC Pressure Monitor typically utilizes an 18-gauge needle, saline air-lock flush, and electronic pressure reader that can be manually calibrated.

TREATMENT/MANAGEMENT

Preoperative Planning

- Review patient history for possible causes.
- Review all relevant imaging and plan for stabilization, if necessary.
- Remove all extrinsic causes of pressure: dressings, splints, and casts.
- Remove invasive lines from the affected extremity.

Patient Positioning

- The patient is placed supine, with the upper extremity on a hand table/arm board.
- The shoulder is placed toward the edge of the operating room table, in order to gain maximum access to the upper extremity, including the axilla.
- A tourniquet does not need to be placed, as the diagnosis of ACS is generally associated with varying degrees of vascular compromise.

Technique

"The goal of treatment is to prevent tissue necrosis, avert neurovascular compromise, and avoid permanent functional deficits."

TIP

Remember that skin is a significant compressive structure. The skin incision should have sufficient length to allow adequate exposure for complete decompression. Staged closure can be planned for the resulting wound.

Fasciotomy Approaches

- Incisions are planned to allow for rapid access, complete decompression, maintenance of coverage for vital structures, and prevention of future contractures that can result in postoperative morbidity secondary to scarring.
- Volar compartment release often decompresses the dorsal compartment; therefore, this compartment should generally be released first. A compartment measuring device can be used to measure dorsal compartment pressure after volar release. Dorsal fasciotomy is indicated if there is no improvement in the pressure measurement.

Volar (Forearm) Approach

- An incision is made 1 cm proximal and 2 cm lateral to the medial epicondyle, which is curved medially and crosses obliquely across the antecubital fossa and over the volar aspect of the mobile wad and reaches midline at the junction of the middle and distal third of the forearm (Fig. 26.1).

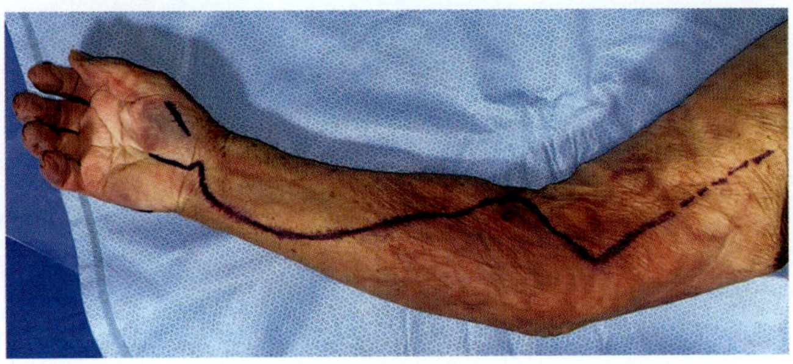

FIGURE 26.1 ▌ Markings for a volar fasciotomy of the upper extremity.

- The incision is continued just ulnar to the palmaris longus tendon to avoid the palmar cutaneous branch of the median nerve. Antebrachial fascia will be encountered deep to subcutaneous tissue in the distal forearm (Fig. 26.2).

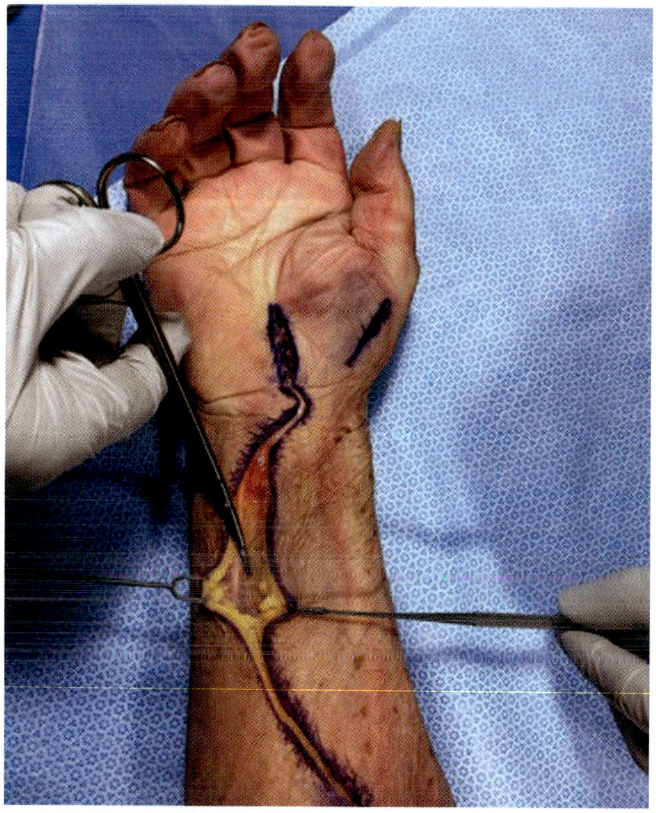

FIGURE 26.2 ▌ Demonstration of antebrachial fascia overlying the flexor tendons.

- For concomitant carpal tunnel release, the incision is designed to cross the wrist crease at an angle and extend into the midpalm (Fig. 26.3).

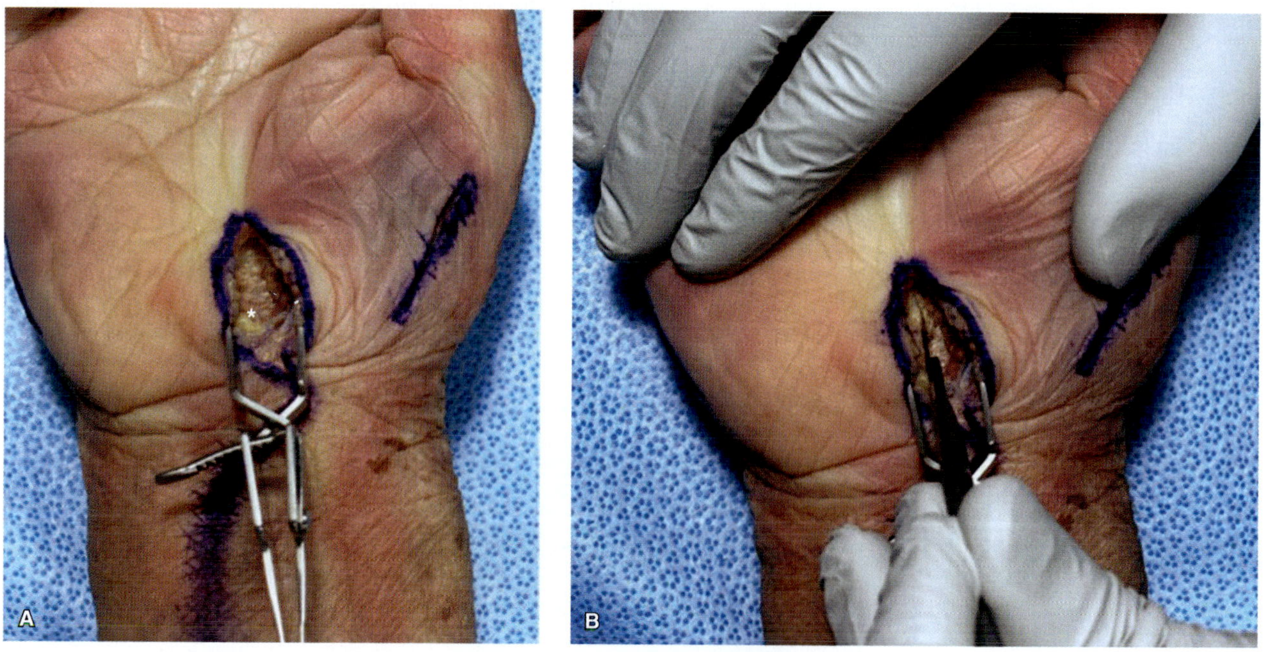

FIGURE 26.3 ▌ Demonstration of the transverse carpal ligament (flexor retinaculum) (*) (**A**), and incising the transverse carpal ligament (**B**).

- The dorsal compartment and mobile extensor wad can be released without need for a dorsal incision.
- In Figure 26.4, the brachioradialis is labeled, with the other two components of the mobile wad of three (mobile wad of Henry), the extensor carpi radialis longus and extensor carpi radialis brevis, deep to this. The dorsal approach to the mobile wad of three is demonstrated below in a separate figure.

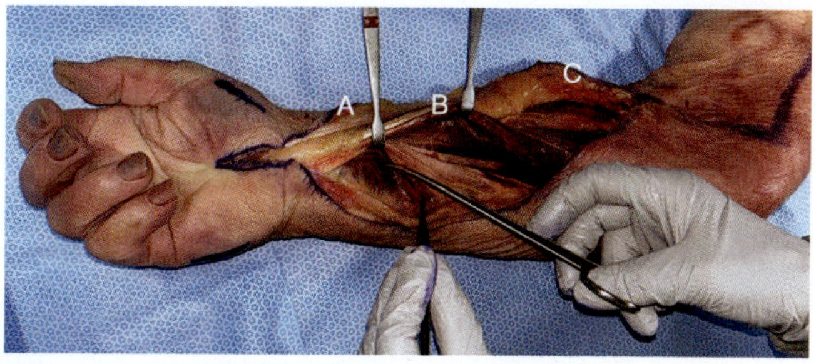

FIGURE 26.4 ▌ **A:** flexor digitorum superficialis muscle, (**B**) flexor digitorum profundus muscle, (**C**) brachioradialis.

Forearm Volar-Ulnar Approach

- A transverse incision is made distal to the antecubital crease on the radial side of the forearm (Fig. 26.5).

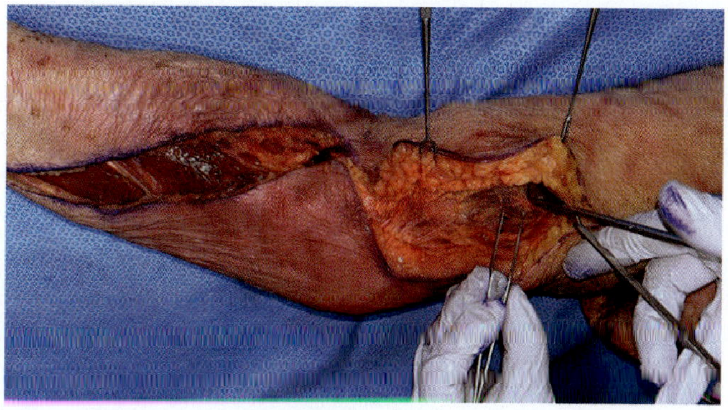

FIGURE 26.5 ▌ Demonstration of a curved incision to release the anterior brachial fascia in an extended volar approach.

- The incision is extended to the ulnar side of the forearm and then turned 90 degrees.
- The longitudinal component of the incision is extended down the ulnar side of the forearm to the wrist and then curved medially to the midaspect of the volar wrist.
- Finally, the incision is curved into the thenar crease of the palm.
- The fascia underlying the space between the flexor carpi ulnaris and flexor digitorum superficialis muscles is separated with retractors to visualize the ulnar nerve and artery in the deep flexor compartment.
- The incision is curved radially in the midforearm and just anterior to the medial epicondyle at the elbow to provide coverage for the median nerve and brachial artery, while preventing a linear incision at the elbow (Fig. 26.6).

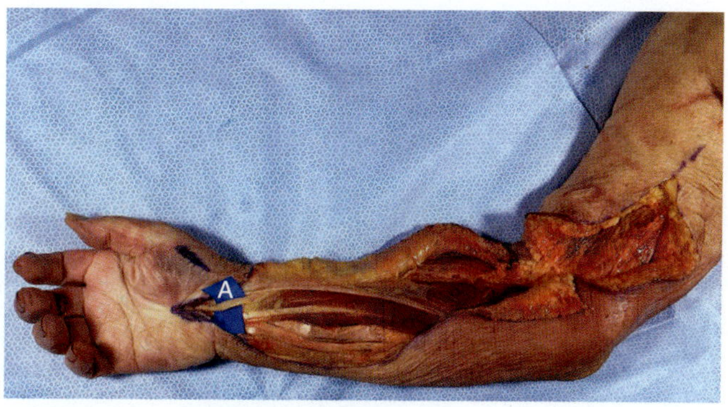

FIGURE 26.6 ▌ Extended volar forearm compartment release, including the carpal tunnel, antebrachial fascia, and anterior brachial fascia. The median nerve is isolated above the blue background (**A**).

Hand Compartment Release

- The hand has 10 compartments.
- Release of all 10 compartments is rarely needed. Therefore, careful intraoperative assessment and measurement of compartment pressures are used to determine which compartments need to be released.

Volar (Hand) Release

- This can be accomplished with an extended carpal tunnel release.
- This incision will usually adequately accommodate for decompression of the ulnar nerve at the level of the wrist, also, at the Guyon canal.
- The thenar and hypothenar spaces can be decompressed through separate incisions, as needed, and/or continued from the original volar incision, onto the thenar space (Fig. 26.7).

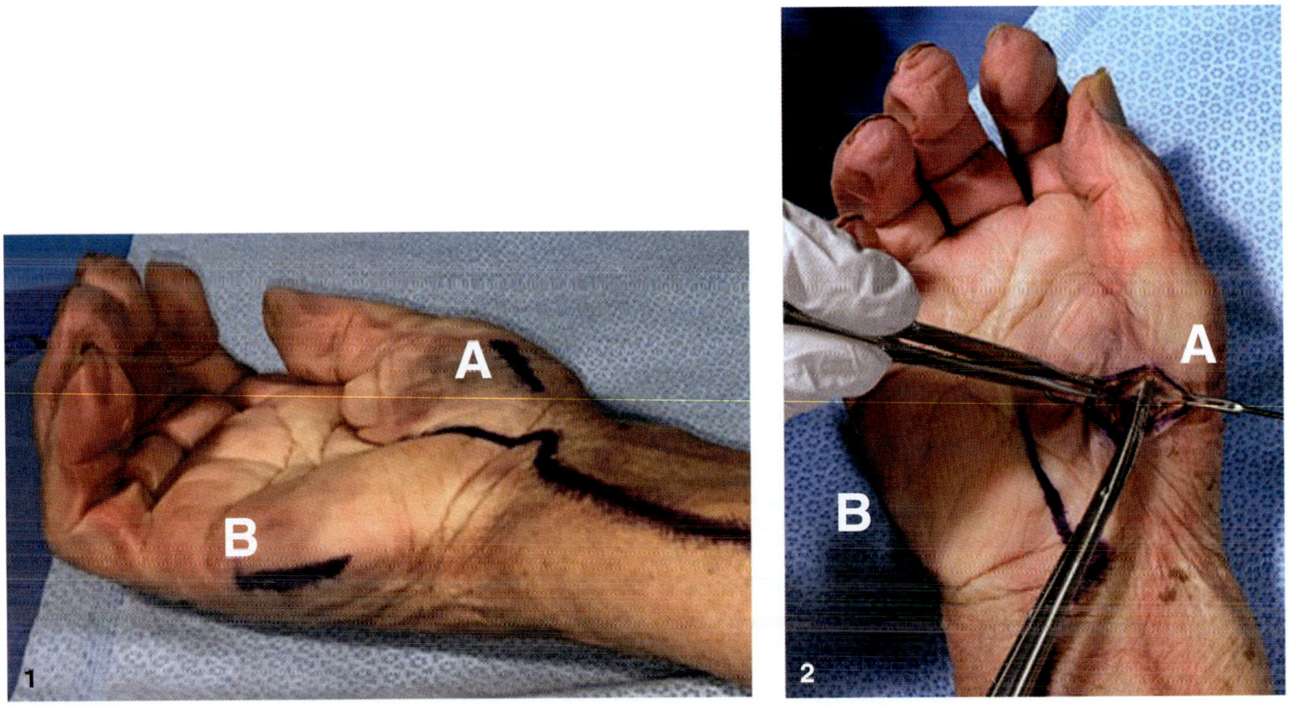

FIGURE 26.7 ▌ (**1**) Markings for (**A**) thenar compartment, and (**B**) hypothenar compartment incisions, and (**2**) release of the thenar compartment fascia (**A**).

- The volar fascia of the adductor pollicis muscle can be released at the distal aspect of the incision. The fascia that extends from the long finger metacarpal to the palmar fascia, which separates the deep radial and ulnar midpalmar spaces, can be released. This allows for adequate decompression of the volar interosseous muscles.

Dorsal (Forearm) Approach

- A dorsal incision is made 2 cm distal to the lateral epicondyle, toward the midline of the wrist. This approach decompresses the mobile wad of Henry (Fig. 26.8).
- Alternatively, a separate incision can be made beginning 3 to 4 cm distal to the lateral epicondyle, on the dorsal forearm, and extending toward Lister's tubercle.

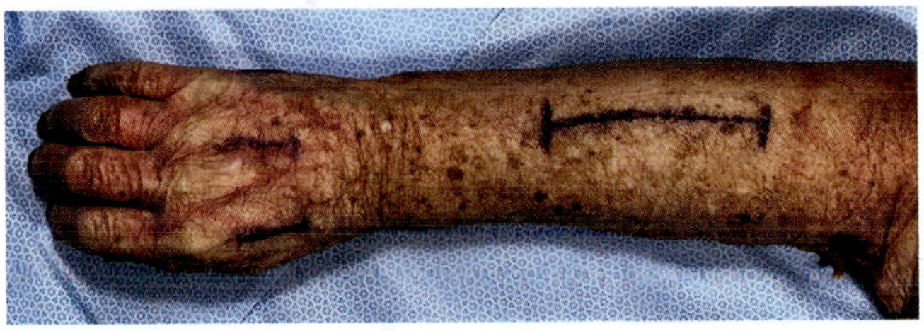

FIGURE 26.8 ▌ Dorsal forearm and hand fasciotomy incision markings.

Dorsal (Hand) Approach

- Dorsal incisions are made between the second and third metacarpals and between the fourth and fifth metacarpals to decompress the dorsal and volar interosseous muscles and dorsal fascia of the adductor pollicis.
- The incisions may be made in a curvilinear fashion, allowing for a wider skin bridge, and preserving blood supply.

Finger Compartment Release

- Subcutaneous tissue and skin necrosis can be prevented by decompressing the digital vessels.
- Grayson and Cleland ligaments can be released with a dermotomy of all involved fingers (as marked above), with a midaxial incision to prevent postoperative contracture scarring (Fig. 26.9).

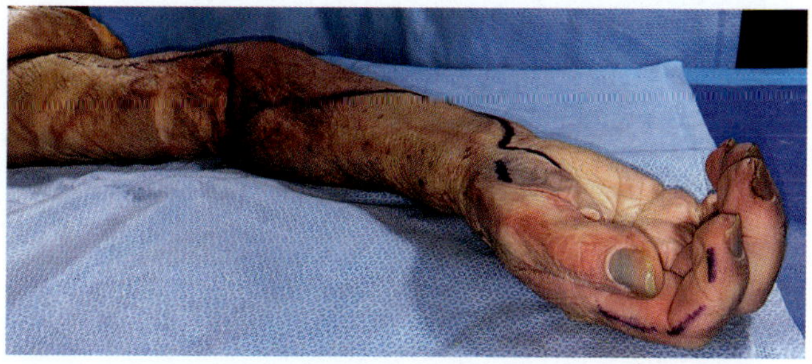

FIGURE 26.9 | Finger fasciotomy incision markings.

- Care should be taken to avoid injury to the neurovascular structures, which are more volar.
- The neurovascular bundle lies volar to the Cleland ligament and dorsal to the Grayson ligament.

TIP

Dermotomy midaxial plane incisions on the finger can be marked by flexing the finger and marking a longitudinal line just dorsal to the flexion creases. This will prevent postoperative contracture scarring.

Closure

- Wounds may be left open and covered in sterile dressings (Fig. 26.10).
- Most patients will need a "second look" intervention at 48 to 72 hours from the index procedure.

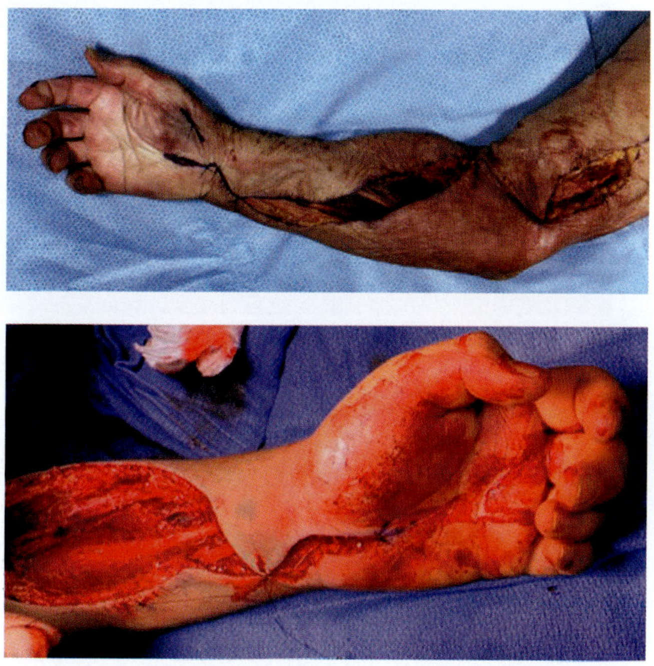

FIGURE 26.10 | Partial closure of the volar fasciotomy incisions.

- At re-evaluation, any additional nonviable tissue must be debrided, and delayed primary closure of the wounds can be attempted.
- Care should be taken to protect vital structures at each procedure. Initial incision, partial closure, and a variety of sterile dressing techniques can be used to ensure this.
- If the wound is unable to be closed primarily, negative pressure dressings, followed by split thickness skin grafting, can be performed at a later stage.
- Definitive closure is delayed until serial debridements are completed, and swelling has decreased.
- Jacob's ladder or shoelace (elastic suture) closure technique can be used to prevent loss of domain in between debridements while awaiting swelling to decrease prior to definitive closure (Figs. 26.11 and 26.12).

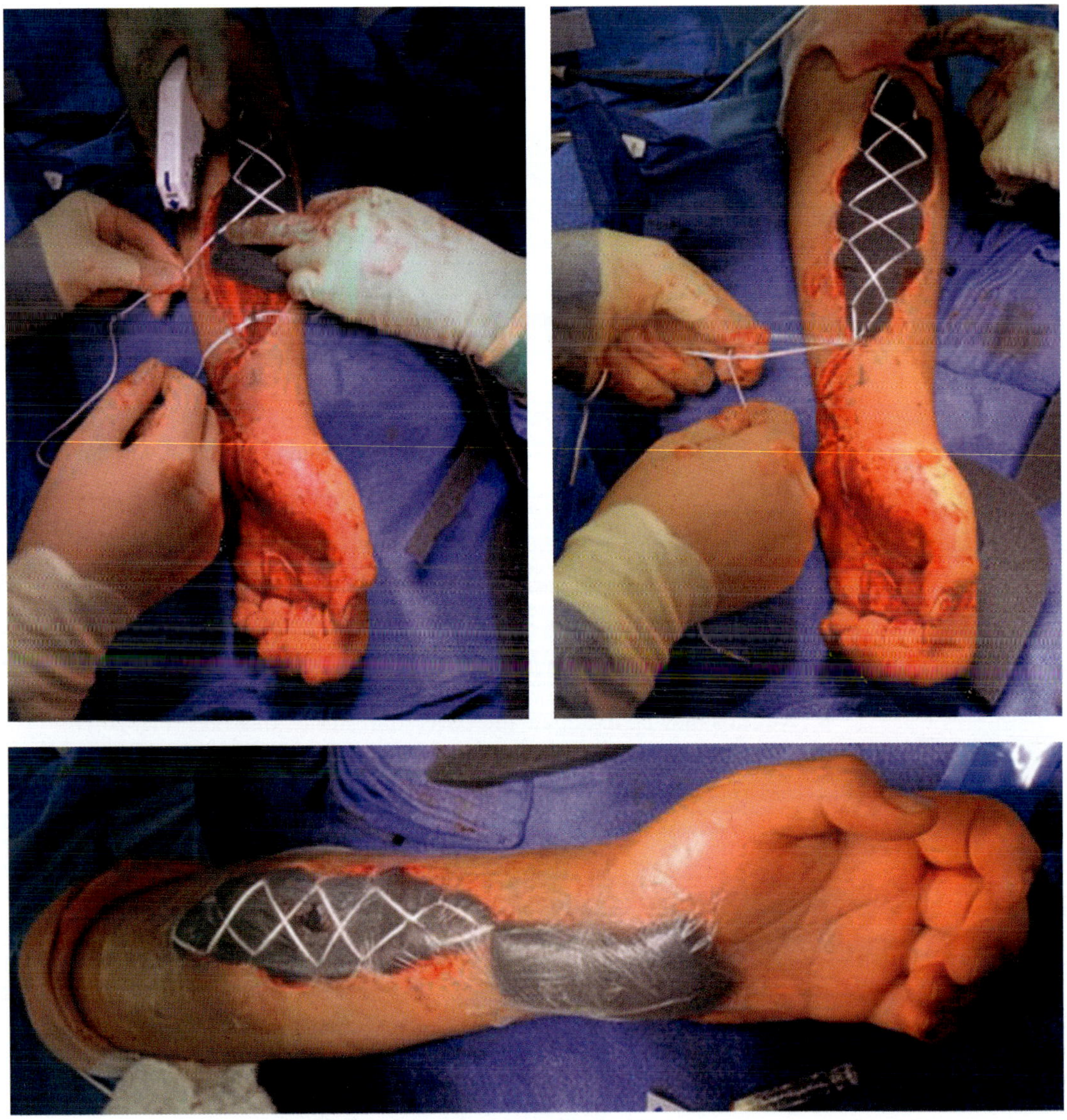

FIGURE 26.11 ▌ Volar Jacob's ladder or shoelace (elastic suture) closure technique.

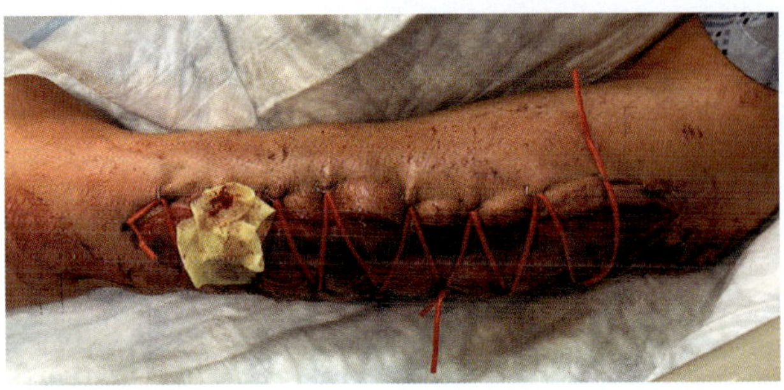

FIGURE 26.12 ▌ Dorsal Jacob's ladder or shoelace (elastic suture) closure technique.

TIP

Partial closure at the index procedure, particularly in areas that cover vital structures, such as nerves, bones, tendons, or other structures that can easily desiccate, can improve postoperative outcomes. Furthermore, this can facilitate better management of inevitable edema, allowing for a staged closure with a smaller defect, and partial primary closure.

POSTOPERATIVE CARE

Elevation

- The affected extremity should be elevated to at least the level of the heart.
- Limb elevation can decrease swelling; however, it can also reduce perfusion to the affected limb, which can exacerbate tissue ischemia.

Splinting

- The upper extremity should be splinted in the intrinsic plus or functional position.
- These positions allow the patient to maintain joint mobility, while protecting the soft tissue, thereby avoiding stiffness and contracture.

Activity

- Gentle active, and passive or assisted range of motion of the hand, wrist, and elbow should be initiated as soon as possible, generally when the swelling has decreased, approximately 2 to 3 days after definitive closure.
- Range of motion may initially be limited postoperatively due to closure, such as skin graft, or flap. Therefore, early range of motion of all joints not requiring immobilization should be considered when placing dressings or splints.

ACKNOWLEDGMENTS

This chapter is dedicated to our families, mentors, and colleagues.

To Alexandra. Thank you for the support and photo editing.

Suggested Readings

Chung KC, Guang Y. *Compartment Syndrome of the Upper Extremity. Grabb and Smith's Plastic Surgery*. Wolters Kluwer; 2020;895–904.

Jones MD, Santamarina R, Warhold LG. Chapter 124: Surgical decompression of the forearm, hand, and digits for compartment syndrome. In: Thomas R. Hunt III, Sam W. Wiesel (eds). *Operative Techniques in Hand, Wrist, and Elbow Surgery*. 2nd ed. Wolters Kluwer; 2016:1121–1128.

Leversedge FJ, Moore TJ, Peterson BC, Seiler JG. Compartment syndrome of the upper extremity. *J Hand Surg Am*. 2011;36(3):544–559. https://doi.org/10.1016/j.jhsa.2010.12.008.

Mailey BA, Neumeister MW. *Hand Surgery: Traumatic and Infectious Emergencies. Fischer's Mastery of Surgery*. Wolters Kluwer; 2019:247–261.

Stevanovic MV, Frances F. *Compartment Syndrome and Volkmann Ischemic Contracture. Green's Operative Hand Surgery*. Elsevier; 2017:1763–1787.

Chapter 27
Lower Extremity Fasciotomy

CHARLES J. FOX

RATIONALE

- Fasciotomy is an important procedure to minimize neuromuscular disability following an ischemia–reperfusion injury and the onset of a compartment syndrome. Compartment syndrome is the local effect of inflammatory processes following reperfusion that results in edema and diffuse swelling of the anterior, lateral, and posterior calf compartments. Rising myofascial pressures will eventually compromise neuromuscular perfusion and result in permanent injury if there is delay in treatment. Compartment syndrome is best determined by careful serial examination (Fig. 27.1).

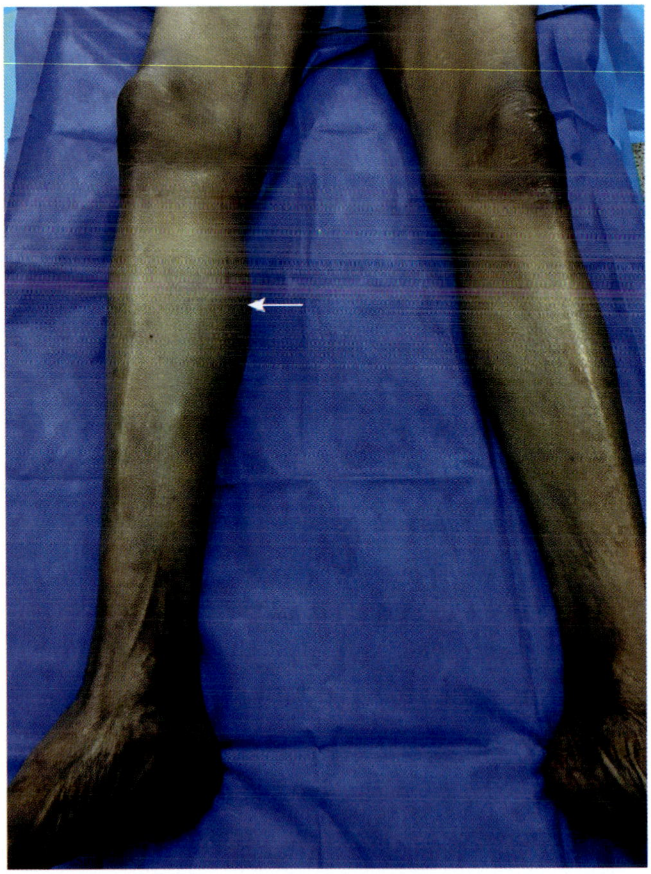

FIGURE 27.1 ❙ A right leg compartment syndrome with swelling of the calf (*arrow*) compared to the left leg.

- A fasciotomy in this setting is considered therapeutic but a fasciotomy can also be done as a prophylactic measure prior to the development of a compartment syndrome. A prophylactic fasciotomy may be necessary following arterial occlusion that may be aggravated by fractures, prolonged ischemic time, venous obstruction, or the absence of collateral circulation. When a patient cannot be serially examined by the same provider following an arterial reconstruction, a fasciotomy is especially encouraged. The optimal ischemic time and threshold for fasciotomy to achieve the best functional outcome remains unknown. Fasciotomy is not without morbidity and can pose significant reconstructive soft tissue challenges. The technique of a two-incision lower extremity fasciotomy is the focus of this chapter.

Essential Equipment

- Electrocautery
- Suction
- No. 10 scalpel blade
- Sutures
  - 3-0 silk plain and stick ties
  - 2-0 silk plain and stick ties
- Metzenbaum scissors (blunt tipped)
- Vessel loops
- Kerlix
- Skin stapler
- Negative pressure wound materials (optional)
- Ioban antimicrobial incise drape

TECHNIQUE

Medial Dissection: Superficial and Deep Posterior Compartments

TIP

During the medial dissection, incise the skin carefully to avoid injury to the saphenous vein. During the lateral incision, the superficial peroneal nerve can be easily injured.

- A two-incision technique is performed by incising the lateral and medial calf.
- A longitudinal incision is made two-finger widths medial to the tibia (Fig. 27.2).
- The skin incision can be shorter but the fascial incision should extend from knee to ankle.
- A skin flap is elevated to identify and preserve the saphenous vein (Fig. 27.3).

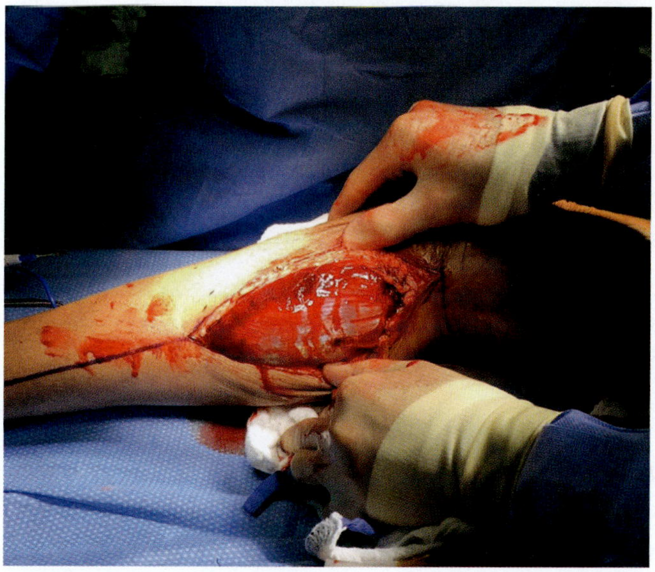

FIGURE 27.2 ▌ A medial skin incision is made and the crural fascia is divided to expose the right superficial posterior compartment. Although the skin incision length can vary, the fascial incision should extend the length of the calf compartment (*surgical ink line*).

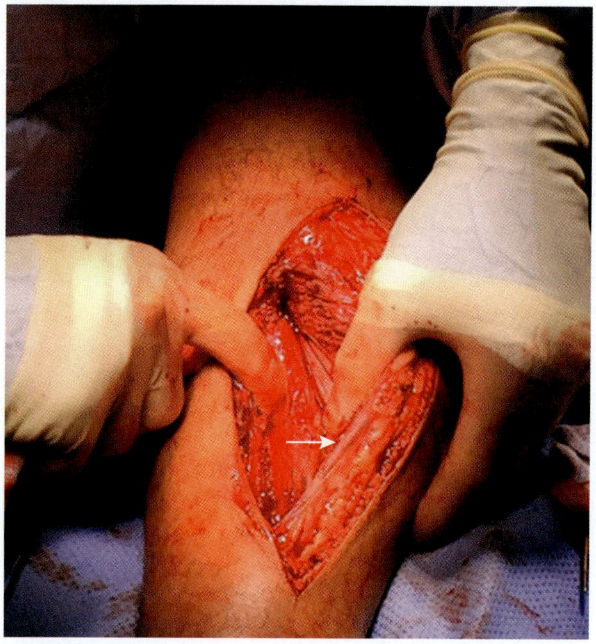

FIGURE 27.3 ▌ The medial approach to the deep posterior compartment should spare the saphenous vein (*arrow*) and requires division of the soleus muscle and opening of a second fascial layer.

- Venous tributaries are ligated and divided to carefully reflect the saphenous posteriorly.
- The crural fascia is opened from knee to ankle with blunt surgical scissors.
- The presence of muscle bulging should be noted.
- The muscular consistency, color, contractility, and capillary perfusion are examined.
- The broad transverse fibers of the soleus are divided with cautery.
- A second layer of fascia is opened, and the deep posterior compartment is entered with scissors.
- Care is taken to avoid injury to posterior tibial artery and its paired segment of veins.
- Bleeding is not uncommon, and hemostasis is achieved with topical agents, cautery, and suture.
- A Kerlix roll or negative pressure device is applied to the surgical site.
- Skin tension is maintained with a Jacob's ladder of vessel loops and a skin stapler.
- A vacuum of 75 to 125 mm Hg is appropriate.
- The Ioban incise drape is useful for obtaining a seal when an external fixator is used.

Lateral Dissection: Anterior and Lateral Compartments

TIP

A transverse incision in the crural fascia will help to identify the transverse intermuscular septum. Opening the fascia on either side of the septum ensures a proper release of both the anterior and lateral compartments. During the lateral incision, the superficial peroneal nerve can be easily injured and should be identified.

- A two-incision technique is performed by incising the lateral and medial calf.
- A longitudinal incision is made two-finger widths lateral to the tibia (Fig. 27.4).
- The skin incision can be shorter but the fascial incision should extend from knee to ankle.
- A generous skin flap is elevated to ensure entry into both anterior and lateral compartments (Fig. 27.5).

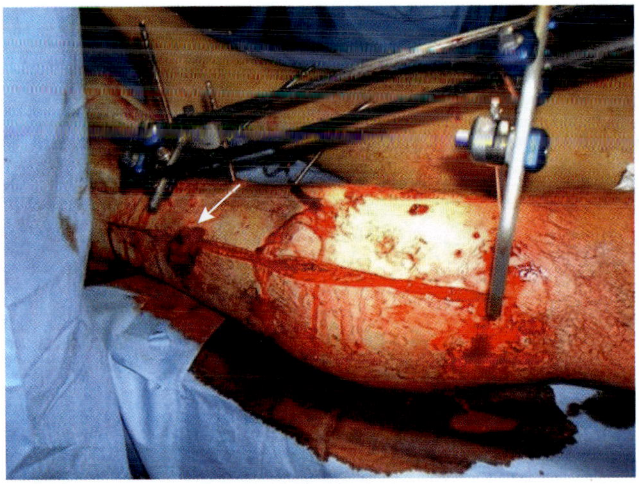

FIGURE 27.4 ▌ A full-length skin incision on the lateral compartment is made through the penetrating wound (*arrow*).

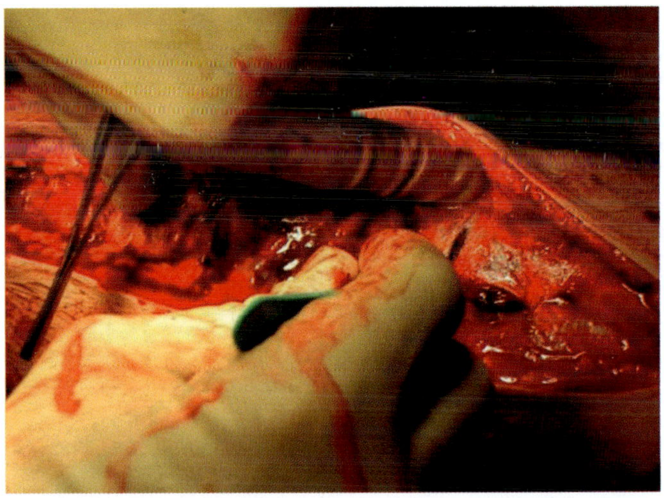

FIGURE 27.5 ▌ Skin flaps are created and a transverse incision on the crural fascia is performed to ensure that both the anterior and lateral compartments are properly identified.

- The transverse intermuscular septum is found by palpation after incision of the crural fascia transversely (Fig. 27.6).
- Metzenbaum scissors are used to open the fascia longitudinally on both sides of the septum preserving the superficial peroneal nerve (Fig. 27.7).

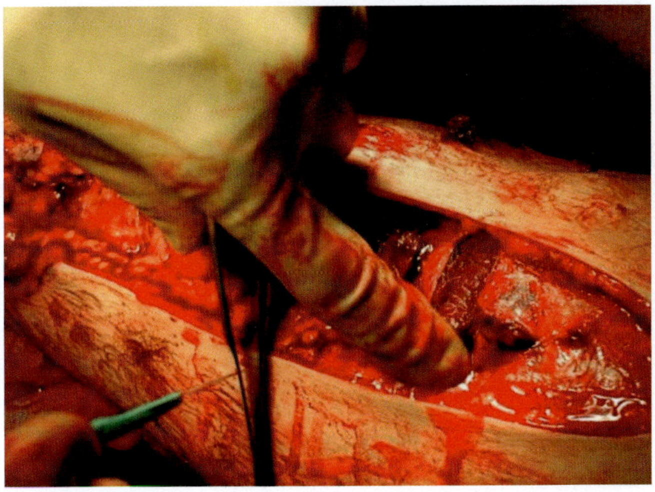

FIGURE 27.6 ▎The transverse intermuscular septum is palpated.

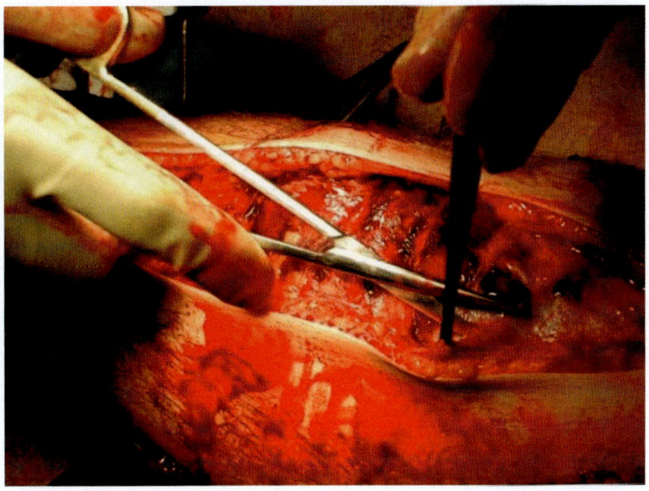

FIGURE 27.7 ▎Metzenbaum scissors are used to open the fascia on either side of the septum to release both the anterior and lateral compartments.

- The position of the superficial peroneal nerve varies and a high transection results in motor as well as sensory loss.
- Apply Kerlix or negative pressure dressing.
- Use a Jacob's ladder technique to maintain skin tension (Fig. 27.8).

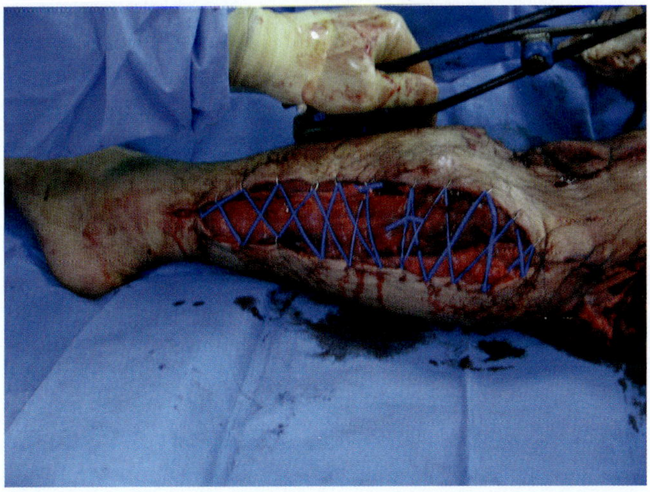

FIGURE 27.8 ▎Jacob's ladder fashioned by vessel loops to prevent skin retraction.

POSTOPERATIVE CONSIDERATIONS

TIP

The medial compartment is closed preferentially because the lateral compartment is easier to place a split-thickness skin graft.

- Return the patient to the OR in 24 to 48 hours.
- Inspect for hemostasis.
- Irrigate the wounds and debride any devitalized tissue.

- Begin a layered closure using interrupted absorbable sutures.
- No. 2 nylon sutures can minimize skin tension.
- Complete the skin closure with vertical mattress sutures or staples.
- Apply Kerlix or negative pressure dressing (Fig. 27.9).

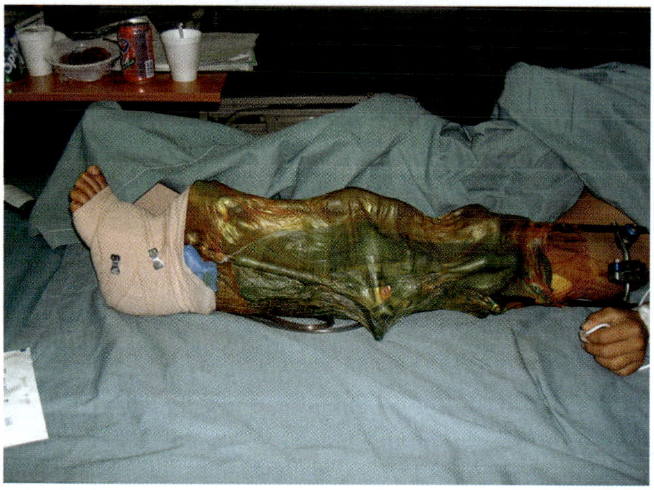

FIGURE 27.9 ▌ Negative pressure wound therapy can be used with external fixation.

Suggested Readings

Dente CJ, Wyrzykowski AD, Feliciano DV. Fasciotomy. *Curr Probl Surg*. 2009;46:779–839.

Feliciano DV, Moore EE, West MA, et al. Western Trauma Association critical decisions in trauma: evaluation and management of peripheral vascular injury, part II. *J Trauma Acute Care Surg*. 2013;75(3):391–397.

Feliciano DV, Moore FA, Moore EE, et al. Evaluation and management of peripheral vascular injury. Part 1. Western Trauma Association/critical decisions in trauma. *J Trauma*. 2011;70(6):1551–1556.

Fox CJ, Holcomb JB. Pathophysiology of vascular trauma, 28–32. In: Rasmussen T, Tai N, eds. *Vascular Trauma*. 3rd ed. Elsevier; 2015.

Matsen FA III. Diagnosis of compartmental syndromes. In: Matsen FA III, ed. *Compartmental Syndromes*. Grune & Stratton; 1980.

Chapter 28
Lower Extremity Amputation

ERIC CAMPION AND CHARLES J. FOX

PERIOPERATIVE CONSIDERATIONS

Procedure Rationale

- The decision to perform lower extremity amputation is often challenging as the outcome will depend on the quality of the amputation performed. While scoring systems exist to aid in decision making for limb salvage no scoring system can replace good surgical judgment. Amputation is generally recommended based on the consensus of a multidisciplinary team, the patient's overall physiologic condition, and supportive family members. In some cases, the physiologic condition may be the result of ongoing myonecrosis from a failed attempt at limb salvage. This chapter is focused on the technical tips on performing a transtibial or transfemoral amputation.

ESSENTIAL EQUIPMENT

TIP

Test the bone saw battery to avoid unnecessary delay. Tourniquets are not necessary and, in some cases, may be harmful when the femoral artery is calcified.

- Basic surgical set
- 10-blade surgical scalpel
- Vascular clamps
- Sutures
  - 3-0 Prolene suture on an SH needle
  - 2-0 and 3-0 silk sutures
  - 2-0 and 3-0 Vicryl sutures
  - 2-0 and 3-0 Nylon sutures
  - 0 Ethibond suture
- Skin Stapler
- Periosteal elevator
- Oscillating bone saw
- Gigli saw
- Rongeur
- Bone rasp
- Bone hook
- Retractors
- Drill
- Jackson-Pratt drain

Positioning

TIP

Always verify the site and check both extremities before starting the operation.

- Supine position.
- Cover genitalia and use a 1010 drape.
- Prep the extremity one anatomic level above and below the amputation.
- Use an extremity drape and surgical towels.
- Elevate the extremity with surgical gowns or an orthopedic stand.

TECHNIQUE

Guillotine Amputation

TIP

The entire operation can be done in 30 seconds using a Gigli saw.

- A supra malleolar amputation done for infectious source control (Fig. 28.1).

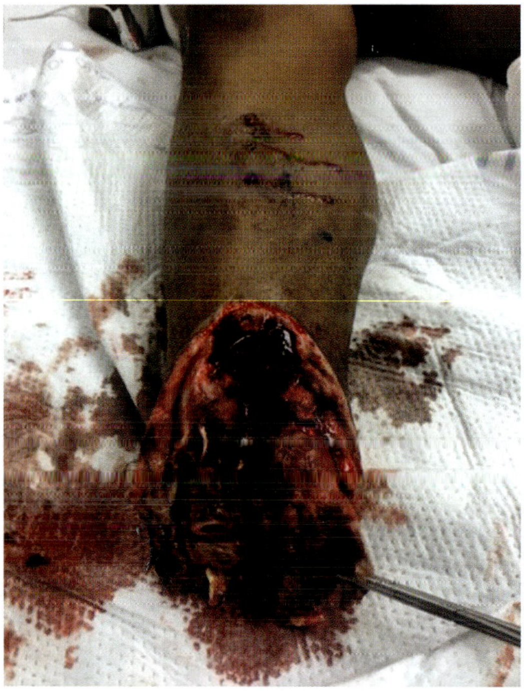

FIGURE 28.1 ▌ A guillotine amputation done for a contaminated mangled foot injury.

- Preserves viable tissue for staged definitive transtibial amputation.
- Use a Gigli saw from posterior to anterior for a hasty operation.
- Circular incision with cautery and identification of tibial and peroneal arteries.
- Stick tie named vessels.
- A power saw should be turned on and gradually approach the bone to avoid jamming of the blade and bone fragmentation.
- Bone wax will help achieve hemostasis.
- Place betadine-soaked dressing over the surgical site.

Definitive Below Knee Amputation (Transtibial)

TIP

Ensure there are sufficient distal skin, viable soft tissue, and blood supply for a posterior flap.

- A careful and methodical operation in a hemodynamically stable patient.

- A long posterior flap is the most common technique (Fig. 28.2)

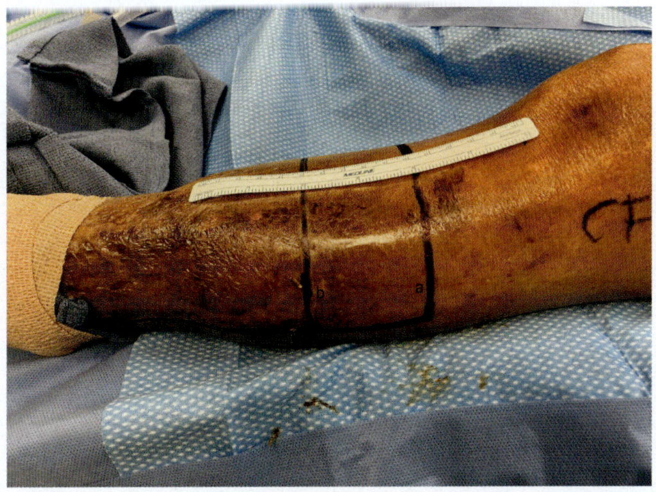

FIGURE 28.2 ▌ Preoperative markings for a transtibial amputation illustrate the long posterior flap and the intended site of bone transection (*a*) relative to the skin incision (*b*).

- Blood supply to the tibioperoneal posterior compartment is crucial.
- Identify the tibial tuberosity.
- The Incision is 10 to 15 cm or a hand measurement distal to the tubercle.
- The transverse incision is extended for about 1/3 of the limb circumference.
- The incision is carried down the long axis of the leg laterally and medially and connects posteriorly.
- The posterior flap is fashioned with a surgical knife to cover the bone without tension.
- The crural fascia and muscles are divided with cautery.
- The tibial and peroneal nerves are retracted, sharply divided, and allowed to retract.
- Arteries are ligated with permanent suture.
- The periosteum is elevated, and the tibia and fibula are cut several centimeters higher than the skin incision (Fig. 28.3).

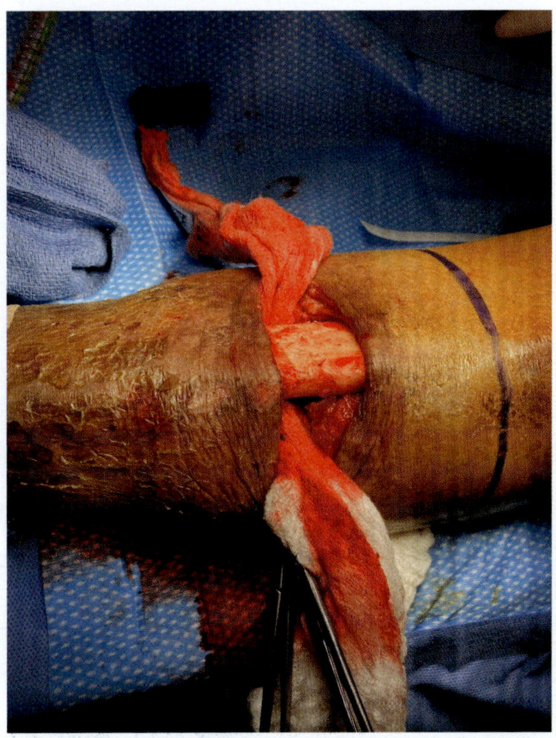

FIGURE 28.3 ▌ Retractors are placed and the vessels are protected before tibial transection. Additional bone is removed if there is any tension on the posterior flap.

- The fibular shaft should be cut shorter than the tibia.
- Bevel the corners of the bone and bone wax is applied.
- The posterior flap is closed in layers (Fig. 28.4).
- The skin is reapproximated with staples or nylon sutures (Fig. 28.5).

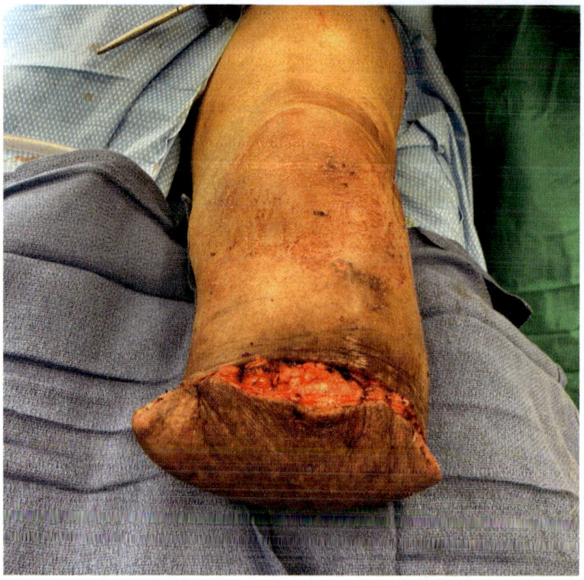

FIGURE 28.4 ▌ Close in layers using fascia to hold sutures.

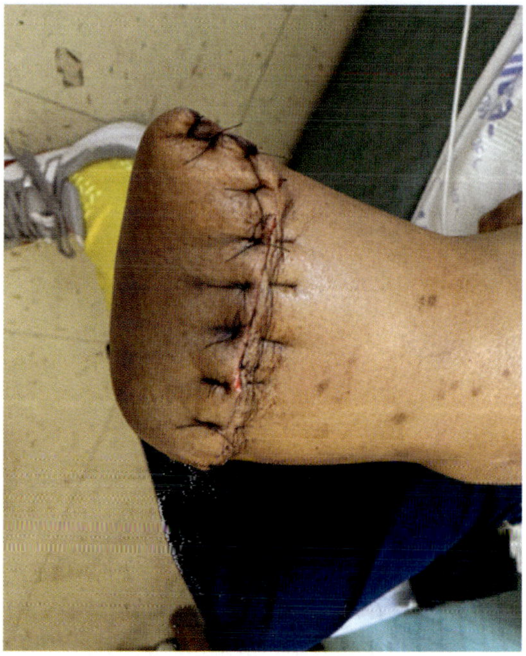

FIGURE 28.5 ▌ Skin closure is done with nylon vertical mattress sutures or skin staples.

Definitive Above Knee Amputation (Transfemoral)

TIP

Plan the skin incision noting the anatomic landmarks with a marking pen (Fig. 28.6).

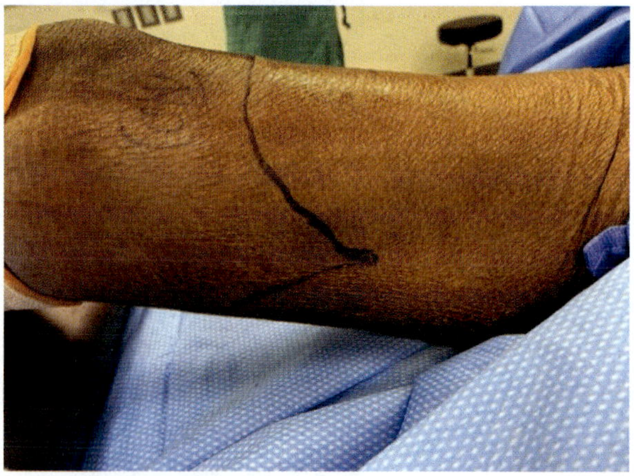

FIGURE 28.6 ▌ Surgical marking in preparation for transfemoral amputation.

- Elevate the extremity.
- A fish mouth incision for anterior and posterior flaps is the most common (Fig. 28.7).

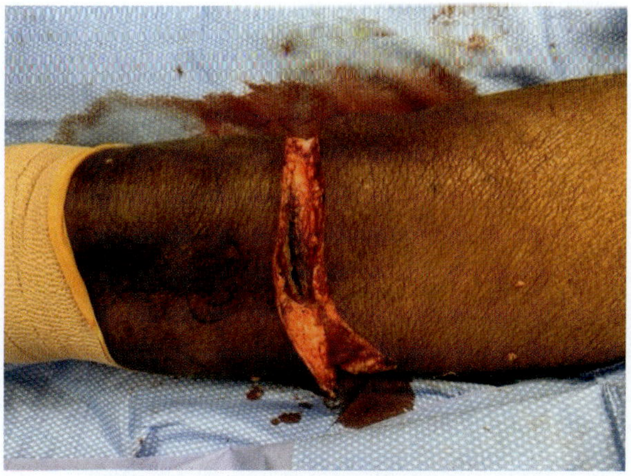

FIGURE 28.7 ▮ Skin incision for transfemoral amputation.

- Medial and lateral flaps are also appropriate.
- In trauma flaps are often dictated by the remaining viable tissues.
- Muscle groups are identified and cut with cautery with meticulous hemostasis.
- Femoral vessels are identified, and suture ligated.
- The sciatic and saphenous nerves are identified and cut under tension to avoid neuroma.
- Ensure the bone is cut high enough to allow for tensionless muscle and skin closure (Fig. 28.8).
- Use a bone rasp to smooth the edge of the transected femur (Fig. 28.9).

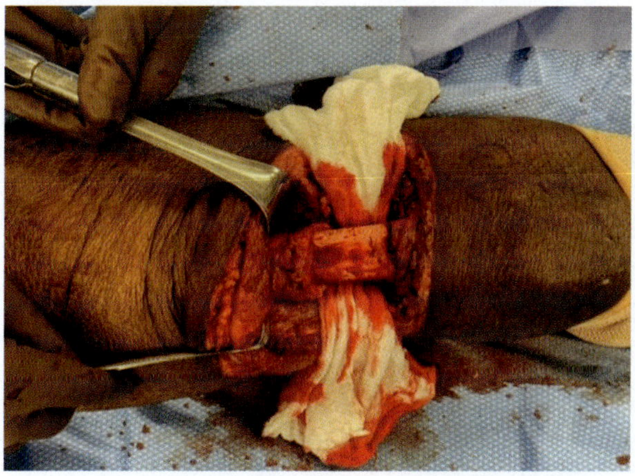

FIGURE 28.8 ▮ Preparation for bone transection.

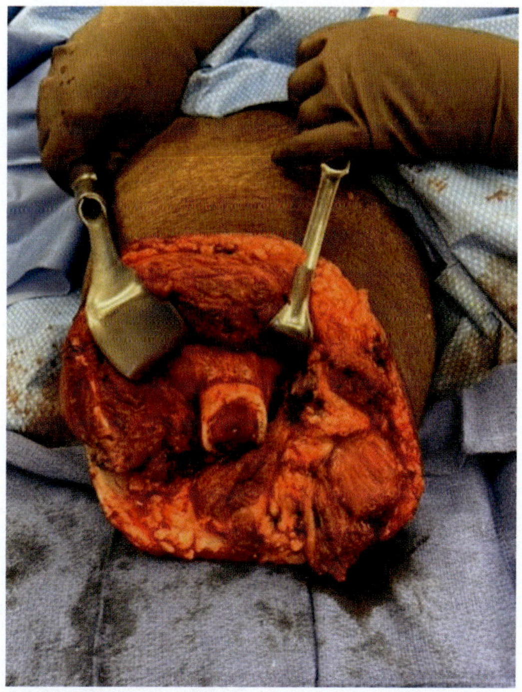

FIGURE 28.9 ▮ Completed transfemoral amputation.

- The adductor magnus can be sutured to the lateral side of the femur to avoid a deformity.
  - Drill holes are made in the lateral and posterior aspects of the distal femur.
  - Secure the adductor magnus tendon with 0 Ethibond suture.
- Reapproximate all muscle layers using fascia to hold sutures (Figs. 28.10 and 28.11).

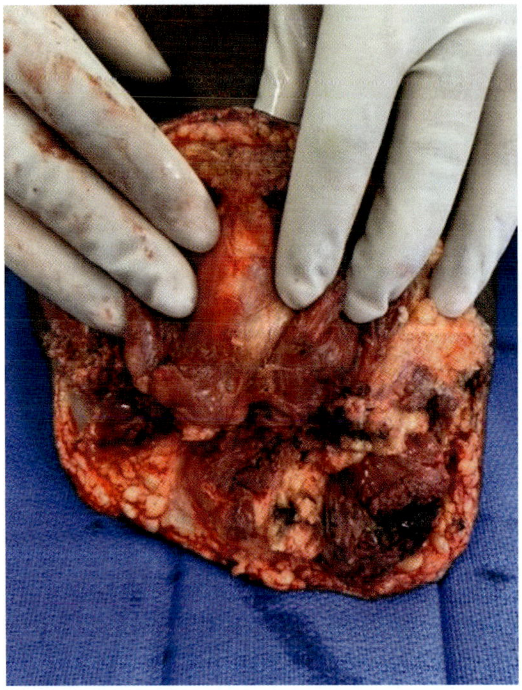

FIGURE 28.10 ▌ Closing deep layers following transfemoral amputation.

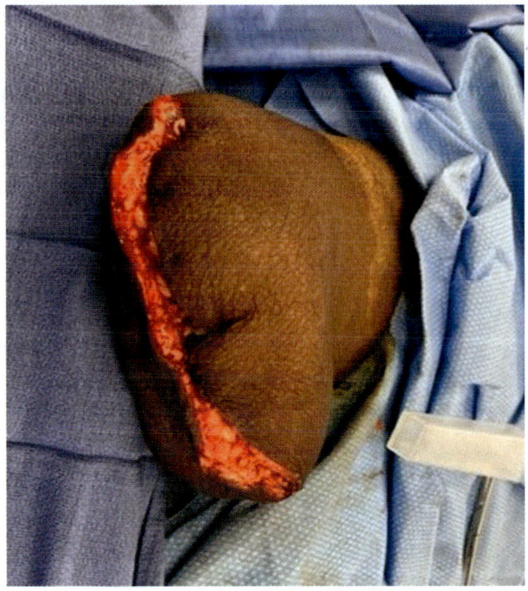

FIGURE 28.11 ▌ Closing superficial layers following transfemoral amputation.

- Staple the skin edges (Fig. 28.12).
- Drains are rarely used.

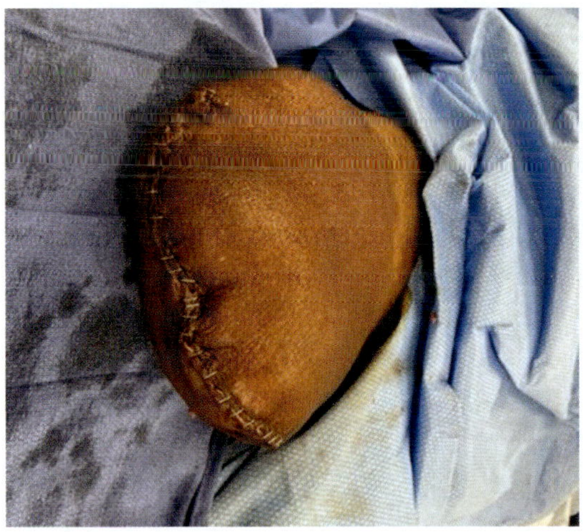

FIGURE 28.12 ▌ Stapled skin incision following transfemoral amputation.

POSTOPERATIVE CARE

TIP

Patients should be referred to a prosthetic company for amputation site protection devices, psychological support, and rehabilitation.

- Remove dressing in 24 hours.
- Inspect every 24 to 48 hours for skin viability and signs of infection.
- Use a Velcro knee immobilizer for transtibial amputees.
- Xeroform, Pads, Kerlix & Stockinette.

- Avoid tape to the skin surround the amputation site.
- DVT prophylaxis.
- Monitor for phantom limb pain and treat with Gabapentin.

Suggested Readings

Scalea TM, DuBose J, Moore EE, et al. Western trauma association critical decisions in trauma: management of the mangled extremity. *J Trauma Acute Care Surg*. 2012;72(1):86–93.

Shawen SB, Keeling JJ, Branstetter J, Kirk KL, Ficke JR. The mangled foot and leg: salvage versus amputation. *Foot Ankle Clin*. 2010;15(1):63–75.

Tisi PV, Than MM. Type of incision for below knee amputation. *Cochrane Database Syst Rev*. 2014;2014(4):CD003749.

Chapter 29
Vascular Techniques

CHARLES J. FOX AND ERNEST E. MOORE

RATIONALE

- Basic techniques in vascular surgery are important steps to master in order to achieve successful restoration of blood flow. Temporary vascular shunts (TVS) are a useful damage control adjunct that allow for distal perfusion to minimize ischemic time during patient transport, extremity fixation, addressing more life-threatening injuries, or assessment of revascularization options including vein harvest.
- Special instruments and suture materials are essential for proper dissection, isolation, and control of hemorrhage.
- Basic anastomotic techniques are important for the trauma surgeon to practice regularly in order to achieve a durable vascular reconstruction. Endovascular techniques are included in this section as they are becoming increasingly essential tools for optimal resuscitation, diagnosis, and hybrid applications in the treatment of vascular injury.

Shunting

TIP

The trauma surgeon should select a shunt that is immediately available, simple to use, and easily guided into the vessel without creating additional injury. The Pruitt-Inahara shunt has the advantage of a T port for infusion.

- Shunts have good early patency, and do not result in extremity loss if reconstruction is accomplished within 6 hours.
- Shunts allow time for fasciotomy, vein harvesting, and skeletal fixation.
- Argyle, Javid, Sundt, and Pruitt-Inahara (PI) shunts are used commonly (Fig. 29.1).

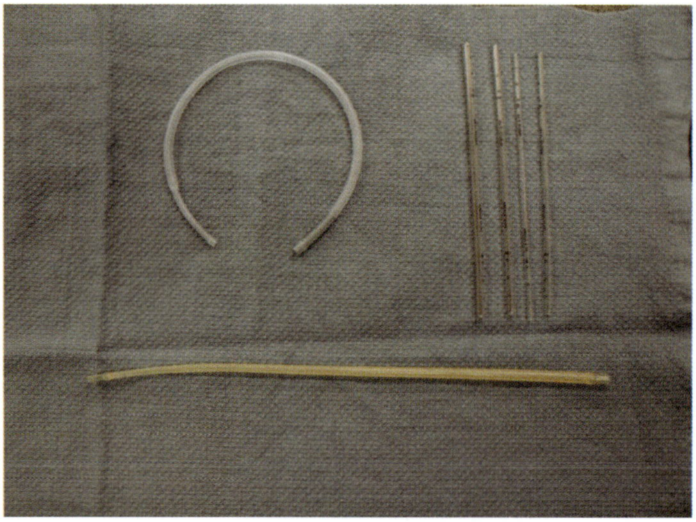

FIGURE 29.1 ❙ Sundt, Javid, and Argyle shunts.

- Argyle shunts are available in 6- or 11-inch lengths with four shunt diameters per package that range from 8 to 14 Fr (Fig. 29.2).
- The Javid shunts are rigid, have a bulged tip, and can be secured with special clamps or sutures.
- Sundt shunts are soft but have a metallic skeleton to prevent external compression (Fig. 29.3).

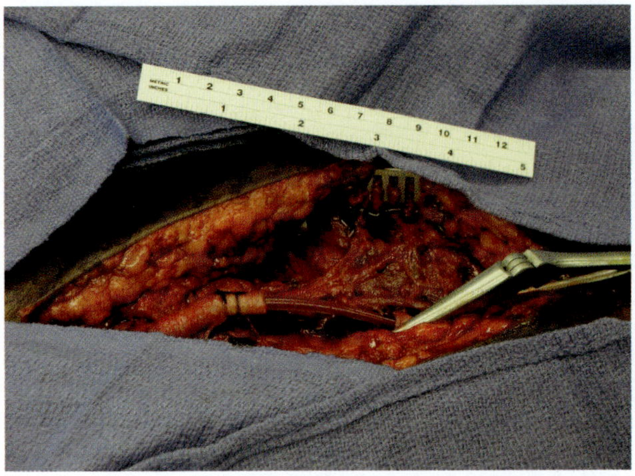

FIGURE 29.2 ❙ Argyle shunt in a femoral artery.

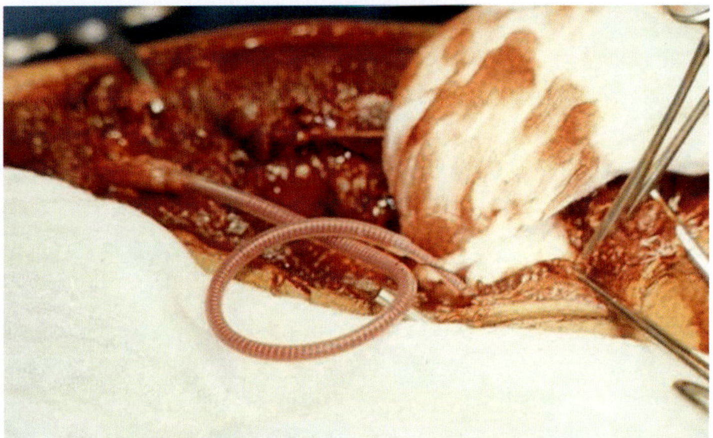

FIGURE 29.3 ❙ Sundt shunt in a femoral artery.

- PI shunts are secured with balloon-expandable tips and have a T port for infusion of saline, contrast, or medications. The PI shunts (with T port) are available in 15- or 31-cm lengths and have an 8- to 14-mm balloon diameter.
- Avoid PI balloon overinflation by using saline syringes and administering the minimal volume to achieve occlusion.
- Insert the shunt after thrombectomy and confirming back bleeding and inflow.
- Shunts should pass easily through the vessel lumen to prevent intimal damage.
- Oversized shunts will cause damage; undersizing will result in bleeding.
- A 10-Fr argyle shunt is a typical size shunt for an internal carotid artery.
- A femoral or popliteal vessel may require a 12- or 14-Fr shunt.
- The shunts are usually secured with a silastic vessel loop or silk suture on either end.
- A PI shunt is advantageous for the following options:
  - Intermittent confirmation of flow.
  - Administration of heparin for regional anticoagulation, papaverine for vasodilation, tissue plasminogen activator (tPA) for fibrinolysis, contrast administration for completion angiography, and measuring perfusion pressure (Fig. 29.4).

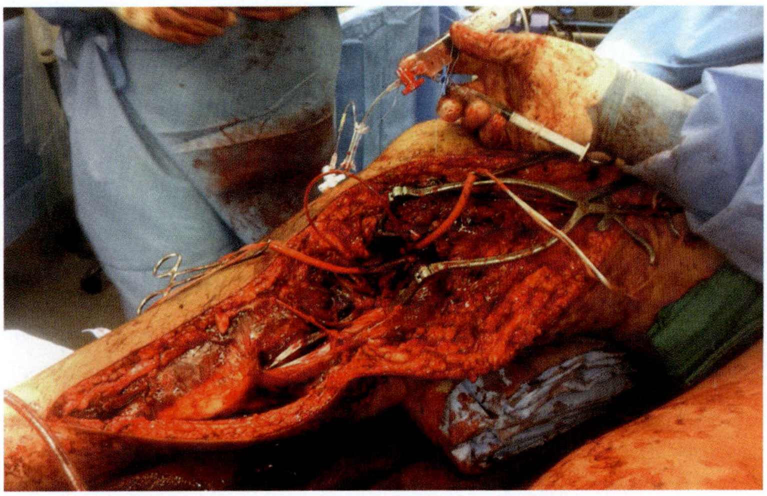

FIGURE 29.4 ❙ Pruitt-Inahara shunt in a popliteal artery.

Essential Equipment

- Shunts as described above
- Metzenbaum scissors (blunt tipped for dissection)
- Potts scissors (for incising and excising vascular wall)
- No. 11 scalpel blade
- Castroviejo needle driver (Fig. 29.5)
- Microvascular forceps (Fig. 29.5)

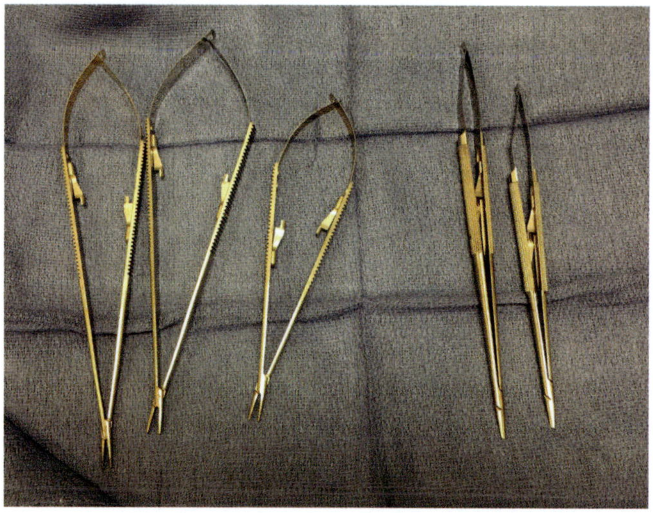

FIGURE 29.5 Essential vascular instruments.

- Profunda vascular clamps (right angled and straight)
- Satinsky shaped clamps (side biting)
- DeBakey clamps (serrated rows of interdigitating teeth)
- Moistened umbilical tape, thin rubber catheters, and silastic vessel loops
- Sutures
  - 5-0, 6-0, 7-0 Prolene on a C1 or BV1 needle
  - 3-0 silk plain and stick ties
  - 0 silk (heavy) for securing shunt
- Sterile 8- to 10-MHz Doppler probe
- Heparinized saline 50 to 100 units in 1,000 mL saline
- Papaverine 60 mg in 20 cc of saline
- Fogarty embolectomy catheters no. 2 and no. 3
- Bulldog soft vascular clamps (small vessels)
- Three-way stopcock and A-line extension tubing
- 10-cc syringes of heparin Saline on 18-gauge blunt tip metal catheters

TECHNIQUE

Dissection Technique

TIP

During the arterial dissection, stay in a plane as close to the adventitia as possible; staying a "safe distance" from the vessel during the dissection is not actually safer.

- Arteries maintain a thin layer of periadventitial loose areolar tissue.
- Look for vasovasorum ("bloodshot eye") as a guide to the proper plane.
- Expose the vessel, taking care to avoid adjacent veins and arterial side branches.
- Passing an umbilical tape under the artery will aid dissection and show branches.

- A double loop (Potts) of tape will control bleeding from the dissected vessel (Fig. 29.6).

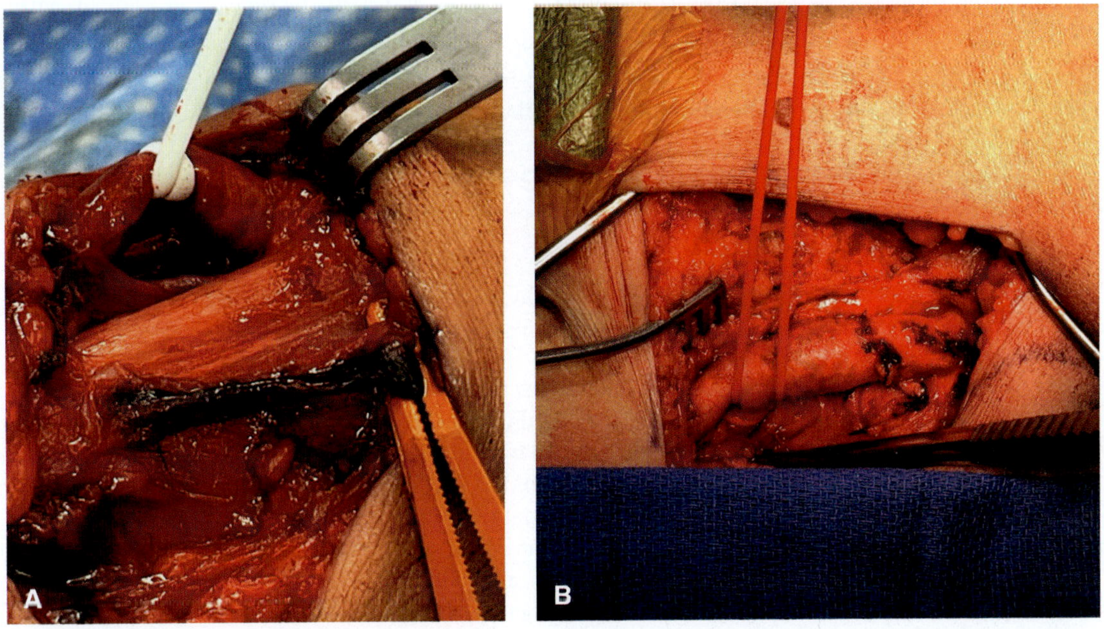

FIGURE 29.6 ▌ Potts tie using a silastic vessel loop around the brachial artery (**A**) and the deep femoral artery (**B**)

- Use angled or perpendicular clamps to reduce the profile and avoid twisting of the artery.
- A Rummel tourniquet is a tape passed around the artery and pulled through a rubber catheter, but it is not ideal for calcified vessels (Fig. 29.7).
- Stay "on top" of the vessel to find the proper plane while working known to unknown.

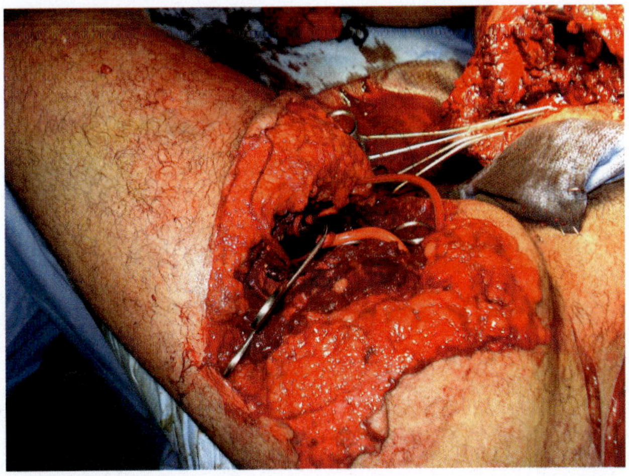

FIGURE 29.7 ▌ Rummel tourniquet using a rubber catheter and umbilical tape.

Suturing

TIP

Inform the scrub technician to always pass the vascular sutures with "double-armed" swaged needles and not to cut any sutures in half or needles off.

- Vascular reconstructions are conducted with monofilament nonabsorbable sutures.
- Suture size ranges from 2-0 to 7-0 progressing from the aorta to the crural arteries.
- The caliber should be fine but without concern for breaking and pseudoaneurysm.
- Five throws are usually placed to secure the knot for monofilament sutures.
- Femoral and popliteal reconstruction is commonly done using 5-0 and 6-0 sutures.

- 4-0 suture is typical for the iliac vessels and 7-0 for tibial repairs.
- Choosing the best needle size and shape is especially important.
- Tapered needles puncture the artery without cutting and avoid tears in the vessel wall.
- Penetrate the vessel wall at 90 degrees and follow the needle curve.
- Pronating the wrist between insertion and withdrawal will eliminate iatrogenic tears.
- Avoid bending the body of the needle during penetration.

Basic Vascular Reconstruction

TIP

A poorly covered vein graft is no better than a prosthetic graft. Always ensure the conduit of any type is properly covered by healthy viable muscle tissue.

- A lateral suture is enough for repairing a small laceration on a large vessel.
- Lacerations should be closed in a direction to minimize restricting the vessel lumen.
- Patch angioplasty is favored over interrupted sutures on small vessels to avoid a stenosis.
- End-to-end anastomosis avoids a conduit and is preferable when repair is tensionless, but adequate vessel mobilization is essential to avoid tension.
- Interposition grafts are reserved for segmental defects when muscle coverage is good.
- For deeper cavitary wounds, a bypass routed around the zone of injury is preferred.
- Know what vessels can be ligated, that is, brachial artery with good distal signals.
- When performing a bypass, do not forget to ligate the native vessel to reduce hemorrhage.

Anastomoses

TIP

A four-quadrant heel-to-toe spatulated anastomosis is the easiest to teach and perform; practice makes perfect.

- End-to-Side Anastomosis
  - The length of the distal anastomosis should be twice the graft diameter.
  - Additional opening of the vessel can be obtained by dividing the vessel at a branch point (Fig. 29.8).
  - Create a sharp arteriotomy with an 11 blade and extend with Potts scissors.
  - The graft should be beveled “spatulated” to match the size of the arteriotomy (Fig. 29.9).

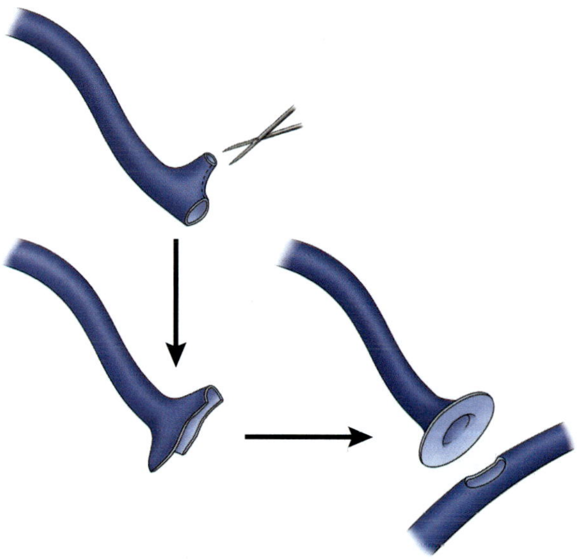

FIGURE 29.8 ▌ The lumen of a vessel can be enlarged by dividing the vessel at a bifurcation.

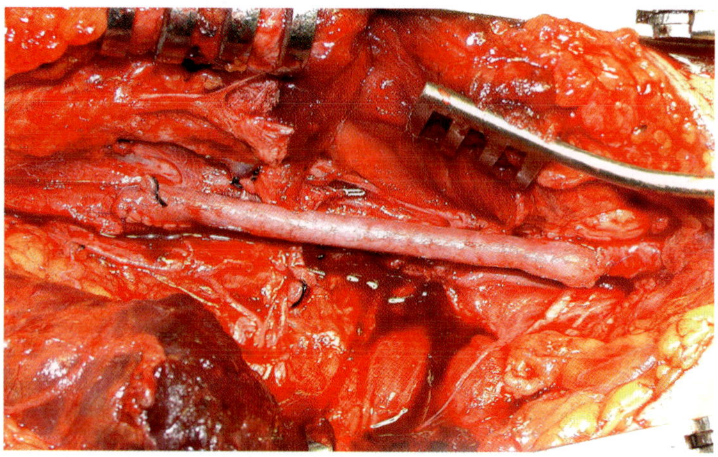

FIGURE 29.9 ▌ Example of a spatulated graft.

- The optimal angle for an end-to-side anastomosis is 45 degrees.
- Anchor Technique (Fig. 29.10)

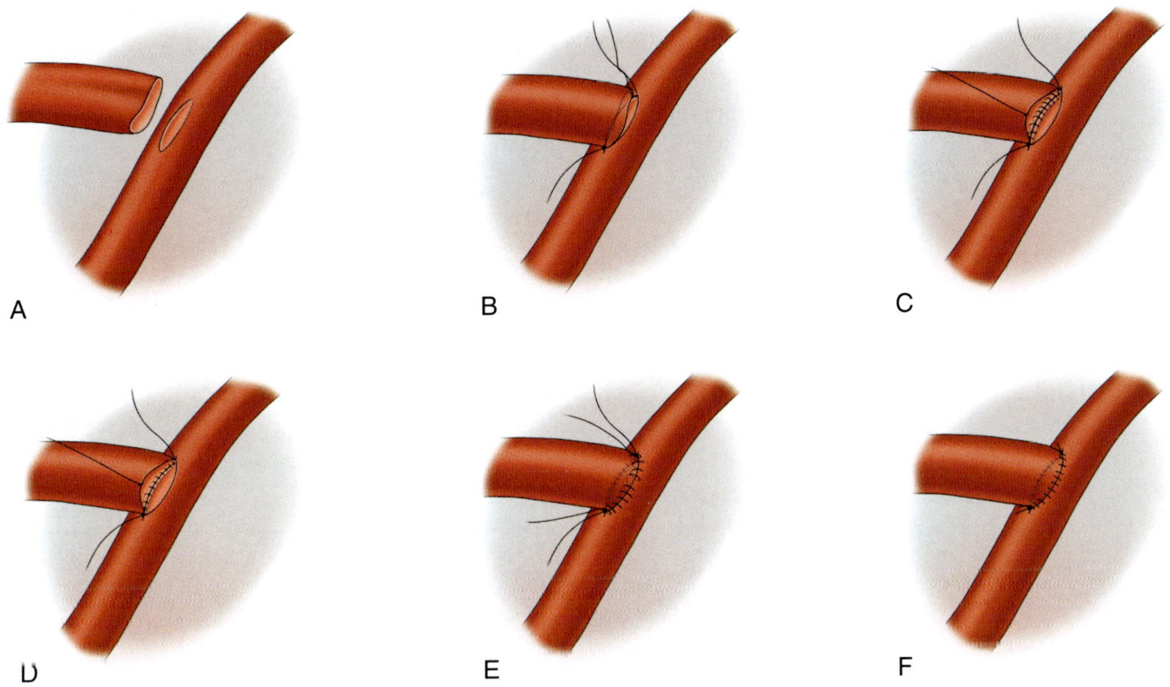

FIGURE 29.10 | Illustration of the anchor anastomotic technique.

  - Starting at the center heel, introduce the needle from out to in on the graft and then from in to out on the artery and tie "anchor" the suture.
  - Place several sutures on one side from heel-to-toe fashion.
  - Dividing the work into four quadrants, tighten the suture line to go to opposite side of the heel and place several more sutures toward the apex.
  - Start a new suture at the apex "toe" and work backward to the other sutures now in the mid-portion of the graft on each side.
  - Flush the graft before securing the running ends of sutures on each side.
  - The suture should be tied as loosely as possible to avoid restricting the anastomosis.
- Parachute Technique (Fig. 29.11)

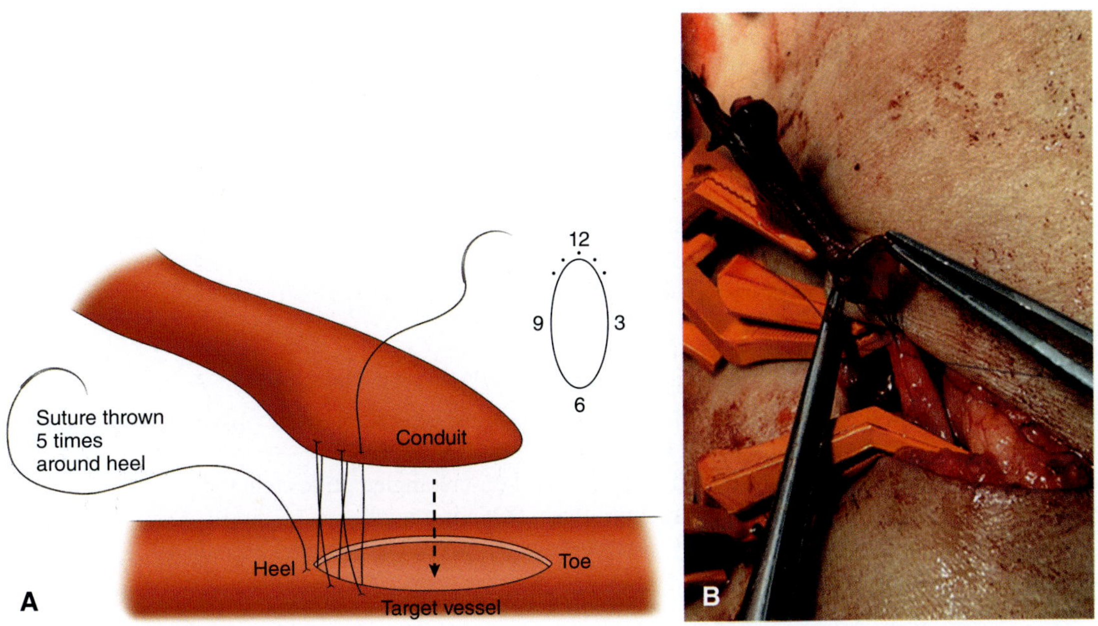

FIGURE 29.11 | Cartoon (A) and photo illustration (B) of the parachuted anastomotic technique.

- Starting at the center heel, introduce the needle from out-in on the graft.
- Introduce the needle into the matching location on the artery in-out.
- Progress with the suturing toward the apex for a few bites, then start the opposite side, going from heel to toe.
- When both sides of the heel are complete, continue to the toe or start a second suture and work back to the heel.
- Tighten the suture line and tie the free ends of sutures.
- Cut the sutures with a 5- to 8-mm tail to avoid unraveling.

- End-to-End Anastomosis
  - Anchor Technique
    - Transected ends should be debrided back to a healthy intimal surface.
    - Start by placing the first suture at equal corners of each vessel and tie.
    - Place an identical suture diametrically opposite to the first suture.
    - Perform a continuous suture starting from either the anterior or posterior wall in a 9 o'clock to 3 o'clock fashion.
    - Start a new suture or continue onto the opposite side until sutures meet.
    - Flush and secure all sutures and cut with a 5- to 8-mm tail.

Basic Endovascular Techniques

TIP

The inguinal skin crease can vary with body habitus and is not a reliable landmark for the common femoral artery. When considering endovascular technical success, "It's all about the access."

- Access
  - Early ultrasound-guided transradial or transfemoral access is crucial for success.
  - Using surface landmarks, the inguinal ligament is identified between the anterior superior iliac spine (ASIS) and the pubic symphysis.
  - The common femoral artery (CFA) is approximately midpoint between these bony landmarks and is accessed 2 cm below the inguinal ligament. (See Chapter 2.)
  - It is important to access the mid-CFA as cephalad entry into the external iliac artery may preclude external compression following sheath removal, and caudal entry into the superficial femoral artery may lead to arterial thrombosis.
  - A useful sonographic landmark for the borders of the CFA is the inferior epigastric artery proximally and profunda/superficial femoral bifurcation distally.
  - Enter the femoral vessel at 75 degrees.

Special Equipment

- A 10 cm 5 French sheath is the workhorse of vascular access.
- An 18-gauge access needle with a 45 cm 0.035-inch stainless steel guidewire or a 21-gauge micropuncture needle with a 45 cm 0.021-inch stainless steel guidewire are acceptable entry tools.
- Contrast agent 50 mL (Omnipaque-240, GE Healthcare, Inc., Chicago, IL) is helpful when there is difficulty and fluoroscopy is available.
- 50 mL injectable saline and heparinized saline (50 U/mL) are prepared for line flushing.
- 5- and 10-cc syringes × 2 each.
- Sutures 2-0 silk or nylon to secure catheters.
- Linear 5- to 15-MHz Doppler probe.
- Ultrasound probe cover.
- Portable ultrasound machine.
- A-line extension tubing to monitor arterial pressure proximal to balloon.
- Scalpel (no. 11 or no. 15).
- .035 in angled glide wire and 65-cm angled glide catheter.
- Flush catheter, Omni flush, SOS, or pigtail.

Angiography

- Use a hybrid room with overhead fixed fluoroscopic imaging or a portable C-arm.
- Bring C-arm in from the door and stand on opposite side for access.
- Keep all endovascular items separate from open surgical instruments (Fig. 29.12).

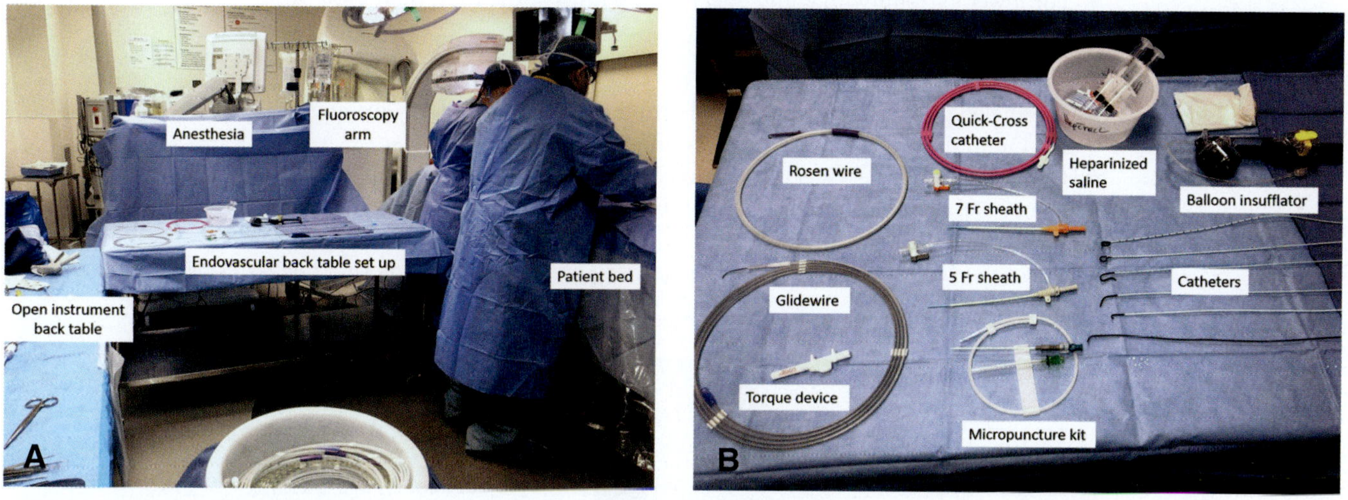

FIGURE 29.12 ❙ A trauma hybrid room (**A**) with a separate table of endovascular equipment (**B**).

- Advance a 035 in guidewire into the abdominal aorta.
- Keep wires "on the screen" to prevent iatrogenic injury or branch cannulations.
- Advance a flush catheter over the guidewire and remove the wire (Fig. 29.13).

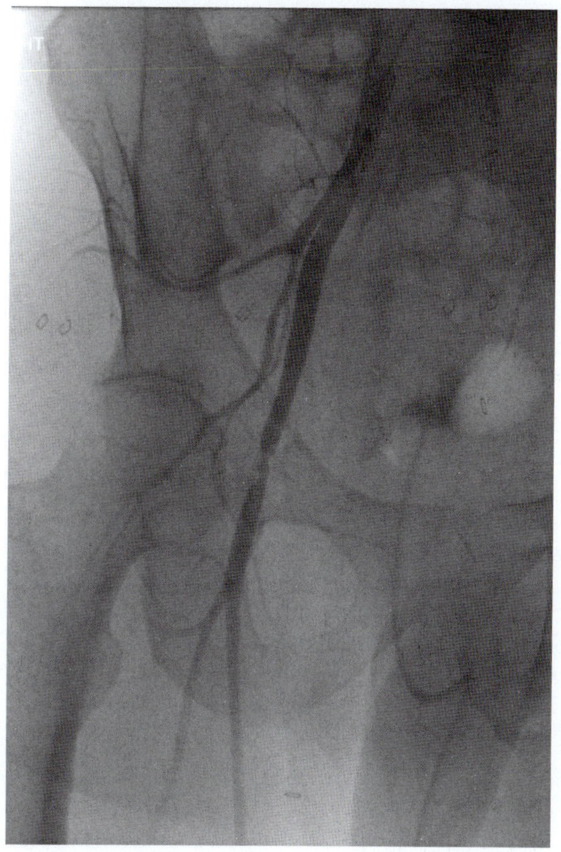

FIGURE 29.13 ❙ Once the glide wire is removed, a flush catheter is used to inject 20 mL of contrast into the common iliac artery demonstrating a right femoral artery dissection.

- Connect power injector to a flush catheter for contrast injection.
- Use digital subtraction angiography (DSA) mode to subtract bones and hardware.
- For abdominal aortic imaging inject "15 for 30," that is, 15 mL/second for 2 seconds or a total volume bolus of 30 milliliters at 1,000 psi.
- For pelvic imaging, inject 10 for 20.
- For lower extremity imaging, inject 3 for 6 until at the foot, then 5 for 10.

Pelvic Embolization

- An angled glide catheter is inserted into the hypogastric artery for angiography.
- An Omni flush or pigtail catheter is often the preferred catheter.
- Gel Foam or stainless steel "tornado coils" are the most common embolic agents.
- Mince Gel Foam into a small cup with mix of contrast into a viscous slurry.
- Aspirate mix into a 10-cc syringe.
- Inject the Gel Foam or coils into the tertiary branches of the internal iliac artery where the blush is noted (Fig. 29.14).

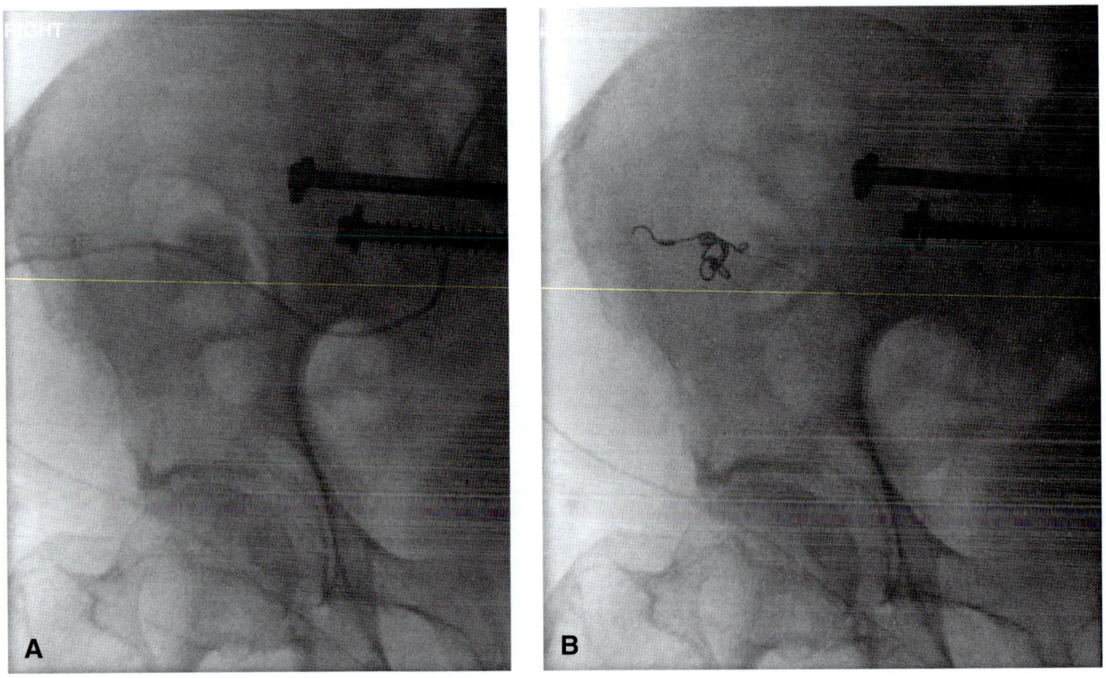

FIGURE 29.14 ▮ Right internal iliac artery angiogram showing a 6-cm pseudoaneurysm of the right gluteal artery (**A**) and coil embolization (**B**).

- Inject slow and steady under fluoroscopic examination to ensure catheter is stable.
- Repeat the angiogram to ensure hemorrhage control.

Suggested Readings

Gifford SM, Aidinian G, Clouse WD, et al. Effect of temporary shunting on extremity vascular injury: an outcome analysis from the Global War on Terror vascular injury initiative. *J Vasc Surg.* 2009;50(3):549–555.

Horer T, DuBose J, Rasmussen T, White J. *Endovascular Resuscitation and Trauma Management.* Springer International; 2019.

Plotkin A, Magee GA, Fox, CJ. A standardized trauma-specific endovascular inventory. *J Trauma Acute Care Surg.* 2020;89(2S Suppl 2):S83–S87.

Rasmussen TE, Clouse WD, Jenkins DH, Peck MA, Eliason JL, Smith DL. The use of temporary vascular shunts as a damage control adjunct in the management of wartime vascular injury. *J Trauma.* 2006;61(1):8–12.

Rutherford RB. *Atlas of Vascular Surgery Basic Techniques and Exposures.* WB Saunders Company; 1993.

Index

Note: Page number followed by f indicates figure only.